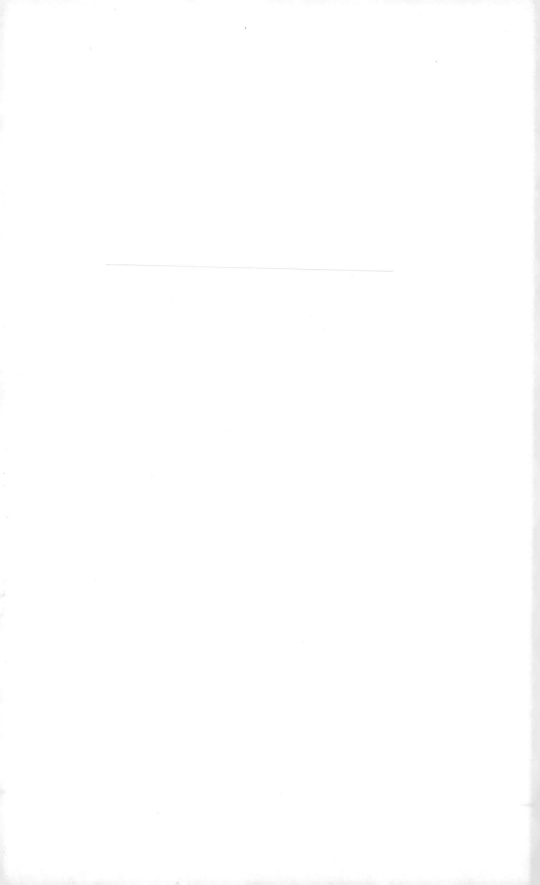

The Behavioral Neurology of
White Matter

THE BEHAVIORAL NEUROLOGY OF WHITE MATTER

Christopher M. Filley

Professor of Neurology and Psychiatry
Director, Behavioral Neurology Section
University of Colorado School of Medicine
Denver Veterans Affairs Medical Center

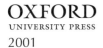
OXFORD
UNIVERSITY PRESS
2001

OXFORD
UNIVERSITY PRESS

Oxford   New York
Athens   Auckland   Bangkok   Bogotá   Buenos Aires   Calcutta
Cape Town   Chennai   Dar es Salaam   Delhi   Florence   Hong Kong   Istanbul
Karachi   Kuala Lumpur   Madrid   Melbourne   Mexico City   Mumbai
Nairobi   Paris   São Paulo   Shanghai   Singapore   Taipei   Tokyo   Toronto   Warsaw

and associated companies in
Berlin   Ibadan

Published by Oxford University Press, Inc.,
198 Madison Avenue, New York, New York, 10016
http://www.oup-usa.org

Library of Congress Cataloging-in-Publication Data
Filley, Christopher M., 1951-
The behavioral neurology of white matter / Christopher M. Filley.
p.; cm.   Includes bibliographical references and index.
ISBN 0-19-513561-X
1. Cognitive neuroscience. 2. Clinical neuropsychology.
3. Neurobehavioral disorders. 4. Higher nervous activity.
5. Neuroanatomy.
I. Title.
[DNLM: 1. Brain Diseases—physiopathology.
2. Brain Diseases—psychology. 3. Behavior—physiology.
4. Brain—physiology. 5. Mental Disorders—physiopathology.
6. Neuropsychology—methods.
WL 348 F485b 2001]   QP360.5.F54 2001   616.8'047— dc21   2001021141

9 8 7 6 5 4 3 2 1

Printed in the United States of America
on acid-free paper

This book is dedicated to all
who seek to understand what is human
through knowledge of the brain.

Foreword

The central nervous system consists of gray matter structures, including the neocortex, basal ganglia, thalamus, and cerebellum, and an extensive array of connecting white matter tracts that allow the integration of the many functions mediated by the gray matter. Neuroscience, neurology, and behavioral neurology have tended to emphasize gray matter function and have left white matter disorders and the essential behavioral functions of white matter relatively unexplored. Individual diseases such as multiple sclerosis have been studied extensively, but an integrated view of the function of white matter and patterns of disfunction occuring when white matter is affected has been lacking. In the current volume, Dr. Filley redresses this imbalance and provides a detailed discussion of the biology of white matter, the phenomenology of white matter diseases, and the pathological disturbances that affect primarily the white matter. When one reads the book, it is impressive how great an effect white matter diseases have, contributing to many disease processes and providing the neurobiological basis for many cognitive disturbances.

The first section addresses the history of white matter neurology, and provides a description of the neuroanatomy and the neurophysiology of white matter tracts. Changes in white matter in the course of development and aging are described, and the neuroimaging of white matter is presented.

Part II deals with the plethora of illnesses that can affect the white matter, including genetic disorders, demyelinating diseases such as multiple sclerosis, infectious diseases such as AIDS and progressive multifocal leukoencephalopathy, inflammatory diseases, toxic disorders such as glue sniffing, metabolic conditions, vascular diseases, traumatic brain injuries, neoplasms, and hydrocephalus.

Part III is devoted to cognitive disorders associated with white matter diseases. Dementias are described and the role of the white matter in focal neurobehavioral syndromes such as amnesia and aphasia is discussed. Neuropsychiatric syndromes arising with white matter dysfunction include depression, mania, psychosis, personality alterations, and fatigue, and they are also presented.

Finally, an overview of the behavioral neurology of white matter, including what is to be learned about distributed neuronal networks and disconnection, is given. Dr. Filley ends by looking ahead to future directions in the study of white matter and white matter diseases, and speculates on the role of white matter in consciousness and self-consciousness.

Clinicians and neurobiologists from many disciplines will find this to be a useful volume. The description of the diseases themselves is a worthwhile contribution, and creating the context for these disorders is an understanding of the neurobiology of white matter provides a unique new perspective on old diseases. Those who make themselves students of Dr. Filley's extensive knowledge of white matter and white matter disorders by reading this book will find themselves richly rewarded for their efforts.

Los Angeles, California   Jeffrey L. Cummings, M.D.

Preface

Every book represents an attempt to discover order from disorder. An area of interest and confusion becomes apparent, study and contemplation proceed, and, with patience and good fortune, a coherent synthesis may emerge from the chaos. In this spirit I have pursued a deeper understanding of white matter. The reader can judge the extent to which I have succeeded.

Behavioral neurology attempts to explain the relationships between brain and behavior, which really means the role of the brain in all mental phenomena. An appropriate first step in this quest is to focus on the cerebral cortex, where astonishingly complex neuronal events play a central role in the variegated and richly textured operations of the mind. One may also look to the subcortical gray matter as making a vital contribution to human behavior. The white matter, however—that tangled collection of tracts coursing everywhere in the brain—is more difficult to understand in neurobehavioral terms. Compared to the adjacent gray matter, white matter may almost seem to be a passive bystander in the extraordinary activities occurring all around it.

This component of the brain has nevertheless proven to be an endless source of fascination. As enticing as cortical structure and function can be for the study of the mind, I have been steadily intrigued by frequent and consistent suggestions from both clinical practice and the neuroscientific literature that the white matter plays a major role in cognition and emotion. I entertain no illusion that my intuition is unique—indeed, experienced neurologists surely have a similar appreciation for this aspect of white matter disease. Yet, it is surprisingly difficult to find comprehensive summary works dealing with the white matter disorders and their effects on higher function.

In this book, therefore, my objective is to examine the role of the brain white matter in the organization of human mental activity. This task is undertaken from the perspective of behavioral neurology, and, as in the description of higher function deficits associated with cortical neuropathology, the lesion method is employed primarily. To begin, a review of relevant background information serves as a broad introduction. Then follows a consideration of white matter disorders that occur across the life span, with special attention to the neurobehavioral syndromes with which they are associated. Finally, by constructing some notion of the behavioral functions that are disrupted by white matter disease or injury, it will be possible to venture tentative speculations about the normal white matter based on these clinical observations. From this process emerges an attempt to establish a behavioral neurology of white matter.

At the conclusion of the book, I hope to have demonstrated that it is most reasonable to regard the white matter as interacting with gray matter in distributed, multifocal neural networks to produce the phenomena of human behavior. There should be no absolute, neophrenological assignment of neurobehavioral functions to discrete brain centers, whether these are individual Brodmann areas, cortical gyri, or the entire cortical mantle. The neural network model of current neuroscience compels a more sophisticated view, and inclusion of the white matter in this theorizing promises to expand our understanding of these networks and how they mediate various neurobehavioral operations. Thus, I attempt to explore how a consideration of the white matter assists in conceptualizing the organization of cognition and emotion in the human brain. The mind, I propose, depends as much on the white matter as on its gray counterpart.

Acknowledgments

This book could not have been written without the valuable assistance of many mentors, colleagues, and advisors. In particular, I am grateful to B. K. Kleinschmidt-DeMasters, C. Alan Anderson, James P. Kelly, Stuart A. Schneck, Kenneth L. Tyler, Jack H. Simon, John R. Corboy, David B. Arciniegas, Bruce H. Price, Neill R. Graff-Radford, S. Rock Levinson, James H. Austin, and M-Marsel Mesulam. My first investigations of the white matter disorders were made possible by Gary M. Franklin, Robert K. Heaton, and Neil L. Rosenberg, without whose help I could not have reached this point. Steven M. Rao has been helpful both for his extensive work with multiple sclerosis and his encouragement of my efforts. Josette G. Harris, C. Munro Cullum, Laetitia L. Thompson, Jose M. Lafosse, John DeLuca, and Elizabeth Kozora have also advised me on many neuropsychological issues that arose in the course of this project. James J. LaGuardia was a trusted source of information on the use of computers and word processing. Michelle LaCasse contributed her talents in medical illustration. Special thanks are due to Joseph B. Green and Jo F. Cembalisty for all they have taught me. I also acknowledge and am grateful for the assistance of Fiona Stevens of Oxford University Press, whose steady support and guidance were critical at all stages of this undertaking.

Contents

I

THE BRAIN, THE MIND, AND WHITE MATTER

1

The Neurologic Background

The title of this book brings together two terms seldom linked in the vocabulary of neuroscience. White matter has not traditionally been emphasized in behavioral neurology, and the higher functions of human beings are generally viewed as implicating the gray matter of the brain, particularly the cerebral cortex. Indeed, the assumption that the singular phenomena of human behavior predominantly require the activities of the cortical gray matter is one of the most pervasive in all of neuroscience. Whereas there is an impressive body of evidence in support of this belief, it is worth recalling that the cerebral cortex consists of only the outermost 3 millimeters of the brain. Moreover, a wealth of clinical experience suggests that disorders affecting structures below the cortex, many of which are white matter tracts, reliably and significantly alter mental functions. Thus, the notion that mental life is *exclusively* represented in the cortical gray matter should be considered an oversimplification.

A wide range of syndromes involving both cognitive decline and emotional dysfunction has been linked with structural involvement of the brain white matter. Clinical observations of patients with white matter disorders generate the essential data to support this claim. Much additional information has been gathered with the help of magnetic resonance imaging (MRI), a powerful neuroimaging technique that has provided unprecedented views of the white matter and permitted correlations with neurobehavioral syndromes. These syndromes may equal or surpass in clinical importance the various deficits in motor and sensory function of white matter lesions well known from classical neurology. Whereas caution is still appropriate in assessing the neurobehavioral importance of white matter changes, it is no longer possible to ignore them.

The goal of this book is to construct a foundation for understanding the relationship of brain white matter and behavior. On this basis, an attempt can then be made to contribute to a larger understanding of how the brain mediates the phenomena of human mental life. The intent is not to diminish the role of the gray matter, but rather to suggest how gray and white matter function together in the elaboration of human behavior. Central to this idea is the concept of distributed neural networks, a widely accepted model of brain function that readily lends itself to an appreciation of the integrated activity of multiple gray and white matter regions. In this light, higher functions can be viewed as resulting from the joint activities of gray and white matter areas that each contribute unique components to the final behavioral product.

By way of introduction, several background issues require attention. The history of the neurobiological understanding of white matter will provide a general orientation to the topic. Next will follow a review of the concept of subcortical dementia, which has provided an organizing framework for considering cerebral white matter disorders. In this context, a discussion of how the white matter may be interpreted as a participant in higher cerebral function will proceed. Finally, an attempt will be made to demonstrate how a conception of the brain as the organ of the mind cannot escape inclusion of the white matter and its many and varied disorders.

White Matter in the History of Neurology

The brain was anatomically recognized in antiquity, and the Greek physican Hippocrates (460–370 B.C.) regarded it as the source of human intelligence, dreams, and thought (McHenry, 1969). The understanding of brain anatomy was long hindered, however, by the reluctance of the Greeks and their successors to open and dissect the human body. Thus, for centuries neuroanatomy made little progress. Although the influential physician Galen of Pergamus (131–201 A.D.) held that the substance of the brain was the site of mental faculties, many authorities throughout the Middle Ages believed that mental functions were localized within the ventricles (McHenry, 1969).

With the arrival of the Renaissance, dissection of the body was undertaken in earnest, and the science of anatomy began to flourish. Neuroanatomy also expanded as never before. In 1543, some of the most remarkable depictions of brain anatomy ever produced were published by the great anatomist Andreas Vesalius (1514–1564; Fig. 1-1) in his monumental *De Humani Corporis Fabrica*. This extraordinary work is one of the most enduring and influential in the history of science, and initiated the objective study of the human body that was encouraged by the humanistic interests of the era in which it appeared. Vesalius himself produced some of the drawings in the *Fabrica*, although most were produced by students working in the studios of the Renaissance master Titian, the most notable of whom was Jan Stephen van Kalkar (Saunders and O'Malley, 1973). The beauty and ele-

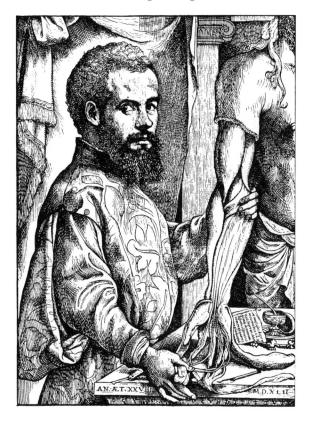

Figure 1-1. Andreas Vesalius. (Reprinted with permission from Saunders and O'Malley, 1973.)

gance of these illustrations, combined with an extraordinary degree of anatomic accuracy, render them superb examples of descriptive science that still impress the observer more than four centuries later.

In the *Fabrica,* the white matter of the brain was identified as a distinct neuro-anatomic structure for the first time. Vesalius clearly distinguished the white matter from the cortical gray matter in drawings from the seventh book of his masterwork (Fig. 1-2). The function of the white matter, however, was not understood, although it was speculated that its purpose was purely mechanical. Vesalius in fact believed that the corpus callosum was primarily a supporting structure in the brain, serving to maintain and protect the integrity of the ventricles (Bogen, 1993).

The observations of Vesalius stimulated others who followed to examine both the structure and the function of white matter. Soon after the appearance of the *Fabrica,* Archiangelo Piccolomini (1526–1586) completed the first successful gross dissection of white from gray matter (Gross, 1998). Piccolomini referred to the cerebral cortex as the "cerebrum" and the white matter as the "medulla," but did not assign functional roles to either structure (Gross, 1998). An early attempt

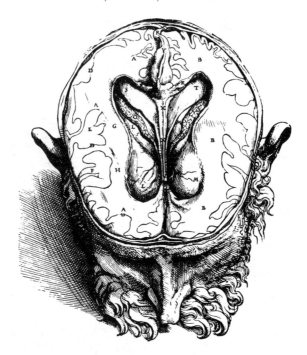

Figure 1-2. Drawing of the brain from the seventh book of Vesalius's *De Humani Corporis Fabrica,* distinguishing cerebral white matter from gray matter. (Reprinted with permission from Saunders and O'Malley, 1973.)

at describing the function of white matter was made in the next century by the noted anatomist Thomas Willis (1621–1675), who thought that the white matter, including the corpus callosum, elaborated sensory signals into perceptions and imaginations that were later stored as memories in the cortex (Gross, 1998). With this speculation, Willis anticipated later understanding of white matter connectivity. After the introduction of the microscope, Marcello Malpighi (1628–1694) was the first to examine the fine structure of brain white matter. Malpighi, the founder of microscopic anatomy, observed that white matter fibers arose from cerebral gyri and travelled to other regions of the brain (Gross, 1998). The philosopher and scientist Emmanuel Swedenborg (1688–1772) then recognized that white matter fibers descended through the brainstem to the spinal cord (Gross, 1998).

Further clarification of the structure and function of white matter in the brain came from the work of Franz Joseph Gall (1758–1828; Fig. 1-3), who, with the help of his student Johann Kaspar Spurzheim (1776–1832), performed credible neuro-anatomic studies before venturing into the fanciful area of organology, later to be known as phrenology (McHenry, 1969). In the early 1800s, Gall and Spurzheim established that white matter did indeed consist of individual fibers, and that these coalesced into tracts that connected cortical gray matter regions they considered the organs of mental activity (McHenry, 1969). Thus, although Gall and Spurzheim

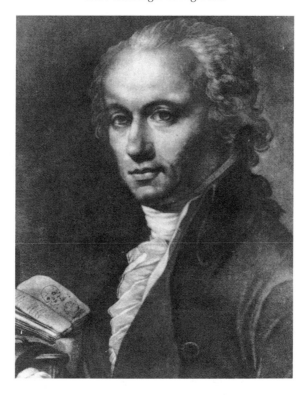

Figure 1-3. Franz Joseph Gall. (Reprinted with permission from McHenry, 1969.)

were primarily neuroanatomists, they speculated on the functional aspects of brain regions. Their emphasis on cortical function strongly influenced subsequent concepts of cerebral localization, but they also laid a foundation for later ideas on the contributions of white matter.

As the nineteenth century progressed, more detail was elucidated on the neuroanatomy of cerebral white matter. Theodor Schwann (1810–1882) was the first to describe the insulating sheath located around the axon in 1838 (McHenry, 1969). Among his many contributions to neuropathology, the noted pathologist Rudolph Virchow (1821–1902) is credited with the introduction of the word myelin to describe the material comprising this sheath (Morell and Norton, 1980). Carl Weigert (1845–1904) developed a stain for myelin in 1882 that advanced the study of white matter tracts and is still in use today (McHenry, 1969). Paul Flechsig (1847–1929) devoted several decades of his long career to the study of white matter and myelinogenesis. Among his many contributions, he described a number of white matter tracts, including the pyramidal tract, the internal capsule, and the auditory radiation (McHenry, 1969). Flechsig also showed that myelinogenesis proceeded in a variable manner depending on the area of the brain involved, and his assertion that cerebral regions are functionally mature only when their myelination is complete has been widely influential (McHenry, 1969). Flechsig's rule, which states that cortical sensory areas are not connected directly with each other but with related association cortices (Flechsig, 1901), played a major role in Geschwind's theorizing about disconnection syndromes many years later (Geschwind, 1965).

In the clinical arena, cerebral localization of function became an object of intense study during the late 1800s (Young, 1970). Neurologists made great strides in understanding disturbed function as a result of cerebral lesions. In terms of cerebral white matter, the leading figure of the era was the French neurologist Jean Marie Charcot (1825–1893; Fig. 1-4). Working at the Salpêtrière Hospital in Paris, Charcot made many seminal contributions to the understanding of multiple sclerosis (MS) that clarified the role of white matter in health and disease (Haymaker, 1953).

Most investigators, however, concentrated on focal lesions of the cerebral cortex, the study of which led to clinical–pathologic correlations that substantially advanced the understanding of the localization of higher functions. From the success of these investigations, it is not surprising that cognitive function came to be increasingly regarded as primarily represented in the cerebral cortex. The seminal studies of Paul Broca (1824–1880), Carl Wernicke (1848–1904), Jules Dejerine (1849–1917), Hugo Liepmann (1863–1925), Heinrich Lissauer (1861–1891),

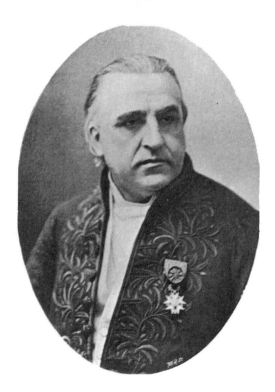

Figure 1-4. Jean Marie Charcot. (Reprinted with permission from McHenry, 1969.)

John Hughlings Jackson (1835–1911), and others provided classic descriptions of syndromes such as aphasia, alexia, apraxia, and agnosia that were based for the most part on lesions in critical cortical areas (Haymaker, 1953). These studies provided the neuroscientific basis for behavioral neurology as understood and practiced today.

The effects of white matter on behavior, however, did attract some attention from neurologists. Charcot, among his many observations of MS patients, clearly recognized that intellectual and emotional faculties could be affected (Charcot, 1877). Others developed elegant brain–behavior relationships based on the study of focal white matter lesions. Dejerine, for example, demonstrated involvement of the splenium of the corpus callosum in pure alexia (Geschwind, 1965). Similarly, Liepmann included the anterior corpus callosum in his explanation of unilateral apraxia (Geschwind, 1965). These focal disorders came to be known as disconnection syndromes, and the disruption of a tract connecting cortical areas was essential for their appearance. Thus, whereas the cortical gray matter was the main interest of classical neurologists, cerebral white matter was included in many formulations of brain–behavior relationships. As the nineteenth century came to a close, one can discern a nascent appreciation of the interaction of multiple cerebral regions in the operations of the mind.

The Concept of Subcortical Dementia

In the twentieth century, a different line of inquiry developed that would prove relevant to the study of cerebral white matter. Whereas it was generally believed that cortical damage was the major neuropathologic substrate of mental dysfunction (Mandell and Albert, 1990), some investigators began to examine the possibility that disorders involving selective lesions of subcortical structures such as the basal ganglia and thalamus could also disrupt cognition and emotion. In 1922, a form of mental impairment called bradyphrenia was described in patients with postencephalitic parkinsonism, who presumably had primary damage to the substantia nigra and related areas (Naville, 1922). The term subcortical dementia was coined 10 years later to describe postencephalitic patients with a similar mental slowness who also had personality and affective disturbances (von Stockert, 1932). These important developments were largely ignored, however, as were concepts of cerebral localization in general during the first half of the century. With the ascendancy of Freudian interpretations of behavior in those years, the neural basis of behavior—cortical or subcortical—received scant attention.

After many decades of neglect, the idea of subcortical dementia was revived in the 1970s. This development evolved from the work of two groups that made remarkably similar clinical observations independent of the other. Martin Albert and colleagues (1974) described a pattern of cognitive impairment consistent with subcortical dementia in five patients with progressive supranuclear palsy, while Paul McHugh and Marshall Folstein (1975) described a nearly identical syndrome in eight patients with Huntington's disease. In general, these investigators empha-sized cognitive slowing, forgetfulness, and personality and emotional changes as typical of subcortical dementias, in contrast to the amnesia, aphasia, apraxia, and agnosia that are traditionally associated with cortical dementias. Subcortical de-mentia was theorized to disrupt the "fundamental" functions of arousal, atten-tion, motivation, and mood that provide for the timing and activation of cortical processes, whereas cortical dementia was seen as interfering with the "instrumen-tal" functions of memory, language, praxis, and perception primarily associated with the neocortex (Albert, 1978). An analogous distinction was also drawn be-tween the concept of "channel" functions, referring to the specific contents of cognition, and "state" functions, those that maintain the state of information pro-cessing in the brain (Mesulam, 2000). Based on these formulations, descriptive clinical work in the dementias flourished, and subcortical dementia became a widely used, if not universally accepted term for the dementia that can be seen in patients with a variety of subcortical diseases (Cummings and Benson, 1984; Whitehouse, 1986). As further studies appeared, the clinical resemblance of sub-cortical with frontal lobe disease was recognized, and the alternate terms fronto-subcortical dementia and frontal systems dementia were suggested (Freedman and Albert, 1985), although subcortical dementia has remained the most common designation of this syndrome.

Cerebral white matter disorders were not initially included in the list of sub-cortical dementias. However, in the years following the reports of Albert, McHugh and their colleagues, disorders of white matter were also recognized as capable of disrupting neurobehavioral function in a similar fashion. Prominent among these was MS, certainly the most familiar disease of cerebral white matter. Considerable effort was concentrated on the neurobehavioral deficits that can accompany MS, and the disease came to be seen as capable of causing many different syndromes and often major disability (Rao, 1986). Other diseases with significant white matter pathology were also found to manifest similar deficits, including Bin-swanger's disease (Babikian and Ropper, 1987) and the acquired immunodefi-ciency syndrome (AIDS) dementia complex (Navia et al., 1986), and cerebral white matter disorders began to be regarded as etiologies of subcortical dementia (Cummings, 1990).

Presently, white matter disorders of the brain are included, albeit somewhat uneasily, in lists of subcortical dementias by most authorities. To some extent, clinical lore persists that white matter disorders do not significantly disturb cog-nition. Subcortical gray matter disorders are more readily accepted as having the potential to disrupt cognition and emotion; white matter disorders are regarded as more likely to cause elementary motor, sensory, and visual deficits than neurobe-havioral disturbances. Although white matter disorders are acknowledged to pro-duce a clinical picture similar to that of subcortical gray matter diseases, whether they have any distinct features remains uncertain. A sign of the lasting emphasis on gray matter function can be seen by perusal of major textbooks in behavioral neurology and neuropsychology, which typically do not specifically address white matter or its disorders (Feinberg and Farah, 1997; Mesulam, 2000).

Does White Matter Contribute to Higher Function?

At the basis of the uncertainty surrounding the role of cerebral white matter in higher function is a long-held belief among neuroscientists that gray matter—cortical and more recently subcortical—is the neural tissue primarily responsible for cognition and emotion. The general public concurs with this opinion, as the popular identification of intelligence with gray matter attests. Indeed, a substantial basis for this view exists. Compelling evidence supporting the neurobehavioral importance of cortical gray matter in particular has been adduced from clinical and experimental studies in humans and experimental animals, and the widely used term "higher cortical function" (Luria, 1980) is used to refer to the interests of behavioral neurologists and neuropsychologists. The white matter, in contrast, is believed to be devoted mainly to motor and sensory systems in the brain and spinal cord. Thus, when cognitive and emotional problems appear in patients with cerebral white matter disorders, there is some reluctance to ascribe these deficits to the white matter lesion(s), and psychological explanations are often invoked to explain them.

The dominance of the concept of higher cortical function results from two centuries of clinical and experimental evidence on the role of cortical gray matter in the activities of the mind. Gall and Spurzheim first concentrated on the cerebral cortex because they believed this was the part of the brain that could exert a physical effect on the conformation of the skull, and identification of palpable surface landmarks of the skull was central to their theories of brain function (Young, 1970). Although they recognized white matter as connecting gray matter areas, Gall and Spurzheim did not include these tracts in their ideas on localization. Despite the errors and excesses of phrenology that were soon recognized, the phrenologists' notion that mental faculties were to be found in the cortex held firm.

Later in the nineteenth century, investigators influenced by Gall and Spurzheim made clinical observations consistent with the idea that higher functions were represented in the cerebral cortex. As the idea of cerebral localizationism gradually gained acceptance during this era (Tyler and Malessa, 2000), the functions of the cortex most often attracted the attention of neurologists. For example, Broca's famous promotion of the role of the left frontal lobe in language production gave strong support to the concept of cortical localization (Young, 1970). In the 1870s, the work of Gustav Fritsch (1838–1927) and Eduard Hitzig (1838–1907) demonstrating the electrical excitability of the motor cortex further focused attention on cortical function (Young, 1970). The more detailed physiological investigations of David Ferrier (1843–1928) confirmed and extended these findings, and he proposed that psychological as well as motor phenomena could be represented in the cortex (Young, 1970). At about the same time, Jackson's clinical observations that irritative cortical lesions could produce psychic phenomena in epileptic patients further supported the role of the cortex in higher functions (McHenry, 1969). As noted above, localizationists in neurology after Broca generally emphasized the role of cortical function in neurobehavioral syndromes. In the mid-twentieth century, the stimulation studies of Wilder Penfield (1891–1976) brought a new level of maturity to these theories, providing direct evidence that mental experiences could be elicited by cortical stimulation (Penfield, 1975). In the last decade, with the arrival of new functional neuroimaging techniques, mental phenomena could be safely and accurately imaged in the living brain, and the major role of the cortex was again abundantly clear (Raichle, 1994). Finally, spectacular advances in molecular biology and neurophysiology have provided major insights into the cortical mediation of memory and other cognitive domains (Kandel and Pittenger, 1999).

The relative underemphasis on white matter in the study of behavior persists despite major contributions from leading clinical neuroscientists. Norman Geschwind (1926–1984), the dominant behavioral neurologist of the twentieth century, influenced a generation of clinicians and investigators with his insights into brain–behavior relationships (Fig. 1-5). In 1965, Geschwind published his famous article on cerebral disconnection syndromes, widely acknowledged to be his most important publication. Among the many features of this tour-de-force, reference is made to the role played by white matter in the cognitive modeling of many classic nineteenth century neurologists. For Geschwind, disconnection of cerebral regions by lesions of association cortices or white matter tracts was central to the classic syndromes of behavioral neurology. It follows from this perspective that interruption of white matter tracts, either intrahemispheric (association) fibers or interhemispheric (callosal) fibers, can disturb neurobehavioral functioning even if the cortical areas connected by these tracts are intact. Although the idea of disconnection has had a substantial impact on behavioral neurology and neuroscience in general (Absher and Benson, 1993), interest in the specific role of white matter lesions has not equalled the attention devoted to lesions of the association cortices.

Disconnection research in the twentieth century has also been focused on the corpus callosum. This structure is the largest white matter tract in the brain, and its obvious importance in connecting the two hemispheres has attracted substantial interest. Geschwind based much of his early theorizing on a patient with cerebral disconnection from a lesion of the anterior corpus callosum (Geschwind and Kaplan, 1962), and additional studies have been undertaken with individuals who have callosal agenesis (Chapter 5) and corpus callosotomy (Chapter 12). In particular, elegant studies supporting a neurobehavioral role of the corpus callosum came from the work of Roger Sperry and Michael Gazzaniga, who used experimental animals and humans with "split brains" following surgical section of the corpus callosum to document commissural white matter contributions to cognitive function (Sperry, 1961; Gazzaniga, 1970). However, because patients with callosal lesions typically have surprisingly few, if any, obvious neurologic deficits, skepticism about the role of the corpus callosum in behavior has persisted (Bogen, 1993). Even today, studies on callosal disconnection are largely of interest to research neuroscientists, and there has been relatively little application of this information to the clinical realm.

The conceptual dominance of gray matter, although still strong, began to be revised in the 1980s with the advent of MRI (Chapter 4). With this development, which made possible the routine imaging of the cerebral white matter with high resolution and without patient exposure to ionizing radiation, clinical detection of

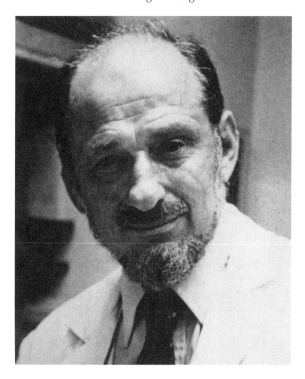

Figure 1-5. Norman Geschwind.

white matter disorders became common. For example, the dementia associated with solvent vapor abuse was somewhat unexpectedly found to be associated with leukoencephalopathy on MRI (Filley et al., 1990), and toluene leukoencephalopathy provided one of the best examples of dementia from white matter disease. Since its introduction, MRI has continued to reveal a variety of cerebral white matter abnormalities in many populations. One of the most intriguing of these is the controversial entity seen in elderly individuals known as leukoaraiosis (Hachinski et al., 1987), a finding that raises many questions about the origin and impact of vascular white matter disease. The study of previously known white matter diseases also advanced rapidly with the arrival of MRI, as the example of MS readily demonstrates. Magnetic resonance imaging has become a major clinical and research tool assisting in the understanding of white matter disorders.

The convergence of considerable clinical and MRI evidence has now prompted a reconsideration of the role of cerebral white matter. The most important syndrome to emerge from early studies was cognitive impairment, and many patients with cognitive loss or frank dementia were increasingly recognized. In an effort to highlight the dementia that could be ascribed specifically to dysfunction of cerebral white matter, the term *white matter dementia* was proposed (Filley et al., 1988). Whereas the main goal of this designation was to call attention to potential neurobehavioral disturbances in these patients, evidence also appeared suggesting that this syndrome has a specific neuropsychological profile that distinguishes it from both cortical and subcortical gray matter dementia (Rao, 1996). Thus, in addition to serving as an exhortation for clinical vigilance in evaluating individuals with white matter disorders, the concept of white matter dementia has a theoretical dimension as well (Filley, 1998).

In the 1990s, further exploration of the role of white matter in behavior was undertaken. The most complete and systematic work has been done on MS, which continues to provide an excellent example of a white matter disorder that disrupts cognition and emotion in a previously intact individual. Multiple sclerosis has come to be recognized as a prototype white matter disorder, with a wide range of neurobehavioral and neuropsychiatric syndromes that may be encountered (Feinstein, 1999). White matter disorders in general began to attract further attention as a group with distinctive neuropsychological features within the broad category of the dementias (Derix, 1994; Rao, 1996). In children and adolescents, a related approach has been the proposal of a model of neuropsychological dysfunction called the "syndrome of nonverbal learning disabilities" (NLD; Rourke, 1995). This model postulates that a pattern of cognitive deficits detectable in a wide range of diverse disorders can be explained by the common feature of white matter dysfunction (Rourke, 1995).

The past decade has thus witnessed several attempts to examine specific disorders, as well as clinical features that can be seen as common to many, in an effort to determine the contribution of white matter to cognition and emotion. With the arrival of the new century, there is an emerging recognition of the importance of white matter in behavioral neurology. Propelled mainly by the remarkable advances of neuroimaging, a specific focus on this portion of the brain has now become feasible.

The Perspective of Behavioral Neurology

This review of the background preceding this book has revealed that the white matter of the brain, while not fully dismissed by behavioral neurologists, merits more attention than it has received. Far from existing only as a supporting structure in the brain, white matter serves to connect cortical and subcortical regions within and between the hemispheres in functionally important ways. White matter in the brainstem and cerebellum may also be relevant to higher function, although information on this possibility is limited. The white matter of the brain necessarily participates in a wide range of neuronal ensembles that subserve capacities of the nervous system as diverse as motor function, visual recognition, and impulse control. Whereas elemental neurologic deficits are clearly a result of white matter lesions, so too are higher functional impairments. Current thinking in behavioral neurology stresses the existence of multifocal distributed neural networks that are dedicated to the higher functions (Mesulam 1990, 1998, 2000). Gray matter areas operate in concert with each other in the mediation of these activities, and white matter forms the connecting tissues that link these areas into coherent neural assemblies. Lesions in these tracts therefore produce dysfunction that reflects the uncoupling of neural networks even when they are not destroyed.

In the tradition of Geschwind, disconnection of neural networks by white matter lesions has been acknowledged as theoretically significant, but many patients with white matter disorders are still evaluated without appropriate regard for potential neurobehavioral syndromes that may exist. This paradoxical situation stems in part from the entrenchment of the idea of higher cortical function, but other factors also influence the thinking of clinicians and researchers in behavioral neurology and related disciplines. First, there is the perplexing occasional patient, usually older, who has extensive white matter changes on MRI but is nonetheless cognitively intact (Fein et al., 1990). Such individuals introduce doubt about whether lesions in the white matter have any neurobehavioral consequences. Second, the neuroanatomy of white matter is complex, and details of white matter connections, well studied in the monkey, are poorly understood in humans (Mesulam, 2000). Thus, unlike cortical or subcortical lesions that can be increasingly well identified by clinical and neuroradiologic methods, discrete white matter tracts cannot be so easily located and analyzed.

Nevertheless, experience with the white matter disorders of the brain is rapidly expanding because of the increasing frequency with which they are encountered, and the weight of clinical evidence supports their impact on cognitive and emotional function (Filley, 1996). The prevalence of neurobehavioral syndromes caused by white matter disorders is difficult to determine, but when the full range of afflictions discussed in Part II of this book is considered, they are clearly not rare. Also, the burden of neurobehavioral disability in patients with these disorders is enormous and underappreciated. Moreover, because white matter lesions often involve damage to myelin alone without axonal damage, the potential for spontaneous improvement or effective treatment is higher than in disorders of gray matter that typically destroy neurons. Substantial clinical benefit may thus accrue from a better understanding of these issues.

To address the role of the brain white matter in neurobehavioral function, the major resource for this book will necessarily be clinical reports of individuals with cerebral white matter disorders. A thorough literature review will provide the basis for considering this question, as there is substantial information in many different contexts that has not been collected in a comprehensive manner to address the topic. As in other areas of behavioral neurology, the lesion method that has proven so useful will be assumed to be equally applicable to the analysis of white matter disorders (Filley, 1995).

In many cases, there will be some ambiguity about whether a given disorder does in fact represent sufficiently selective white matter involvement to allow for correlation with neurobehavioral observations. The problem of neuroanatomic specificity, though not trivial, has long bedeviled behavioral neurology and should not deter an attempt such as this. The cerebral localization of many well-known neurobehavioral disorders is in fact still debated, and this process energizes and refines our understanding of brain–behavior relationships. The intent here is to provide a preliminary survey of white matter disorders that can introduce the possibility of significant neurobehavioral correlations. If further work either confirming or denying such correlations is accomplished, this book will have served a useful purpose.

A recurring theme will be the remarkable frequency with which important and similar neurobehavioral features of white matter disorders appear in clinical observations, even when they are not the focus of the report. Findings from MRI will also play a central role in this undertaking. The specific objectives are to explore what information is available, consider how can it be employed clinically and theoretically, and suggest ways in which further useful data can be gathered. Throughout what follows, a conceptual scheme for how the white matter functions to assist in elaborating human mental activity will be developed. As the organ of the mind, the brain in all of its structural and functional complexity deserves meticulous scrutiny.

References

Absher JR, Benson DF. Disconnection syndromes: an overview of Geschwind's contributions. Neurology 1993; 43: 862–867.

Albert ML. Subcortical dementia. In: Katzman R, Terry RD, Bick KL, eds. Alzheimer's disease: senile dementia and related disorders. New York: Raven Press, 1978: 173–180.

Albert ML, Feldman RG, Willis AL. The "subcortical dementia" of progressive supranuclear palsy. J Neurol Neurosurg Psychiatry 1974; 37: 121–130.

Babikian V, Ropper AH. Binswanger's disease: a review. Stroke 1987; 18: 2–12.

Bogen JE. The callosal syndromes. In: Heilman KM, Valenstein E, eds. Clinical neuropsychology. 3rd ed. New York: Oxford University Press, 1993: 337–407.

Charcot JM. Lectures on the diseases of the nervous system delivered at La Salpêtrière. London: New Sydenham Society, 1877.

Cummings JL, ed. Subcortical dementia. New York: Oxford University Press, 1990.

Cummings JL, Benson DF. Subcortical dementia. Review of an emerging concept. Arch Neurol 1984; 41: 874–879.

Derix MMA. Neuropsychological differentiation of dementia syndromes. Lisse: Swets and Zeitlinger, 1994.

Fein G, Van Dyke C, Davenport L, et al. Preservation of normal cognitive functioning in elderly subjects with extensive white-matter lesions of long duration. Arch Gen Psychiatry 1990; 47: 220–223.

Feinberg TE, Farah MJ, eds. Behavioral neurology and neuropsychology. New York: McGraw-Hill, 1997.

Feinstein A. The clinical neuropsychiatry of multiple sclerosis. Cambridge: Cambridge University Press, 1999.

Filley CM. Neurobehavioral anatomy. Niwot, CO: University Press of Colorado, 1995.

Filley CM. Neurobehavioral aspects of cerebral white matter disorders. In: Fogel BS, Schiffer RB, Rao SM, eds. Neuropsychiatry. Baltimore: Williams and Wilkins, 1996: 913–933.

Filley CM. The behavioral neurology of cerebral white matter. Neurology 1998; 50: 1535–1540.

Filley CM, Franklin GM, Heaton RK, Rosenberg NL. White matter dementia. Clinical disorders and implications. Neuropsychiatry Neuropsychol Behav Neurol 1988; 1: 239–254.

Filley CM, Heaton RK, Rosenberg NL. White matter dementia in chronic toluene abuse. Neurology 1990; 40: 532–534.

Flechsig P. Developmental (myelogenetic) localisation of the cerebral cortex in the human subject. Lancet 1901; 2: 1027–1029.

Freedman M, Albert ML. Subcortical dementia. In: Vinken PJ, Bruyn GW, Klawans H, Frederiks JAM, eds. Handbook of clinical neurology. Vol. 46: Neurobehavioral disorders. Amsterdam: Elsevier 1985: 311–316.

Gazzaniga M. The bisected brain. New York: Appleton Press, 1970.

Geschwind N. Disconnexion syndromes in animals and man. Brain 1965; 88: 237–294, 585–644.

Geschwind N, Kaplan E. A human cerebral deconnection syndrome: a preliminary report. Neurology 1962; 12: 675–685.

Gross CG. Brain, vision, memory. Tales in the history of neuroscience. Cambridge: MIT Press, 1998.

Hachinski VC, Potter P, Merskey H. Leuko-araiosis. Arch Neurol 1987; 44: 21–23.

Haymaker W. The founders of neurology. Springfield, IL: Charles C. Thomas, 1953.

Kandel ER, Pittenger C. The past, the future and the biology of memory storage. Phil Trans R Soc Lond B 1999; 354: 2027–2052.

Luria AR. Higher cortical functions in man. New York: Consultants Bureau, 1980.

Mandell AM, Albert ML. History of subcortical dementia. In: Cummings JL, ed. Subcortical dementia. New York: Oxford University Press, 1990: 17–30.

McHenry LC. Garrison's history of neurology. Springfield, IL: Charles C. Thomas, 1969.

McHugh PR, Folstein MF. Psychiatric syndromes of Huntington's chorea: a clinical and phenomenologic study. In: Benson DF, Blumer D, eds. Psychiatric aspects of neurologic disease. Vol. 1. New York: Grune and Stratton, 1975: 267–285.

Mesulam M-M. Large-scale neurocognitive networks and distributed processing for attention, language, and memory. Ann Neurol 1990; 28: 597–613.

Mesulam M-M. From sensation to cognition. Brain 1998; 121: 1013–1052.

Mesulam M-M. Behavioral neuroanatomy. Large-scale neural networks, association cortex, frontal systems, the limbic system, and hemispheric specializations. In: Mesulam M-M. Principles of behavioral and cognitive neurology. 2nd ed. New York: Oxford University Press, 2000: 1–120.

Morell P, Norton WT. Myelin. Sci Am 1980; 242: 88–118.

Navia BA, Cho E-S, Petito CK, Price RW. The AIDS dementia complex: II. Neuropathology. Ann Neurol 1986; 19: 525–535.

Naville F. Etudes sur les complications et les séquelles mentales de l'encéphalite épidémique. La bradyphrénie. L'Encéphale 1922; 17: 369–375, 423–436.

Penfield W. The mystery of the mind. Princeton, NJ: Princeton University Press, 1975.

Raichle M. Visualizing the mind. Sci Am 1994; 270: 58–64.

Rao SM. Neuropsychology of multiple sclerosis. A critical review. J Clin Exp Neuropsychol 1986; 8: 503–542.

Rao SM. White matter disease and dementia. Brain Cogn 1996; 31: 250–268.

Rourke BP, ed. Syndrome of nonverbal learning disabilities. New York: Guilford Press, 1995.

Saunders JBDM, O'Malley CD. The illustrations from the works of Andreas Vesalius of Brussels. New York: Dover, 1973.

Sperry RW. Cerebral organization and behavior. Science 1961; 133: 1749–1757.

Tyler KL, Malessa R. The Goltz-Ferrier debates and the triumph of cerebral localizationist theory. Neurology 2000; 55: 1015–1024.

Von Stockert FG. Subcorticale demenz. Arch Psychiatry 1932: 97: 77–100.

Whitehouse PJ. The concept of subcortical and cortical dementia: another look. Ann Neurol 1986; 19: 1–6.

Young RM. Mind, brain, and adaptation in the nineteenth century. London: Oxford University Press, 1970.

2

White Matter Structure and Function

The white matter forms a major constituent of the brain. In the adult human, white matter makes up more than 40% of the brain's cross-sectional area (Morell and Norton, 1980), and 40%–50% of the adult cerebral volume is occupied by white matter (Miller et al., 1980). The remainder of the brain parenchyma comprises the cerebral cortex, a number of subcortical and posterior fossa gray matter structures, and the blood vessels. White matter is made up of axons invested with myelin, millions of which combine to form the many tracts that travel within and between the hemispheres as well as to more caudal brainstem and cerebellar regions. Myelinated fibers perform a critical role in normal brain function by virtue of this vast and intricate connectivity. Although the great majority of the white matter is located within these tracts, myelinated fibers can also be found in gray matter areas. Smaller numbers of white matter fibers course within cortical and subcortical gray matter structures en route to their final destinations. Thus, the distinction between gray and white matter is only relative, and disorders of myelin can affect gray matter regions to some extent. This chapter reviews clinically relevant details of the structure and function of the brain white matter.

Neuroanatomy

The human brain is a collection of nervous tissue, glial cells, and vasculature weighing about 1400 grams in the adult (range 1100–1700), or roughly 2% of the total body weight (Nolte, 1999). It contains an estimated 100 billion neurons, each of which makes contact with at least 10,000 others, and many times the same number of glial cells (Kandel et al., 2000). The great majority of neurons (more than 99%) are classified as interneurons, meaning that most brain neurons are interposed between the afferent sensory systems concerned with the acquisition of external information, and the efferent systems concerned with the generation of motor output (Nolte, 1999). Many of these interneurons include long, myelinated axons that course through the brain and constitute roughly half of its volume. The white matter of the brain consists of myelinated axons, a large number of glial cells, and the blood vessels that nourish this portion of the central nervous system.

Myelin

The word myelin derives from the Greek word for marrow (*myelos*), and was coined by Rudolph Virchow to indicate the abundance of white matter in the core or marrow of the brain (Morell and Norton, 1980). This complex lipid-rich substance is now known to surround axons in both the peripheral and the central nervous systems, and although structural differences exist between central and peripheral myelin, its universal function is to insulate axons and thereby dramatically affect their electrical properties. The structure of myelin consists of multiple lipid bilayers with which proteins are closely related. Myelin in the freshly cut brain is easily visible because of its glistening white appearance that derives from its preponderance of lipid. In the brain, lipid accounts for approximately 70% of the dry weight of myelin, and protein for approximately 30% (McLaurin and Yong, 1995). Cholesterol is the most abundant lipid in brain myelin (40%), followed by cerebrosides (20%), phosphatidylserine and phosphatidylcholine (16%), ethanolamines (13%), phosphoglycerides (5.5%), sphingomyelin (4%), gangliosides (1%), and inositides (0.5%) (McLaurin and Yong, 1995). Proteins in the myelin of the brain include proteolipid protein (30%), myelin basic protein (25%), Wolfgram proteins (4%), myelin associated glycoproteins (1%), myelin/oligodendrocyte glycoprotein (0.05%), and a variety of other enzymes and glycoproteins (40%) (McLaurin and Yong, 1995).

Glial Cells

Of the four types of glial cells in the central nervous system (CNS)—oligodendrocytes, astrocytes, ependymal cells, and microglia—the first two are important in determining the structure and function of white matter. Oligodendrocytes are responsible for the formation of myelin, in a manner analogous to the Schwann cells of the peripheral nervous system. These cells originate from neuroectodermal cells in the ependymal germinal matrix that migrate into both white and gray matter to complete their maturation. Myelin is deposited concentrically along the axon by oligodendrocytes, which perform this task by laying down their membranes in a manner permitting the circumferential encircling of the axon (Fig. 2-1). The oligodendrocyte extends its process to the axon, and then wraps its plasma membrane

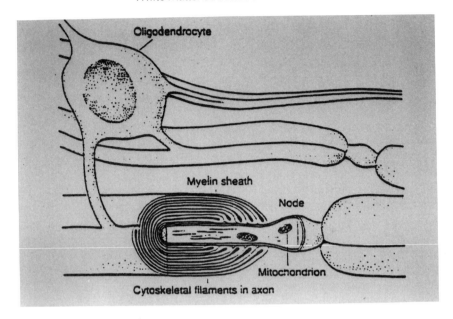

Figure 2-1. Drawing of an oligodendrocyte and the myelination of axons in the brain. (Reprinted with permission from Kandel et al., 2000.)

around the axon several times to form a compact myelin sheath. Each oligodendrocyte is capable of investing up to 60 neighboring axons with myelin, although this process is always limited to a specific segment of the axon (McLaurin and Yong, 1995). Thus, the myelin sheath is discontinuous, leaving uncovered short segments of the axon between areas of myelin. These regions, called nodes of Ranvier, permit much more efficient axonal transmission, as discussed below.

Astrocytes are star-shaped glial cells found throughout the CNS. These abundant cells are closely associated with neurons, for which they provide structural support, and they also contribute to metabolic homeostasis. In the white matter, astrocytic processes make numerous contacts with nearby axons at the nodes of Ranvier, and these connections enable the involvement of astrocytes in the regulation of the ionic microenvironment (Vernadakis, 1988). In addition, it is thought that astrocytes participate in synthesizing sodium channels for the nodal axon membrane (Waxman and Ritchie, 1993; see below).

White Matter Tracts

White matter consists of large collections of myelinated fibers that travel together between various cortical and subcortical destinations. Axons of these fibers may be as short as 1 mm (if they are strictly intracortical), or as long as 1 meter (if they travel from the brain to the caudal spinal cord) (Kandel et al., 2000). The diameter of brain axons ranges from 0.2 to 20 micrometers, and the myelin sheath substantially increases this figure (Kandel et al., 2000). In their aggregate form, white matter tracts are large enough to be grossly discernible, although they are extensively interwoven with each other so that identification of a single tract from its origin to its destination is not a simple task.

The word tract is the most commonly used descriptor for white matter pathways in the brain, but other similar words are fasciculus, funiculus, lemniscus, peduncle, and bundle (Nolte, 1999). Whereas these various terms find use in specific neuroanatomic contexts, all refer to discrete collections of white matter fibers. Three major groups of cerebral white matter pathways are recognized (Table 2-1). These are the projection, commissural, and association fibers.

Projection fibers consist of long ascending (corticopetal) and descending (corticofugal) tracts. Corticopetal (efferent) tracts connect structures lower in the brain and the spinal cord with the cortex, whereas corticofugal (afferent) tracts proceed in the opposite direction. Well-known projection fiber systems include the thalamocortical radiations linking thalamic nuclei with somatosensory and visual cortices, and the corticospinal and corticobulbar tracts connecting motor cortices with lower motor areas via the internal capsule and cerebral peduncle.

Commissural fibers connect the two hemispheres of the cerebrum. The most important commissural tract is the corpus callosum, a prominent structure containing some 300 million myelinated axons (Nolte, 1999; Fig. 2-2). The corpus callosum connects cortical regions in one hemisphere with homologous areas in the other, and consists of the posterior splenium, the central body, the anterior genu, and the ventrally directed rostrum, which merges with the lamina terminalis. Other commissures are also recognized: the anterior commissure, which connects olfactory and temporal regions, and the hippocampal or fornical commissure, which links the two crura of the fornices. Two other small commissures are the habenular commissure in the posterior thalamus and the posterior commissure at the junction of the midbrain and diencephalon.

Table 2-1. White Matter Tracts in the Brain

Projection
   Corticopetal
   Corticofugal
Commissural
   Corpus callosum
   Anterior commissure
   Hippocampal (fornical) commissure
Association
   Short—U (arcuate) fibers
   Long
      Arcuate fasciculus
      Superior occipitofrontal fasciculus
      Inferior occipitofrontal fasciculus
      Cingulum
      Uncinate fasciculus

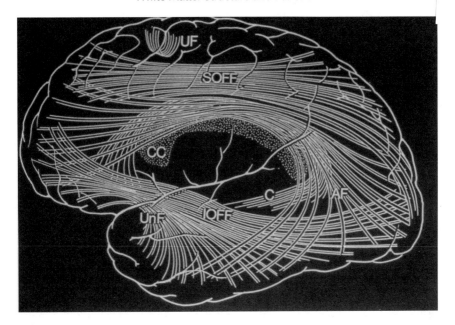

Figure 2-2. Drawing of association and commissural white matter tracts. UF, U fibers; CC, corpus callosum; SOFF, superior occipitofrontal fasciculus; IOFF, inferior occipitofrontal fasciculus; AF, arcuate fasciculus; UnF, uncinate fasciculus; C, cingulum (Reprinted with permission from Filley, 1995).

Association fibers connect cerebral areas within each hemisphere (Table 2-2; Fig. 2-2). First, there are short association fibers, the U or arcuate fibers, that link adjacent cortical gyri. Second, a large number of long association fibers connect more distant cerebral areas: the arcuate (superior longitudinal) fasciculus, the superior occipitofrontal fasciculus (subcallosal bundle), the inferior occipitofrontal fasciculus, the cingulum, and the uncinate fasciculus. These tracts are known primarily from gross dissection, and many details of their origin and termination have yet to be established (Nieuwenhuys et al., 1988). However, it is clear that association systems are generally arranged so as to be bidirectional (Nieuwenhuys et al., 1988),   which allows for extensive reciprocal communication between cerebral regions.

Long association fibers also share the interesting feature that they all have one terminus in the frontal lobe. No other lobe of the brain enjoys such rich connectivity. The white matter is therefore structurally organized to facilitate frontal lobe interaction with all other regions of the cerebrum. Although the means by which the frontal lobes exert their prominent influence remain obscure, this pattern of connectivity provides a neuroanatomic basis for their essential role in human behavior (Weinberger, 1993; Filley, 1995; Mesulam, 2000).

White matter tracts coalesce with each other in the cerebrum, forming a richly interdigitated mass of white matter within each hemisphere. Above the internal capsule, through which nearly all the neural traffic to and from the cerebral cortex

Table 2-2. Connections of the Association Fiber Systems

Tract	Structures Connected
Short (U or Arcuate Fibers)	Adjacent cortical gyri
Long	
Arcuate fasciculus	Frontal, parietal, temporal, occipital lobes
Superior occipitofrontal fasciculus	Frontal, parietal, occipital lobes
Inferior occipitofrontal fasciculus	Frontal, temporal, occipital lobes
Cingulum	Frontal, parietal, temporal lobes
Uncinate fasciculus	Frontal, temporal lobes

passes, lies a collection of fibers that fans out laterally called the corona radiata (Nolte, 1999). Still higher is found the centrum semiovale, the white matter located subjacent to the cortical mantle (Nolte, 1999). Other descriptive terms are also used to describe the white matter of the hemispheres. The periventricular white matter conveniently refers to that which lies immediately adjacent to the lateral ventricles. Less specific is the subcortical white matter, used by some authors to refer to the white matter just below the cortex, or by others to designate the aggregate of all major tracts found within the hemispheres. Although these terms all have a useful role for descriptive purposes, their imprecision underscores the fact that white matter structures in the human brain are understood only in general terms.

A number of smaller tracts can be found deep within the brain, the clinical significance of which remains largely obscure. Some of these deserve mention, however, because of evolving knowledge of their application to clinical syndromes: the fimbria-fornix, the medial forebrain bundle, the external capsule, and the extreme capsule. The fimbria emanates from the hippocampus and merges into the fornix as it curves posteriorly and dorsally to terminate in a nucleus of the hypothalamus called the mammillary body (Nolte, 1999). This tract serves as an important link in the limbic system, and has a role in both memory and emotion. The medial forebrain bundle connects the hypothalamus with the brainstem below and the cerebral cortex above (Kandel et al., 2000), and contains neurons conveying various biogenic amines (dopamine, norepinephrine, and serotonin) to their cortical destinations. The external capsule courses lateral to the lenticular nucleus (putamen and globus pallidus), and contains cholinergic fibers also destined for the cerebral cortex (Selden et al., 1998). The neurotransmitters carried within these tracts enable the major modulatory influences on the cortex that originate from the ascending reticular activating system in the brainstem (Mesulam, 1998). The extreme capsule lies lateral to the claustrum and subjacent to the insula, and its fibers connect the temporal and frontal lobes in addition to those of the arcuate fasciculus (Damasio and Damasio, 1980).

Other details of white matter neuroanatomy deserve comment. One intriguing observation pertains to data on laterality differences in the distribution of white matter. Some evidence exists to support the idea that the right hemisphere contains a larger relative proportion of white matter than the left, with a particularly marked difference in the frontal lobes (Gur et al., 1980). In contrast, the left hemisphere, or at least some areas within it, may contain a relatively larger proportion of gray matter (Geschwind and Levitsky, 1968). Just as interhemispheric cortical gray matter differences may represent differential functional affiliations, this discrepancy in the distribution of white matter may have significant implications in terms of the functional specializations of the two hemispheres, and even of individual regions within the hemispheres.

Another area of interest concerns gender differences. Although males have larger brains at all ages (Dekaban and Sadowsky, 1978), volumetric magnetic resonance imaging (MRI) studies indicate that women have a higher percentage of gray matter, whereas men appear to have proportionately more white matter and cerebrospinal fluid (Gur et al., 1999). The increase in gray matter among females may be particularly notable in the language regions of the left hemisphere, as autopsy studies indicate that women have proportionally larger Broca's and Wernicke's areas than do men (Harasty et al., 1997). These differences may have several important functional implications. First, the relative increase in left hemisphere gray matter in women may help explain the well-documented superiority of females in language tasks (Mann et al., 1990). Second, the relative increase in white matter among males, presumably more in the right than the left hemisphere (see above), may account in part for the superiority of males on visuospatial tasks (van Vugt et al., 2000). Finally, the larger percentage of white matter in males raises the possibility that disorders of white matter may be more clinically apparent in males than in females.

Knowledge of the neuroanatomy of cerebral white matter, however, is still limited by the fact that almost all of the research on corticocortical and corticosubcortical connectivity has been conducted using the monkey brain, and little corresponding information is available for humans (Mesulam, 2000). Studies using neuroanatomic, neuroimaging, electrophysiological, and computational methods to address this issue are underway but are still in their infancy (Mesulam, 2000). From a clinical point of view, the typical absence of precise delineation of white matter tracts renders brain–behavior correlations in this area difficult. Analysis of white matter lesions approaching the accuracy with which cortical damage can be localized must await a more complete understanding of the brain's intricate connectivity. One of the emerging challenges for neuroscientists is to develop a more sophisticated understanding of white matter neuroanatomy so that clinical lesions can be more confidently localized and appropriately treated.

Blood Supply

The arterial supply of the cerebral white matter comes from many perforating arteries that arise from larger arteries at the base of the brain. The most prominent of these are the lenticulostriate arteries that originate from the middle cerebral artery and follow a long course as they penetrate the deep structures of the cerebrum (Nolte, 1999). Autopsy studies of the brain microvasculature have shown some exceptions to this rule. The U or arcuate fibers, the external capsule, and the extreme capsule receive a rich blood supply provided by many short and interdigitated cortical arterioles (Moody et al., 1990). The corpus callosum is supplied by short, small caliber arterioles that arise from the pial plexus (Moody et al., 1988). The blood supply of the brainstem white matter comes from penetrating arteries arising from the basilar artery, and the cerebellar white matter is supplied by penetrating branches of the superior cerebellar, posterior inferior cerebellar, and anterior inferior cerebellar arteries (Nolte, 1999).

Neurophysiology

The brain is an electrical organ, and its function depends on the capacity to transmit electrical signals. Neurons are excitable cells that serve as the basic functional units of the nervous system. Each neuron, whether in the central or peripheral nervous system, operates by conducting an electrical impulse. This impulse, or action potential, is propagated along the axon in an all-or-none fashion, and the neuron can then influence another to which it is connected by synaptic transmission. All neurons in the brain, whether they are motor, sensory, or interneuronal, function in a similar manner. The speed and efficiency of this process, however, is significantly influenced by the degree of myelination of the axons. In the absence of normal myelination and white matter integrity, brain function is dramatically compromised.

The Action Potential

The axon of a neuron is constructed so that it may propagate a nerve impulse called the action potential. This event represents a departure from the normal resting membrane potential of the neuron, which is typically about -65 mV in humans (Kandel et al., 2000). The resting potential is determined by the separation of extracellular positive charges from intracellular negative charges that is maintained by the activity of the adenosine triphosphate (ATP)-dependent sodium-potassium pump. The action potential, or spike, is generated by the rapid influx of positively charged sodium ions through voltage-gated sodium channels that temporarily depolarizes the membrane so that the membrane potential briefly becomes positive (Fig. 2-3). The depolarization so produced is then quickly reversed by a rapid efflux of potassium ions that restores the resting potential. After a refractory period during which no action potential can be propagated, the axon is again prepared to conduct another impulse.

Neurons in the brain conduct electrical impulses at a velocity ranging from 1 to 120 meters per second. This variability is in part due to differences in axon diameter because smaller fibers conduct the impulse more slowly than larger ones. Very small axons, therefore, have very slow conduction velocity (Kandel et al., 2000).

Saltatory Conduction

An increase of neuronal conduction velocity is also conferred by the phenomenon of saltatory conduction. The myelin sheath is interrupted every 1–2 millimeters by unmyelinated segments of the axon called nodes of Ranvier, which are themselves

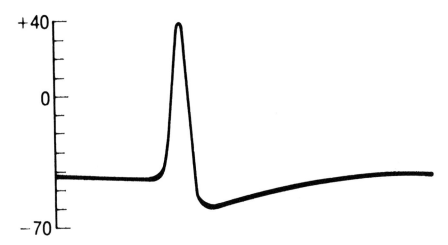

Figure 2-3. Action potential recorded from a squid giant axon. The "spike" represents a brief depolarization of the axonal membrane. (Reprinted with permission from Smith CUM. Elements of molecular neurobiology. 2nd ed. Chichester: John Wiley and Sons, 1996.)

about 2 micrometers in length (Kandel et al., 2000). The nodal axon membrane contains a higher density of sodium channels than the membrane of the internodal axon (Waxman and Ritchie, 1993). This arrangement permits the action potential to jump from one node to the next without the need for the entire axonal membrane to be depolarized. This kind of conduction is known as saltatory because of its derivation from the Latin verb *saltare,* meaning to leap (Fig. 2-4).

It is estimated that large myelinated fibers conduct impulses as much as 100 times faster than small unmyelinated fibers (Kandel et al., 2000), an increase largely due to myelination and the advantage of saltatory conduction. In addition, because the ionic current in myelinated axons flows only at the nodes of Ranvier, saltatory conduction reduces the energy expenditure required for restoring the sodium–potassium concentration gradient necessary for another action potential to follow (Kandel et al., 2000).

Clinical Neurophysiology

In clinical practice, the function of white matter tracts can be assessed to some extent with the use of in vivo neurophysiological techniques. In contrast to electroencephalography (EEG), which yields primarily an index of cortical function, evoked potentials (EPs) can offer insights into the integrity of white matter tracts.

The most familiar EPs are the conventional visual (VEP), auditory (AEP) or brainstem auditory (BAEP), and somatosensory (SEP) evoked potentials (Chiappa, 1980). These are potentials recorded at the scalp that reflect the function of primary sensory pathways as they traverse the CNS. Initially, evoked potentials found the most utility in the evaluation of suspected multiple sclerosis (MS), but

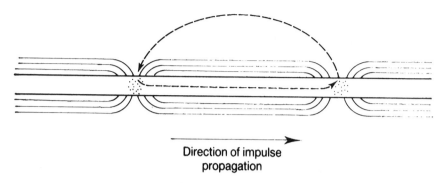

Direction of impulse
propagation

Figure 2-4. Saltatory conduction. The impulse rapidly "jumps" from one node of Ranvier to the next. (Reprinted with permission from Smith CUM. Elements of molecular neurobiology. 2nd ed. Chichester: John Wiley and Sons, 1996.)

their usefulness for this purpose has been considerably diminished by MRI, which has improved the depiction of normal and pathologic neuroanatomy and facilitated diagnosis of MS and other white matter disorders. The application of conventional EPs to behavioral neurology has not proven feasible because of the complex representation of cognition and emotion in comparison to elemental sensory function.

A special variety of EP, however, is the event-related potential (ERP), in which cognition is engaged in the generation of the electrophysiological response (Knight, 1997). Event-related potentials are also known as "endogenous" potentials to distinguish them from "exogenous" conventional EPs, and their promise for the study of behavior is considerable. In general, ERPs are long-latency waves related to the cognitive processing of stimuli (Hillyard and Kutas, 1983). The most familiar ERP is the P300 or P3, and this and other ERPs have been studied in neurologic (Puce et al., 1991) and psychiatric disorders (Egan et al., 1994), as well as in normal aging (Oken and Kaye, 1992). Because of the multiple neuroanatomic levels of processing that are involved, both gray and white matter structures are presumed to contribute to the generation of ERPs. Thus, whereas ERP abnormalities may reflect disturbances in neural systems relevant to behavior, these potentials are limited in the degree to which they can localize areas of dysfunction. It is therefore not surprising, for example, that prolonged P300 latencies can be found in a variety of different dementing diseases, including Alzheimer's disease, vascular dementia, and Parkinson's disease (Ito, 1994). In addition, controversy has surrounded the ERP technique because of technical difficulties that can complicate interpretation. Thus, the P300 and other ERPs are of research interest but have no routine clinical applications as yet.

Preliminary studies of ERPs have been performed in patients with white matter disorders. In MS, several groups have found that P300 abnormalities correlate with cognitive dysfunction and MRI lesion burden (Newton et al., 1989; Honig et al., 1992; Giesser et al., 1992), although there has been some evidence to the contrary (van Dijk et al., 1992). In children with cancer who developed treatment-related white matter changes, prolonged P300 latency has been correlated with cognitive impairment (Moore et al., 1992). Another cognitive evoked potential, the P50 (Freedman et al., 1996), has been found to be abnormal in traumatic brain injury patients (Arciniegas et al., 1999), and may prove to be particularly reflective of attentional dysfunction (Cullum et al., 1993; Erwin et al., 1998). Although it remains difficult to establish the neuroanatomy responsible for the generation of ERP data, the technique appears to have a potential contribution to the study of cognitive function in patients with white matter disorders.

White Matter and Neural Networks

A consideration of axonal transmission makes it clear that white matter plays a central role in efficient interneuronal communication. Without normal myelin, neurons can signal to each other, but the speed with which this process occurs is greatly reduced. In the brain, where the operations of the many distributed neural networks depend critically on normal communication between widely dispersed regions, integrity of the white matter tracts is a necessary condition for normal function. As discussed at more length later in this book, distributed neural networks are currently believed to form the foundation of a variety of neurobehavioral functions, such as attention, memory, language, and emotional competence (Mesulam, 1990, 1998, 2000). In terms of both structure and function, the cerebral white matter provides an essential component of these networks.

References

Arciniegas D, Adler L, Topkoff J, et al. Attention and memory dysfunction after traumatic brain injury: cholinergic mechanisms, sensory gating, and a hypothesis for further investigation. Brain Inj 1999; 13: 1–13.

Chiappa KH. Pattern shift visual, brainstem auditory, and short-latency somatosensory evoked potentials in multiple sclerosis. Neurology 1980; 30: 110–123.

Cullum CM, Harris JG, Waldo MC, et al. Neurophysiological and neuropsychological evidence for attentional dysfunction in schizophrenia. Schizophr Res 1993; 10: 131–141.

Damasio H, Damasio AR. The anatomical basis of conduction aphasia. Brain 1980; 103: 337–350.

Dekaban AS, Sadowsky D. Changes in brain weights during the span of human life: relations of brain weights to body heights and body weights. Ann Neurol 1978; 4: 345–356.

Egan MF, Duncan CC, Suddath RL, et al. Event-related potential abnormalities correlate with structural brain alterations and clinical features in patients with chronic schizophrenia. Schizophr Res 1994; 11: 259–271.

Erwin RJ, Turetsty BI, Moberg P, et al. P50 abnormalities in schizophrenia: relationship to clinical and neurophysiological indices of attention. Schizophr Res 1998; 33: 157–167.

Filley CM. Neurobehavioral anatomy. Niwot, CO: University Press of Colorado, 1995.

Freedman R, Adler LE, Myles-Worsley M, et al. Inhibitory gating of an evoked response to repeated auditory stimuli in schizophrenic and normal subjects. Human recordings, computer simulation, and an animal model. Arch Gen Psychiatry 1996; 53: 1114–1121.

Geschwind N, Levistsky W. Human brain: left-right asymmetry in temporal speech region. Science 1968; 161: 186–187.

Giesser BS, Schroeder MM, LaRocca NG, et al. Endogenous event-related potentials as indices of dementia in multiple sclerosis patients. Electroenceph Clin Neurophysiol 1992; 82: 320–329.

Gur RC, Packer IK, Hungerbuhler JP, et al. Differences in the distribution of gray and white matter in the human cerebral hemispheres. Science 1980; 207: 1226–1228.

Gur RC, Turetsky BI, Matsui M, et al. Sex differences in brain gray and white matter in healthy young adults: correlations with cognitive performance. J Neurosci 1999; 19: 4065–4072.

Harasty J, Double KL, Halliday GM, et al. Language-associated cortical regions are proportionally larger in the female brain. Arch Neurol 1997; 54: 171–176.

Hillyard SA, Kutas M. Electrophysiology of cognitive processing. Ann Rev Psychol 1983; 34: 33–61.

Honig LS, Ramsay RE, Sheremata WA. Event-related potential P300 in multiple sclerosis. Relation to magnetic resonance imaging and cognitive impairment. Arch Neurol 1992; 49: 44–50.

Ito J. Somatosensory event-related potentials (ERPs) in patients with different types of dementia. J Neurol Sci 1994; 121: 139–146.

Kandel ER, Schwartz JH, Jessell TM, eds. Principles of neural science. 4th ed. New York: McGraw-Hill, 2000.

Knight RT. Electrophysiologic methods in behavioral neurology and neuropsychology. In: Feinberg TE, Farah MJ, eds. Behavioral neurology and neuropsychology. New York: McGraw-Hill, 1997: 101–119.

Mann VA, Sasanuma S, Sakuma N, Masaki S. Sex differences in cognitive abilities: a cross-cultural perspective. Neuropsychologia 1990; 10: 1063–1077.

McLaurin J, Yong VW. Oligodendrocytes and myelin. Neurol Clin 1995; 13: 23–49.

Mesulam M-M. Large-scale neurocognitive networks and distributed processing for attention, language, and memory. Ann Neurol 1990; 28: 597–613.

Mesulam M-M. From sensation to cognition. Brain 1998; 121: 1013–1052.

Mesulam M-M. Behavioral neuroanatomy. Large-scale neural networks, association cortex, frontal systems, the limbic system, and hemispheric specializations. In: Mesulam M-M. Principles of behavioral and cognitive neurology. 2nd ed. New York: Oxford University Press, 2000: 1–120.

Miller AKH, Alston RL, Corsellis JAN. Variation with age in the volumes of grey and white matter in the cerebral hemispheres of man: measurements with an image analyser. Neuropathol Appl Neurobiol 1980; 6: 119–132.

Moody DM, Bell MA, Challa VR. The corpus callosum, a unique white-matter tract: anatomic features that may explain sparing in Binswanger disease and resistance to flow of fluid masses. AJNR 1988; 9: 1051–1059.

Moody DM, Bell MA, Challa VR. Features of the cerebral vascular pattern that predict vulnerability to perfusion or oxygenation deficiency: an anatomic study. AJNR 1990; 11: 431–439.

Moore BD, Copeland DR, Reid H, Levy B. Neurophysiological basis of cognitive deficits in long-term survivors of childhood cancer. Arch Neurol 1992; 49: 809–817.

Morell P, Norton WT. Myelin. Sci Am 1980; 242: 88–118.

Newton MR, Barrett G, Callanan MM, Towell AD. Cognitive event-related potentials in multiple sclerosis. Brain 1989; 112: 1637–1660.

Nieuwenhuys R, Voogd J, van Huijzen C. The human central nervous system. A synopsis and atlas. 3rd ed. Berlin: Springer-Verlag, 1988.

Nolte J. The human brain. 4rd ed. St Louis: Mosby, 1999.

Oken BS, Kaye JA. Electrophsyiologic function in the healthy, extremely old. Neurology 1992; 42: 519–526.

Puce A, Andrewes DG, Berkovic SF, Bladin PF. Visual recognition memory. Neurophysiological evidence for the role of temporal white matter in man. Brain 1991; 114: 1647–1666.

Selden NR, Gitelman DR, Salamon-Murayama N, et al. Trajectories of cholinergic pathways within the cerebral hemispheres of the human brain. Brain 1998; 121: 2249–2257.

van Dijk JG, Jennekens-Schinkel A, Caekebeke JFV, Zwinderman AH. Are event-related potentials in multiple sclerosis indicative of cognitive impairment? Evoked and event-related potentials, psychometric testing and response speed: a controlled study. J Neurol Sci 1992; 109: 18–24.

van Vugt P, Fransen I, Creten W, Pasquier P. Line bisection performances of 650 normal children. Neuropsychologia 2000; 38: 886–895.

Vernadakis A. Neuron-glia interrelations. Int Rev Neurobiol 1988; 30: 149–224.

Waxman SG, Ritchie JM. Molecular dissection of the myelinated axon. Ann Neurol 1993; 33: 121–136.

Weinberger DR. A connectionist approach to the prefrontal cortex. J Neuropsychiatry Clin Neurosci 1993; 5: 241–253.

3

Development and Aging

The human brain is a dynamic organ that undergoes a constant process of structural change during the life span. As development, maturity, and aging occur, the brain continually remodels both its fine and its gross structure. Microscopically, this remodeling occurs in the gray matter at the level of the synapse, where constant coupling and uncoupling of dendrites takes place in parallel with the processes of learning and cognition. At the macroscopic level, the changes in the brain appear to be more evident in the white matter. Whereas the gray matter remains relatively constant in volume throughout life, white matter volume fluctuates significantly at different stages. This chapter reviews the development and aging of white matter from a neurobiological perspective, with an emphasis on the potential clinical relevance of these phenomena.

Development of White Matter

Most of the axons in the adult brain are myelinated. The process by which myelination is accomplished, however, requires a prolonged period that begins in utero and continues for decades thereafter. The first information on this topic was derived from classic neuroanatomic studies on the sequence of myelination (Flechsig, 1901; Yakovlev and Lecours, 1967), followed by more recent investigations (Benes et al., 1994). The magnetic resonance imaging (MRI) era of the last two decades has added substantially to this field by enabling the noninvasive and sensitive in vivo brain imaging of normal neonates, infants, and children (Byrd et al., 1993), and MRI has become a powerful tool for the assessment of the myelination—and hence maturation—of the young brain (Barkovich et al., 1988). The findings of neuroanatomy and neuroradiology have largely been consistent in describing an orderly progression of brain myelination.

Gray matter and white matter differ significantly in their patterns of development. Nerve cells begin to develop early in gestation, and the entire complement of central nervous system neurons is formed before birth (Nolte, 1999). The embryonic development of gray matter involves continual pruning of inessential neurons by programmed cell death and the simultaneous establishment of synaptic contacts between the ones that remain (Kandel et al., 2000). In contrast, the white matter does not begin to form until the middle trimester of gestation (Nolte, 1999). The process is only partially completed at birth, and even by 2 years of age, it is still just 90% complete (Byrd et al., 1993). The remainder of myelination then requires many years (Yakovlev and Lecours, 1967; Klingberg et al., 1999; Fig. 3-1). The exact duration of this process is unclear, but recent evidence from a series of normal brains studied postmortem suggests that myelination proceeds throughout the end of the 6th decade (Benes et al., 1994).

As a general rule, myelination follows a pattern that begins with more caudal regions and advances to more rostral structures in the brain (Barkovich et al., 1988). As myelination progresses, the water content of white matter decreases and the MRI appearance of the brain approaches that of the normal adult (Bird et al., 1989). Thus, the brainstem and cerebellum are myelinated first, followed by the diencephalon and the cerebral hemispheres. This ontogenetic sequence mirrors the phylogenetic background of the brain, as more recently acquired brain structures require a longer time to myelinate than more ancient ones. Moreover, the occipital and parietal lobes mature sooner than the temporal and frontal lobes (Byrd et al., 1993; Klingberg et al., 1999), again in keeping with this principle. Among the major white matter tracts, the association and commissural fibers are the last to myelinate (Yakovlev and Lecours, 1967; Fig. 3-1).

The clinical significance of the sequence of brain myelination has long been debated. Flechsig (1901) first speculated that myelination reflected functional maturity of the cerebral areas involved, and the observations of Yakovlev and Lecours (1967) supported this idea. However, the relative importance of white matter versus gray matter development has not been entirely clear. More recently, neuroradiologists have increasingly interpreted delayed myelination on MRI as indicating a neurologic abnormality (Byrd et al., 1993). In clinical studies, there have been many suggestions that intact white matter contributes to cognitive development. In MRI studies of children with congenital hydrocephalus, for example, cognitive impairment has been correlated with delayed myelination (van der Knaap et al., 1991) and with reduced size of the corpus callosum and other cerebral white matter tracts (Fletcher et al., 1992).

One of the intriguing notions to arise from study of this area is the possibility that the acquisition of the mature personality in young adulthood depends to a substantial extent on frontal lobe myelination (Filley, 1998). Normal personality de-

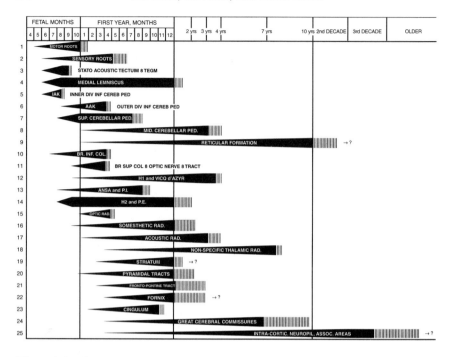

Figure 3-1. The sequence of myelination in the human brain. (Reprinted with permission from Yakovlev and Lecours, 1967.)

velopment requires the acquisition of traits such as reasoning, impulse control, and judgement that are traditionally associated with frontal lobe function. Because myelination of the frontal lobes occurs quite late in development—at a time when gray matter is relatively stable—the arrival of the adult personality may require the completion of this myelogenetic phase. Moreover, subtle modifications in personality with later adulthood may conceivably relate to continuing myelination in the 5th and 6th decades (Benes et al., 1994). The understanding of these potential correlations could help establish a foundation for considering the neural organization of personality throughout the life span.

White Matter Changes in Aging

Until recently, it was widely held that aging in the brain was characterized by the extensive and inevitable death of neurons in the neocortex and hippocampus (Morrison and Hof, 1997). In recent years, however, improvements in estimating neuron number have led to a reconsideration of this view (Morrison and Hof, 1997). The data at present suggest that cortical gray matter loss in aging is less pronounced than previously thought, and this insight has helped stimulate a search for other neuroanatomic changes in aging. Several different lines of evidence now support the idea that cerebral white matter undergoes significant alterations in aging, and that these changes have important functional consequences.

Much has been written about the possibility of brain cell loss in aging and its potential impact on cognition in older people. The issue of age-related cognitive changes is important because of widespread concern about the problem of dementia in the elderly. One of the crucial distinctions to be made in the practice of behavioral neurology, for example, is whether an older individual with memory or cognitive complaints has neurologic disease—the most ominous example of which is Alzheimer's disease (AD)—or is simply manifesting normal cognition that is appropriate for age. It is generally recognized that cognitive changes occur in aging that do not meet criteria for dementia, and this somewhat vague clinical area is currently receiving much attention (Chapter 14). However, the neurobiological basis for the mental status changes of normal aging remains obscure.

A natural point from which to begin studying this question is the gross structure of the brain, and post-mortem studies generally leave little doubt that the brain does indeed show reductions in weight and volume with advancing years (Creasey and Rapoport, 1985). However, the assumption that this phenomenon, often called "cortical atrophy," results from gray matter cell loss may be premature. More refined studies have added to knowledge of this topic. Two decades ago, image analyzer techniques were used to demonstrate that the relative proportion of cerebral white matter to gray matter varies considerably at different ages (Miller et al., 1980). These findings suggested that, in comparison to gray matter, there appears to be an early deficiency of white matter, followed by relative parity in midlife, and then again a deficiency in old age (Miller et al., 1980; Table 3-1). The impact of these observations was minimal, however, until more detailed neuroimaging and postmortem studies were undertaken in subsequent years.

Neuroimaging studies with MRI in normal individuals consistently indicate a loss of white matter in the aging brain that exceeds loss of cortical gray matter (Albert, 1993; Guttmann et al., 1998; Salat et al., 1999). When AD is present, gray matter loss also contributes to a decline in brain volume (Salat et al., 1999). Other investigators have found that loss of white matter, not gray matter, predicts an increase in sulcal fluid volume in aging (Symonds et al., 1999), supporting the notion that "cortical atrophy" in aging may in fact relate to white matter loss alone. More sophisticated neuroimaging studies using advanced MRI techniques (Chapter 4) have supported these observations. Increased diffusivity of water (diminished anisotropy) in the cerebral white matter has been shown in children with the use of diffusion-weighted MRI (Nomura et al., 1994) and the more advanced diffusion tensor MRI (Klingberg et al., 1999), and in older adults with these techniques (Chun et al., 2000; Engelter et al., 2000; Pfefferbaum et al., 2000). These findings have been interpreted as reflecting incomplete myelination among normal individuals in these age groups.

The hypothesis that neuronal loss explains cognitive changes in aging has also been challenged by recent research at the microscopic level. For most of the past century, it has been widely believed that as many as 50% of neocortical cells are

Table 3-1. Ratio of Cerebral
Gray Matter to White Matter
at Various Ages

Age	Ratio
20	1.3
50	1.1
100	1.5

Source: Miller et al., 1980

lost over the life span (Brody, 1955). However, methodological problems with counting neurons have rendered this gloomy picture suspect (Coleman and Flood, 1987), and recent studies using improved stereoscopic methods have suggested a more modest number of 10% (Pakkenberg and Gunderson, 1997). Moreover, the functional implication of the neuronal cell loss that does occur is unclear. There is, for example, no evidence of a correlation between neuron number in the aging human brain and any cognitive test result, be it global intellectual function or a specific cognitive domain (Uylings et al., 2000). Studies examining dendritic extent and synaptic density in aging have also been conflicting, and it is uncertain if any notable changes in these parameters can be detected (Uylings et al., 2000). Thus, neither cell loss nor synaptic change has been confirmed as regular and significant features of normal aging.

Other lines of evidence support the hypothesis that white matter loss is more characteristic of normal brain aging than neuronal dropout. Neurophysiological studies in aged laboratory animals have demonstrated a slowing of conduction velocity between the basal forebrain and the neocortex, suggesting that aging produces a decrement in subcortical myelin (Aston-Jones et al., 1985). More recently, postmortem studies of normal older humans consistently indicate a loss of white matter in the brain with aging that exceeds loss of cortical gray matter (Meier-Ruge et al., 1992; Double et al., 1996; Tang et al., 1997).

The origin of this white matter loss is uncertain but several possibilities have been proposed. One immediately appealing idea is that the near ubiquitous white matter hyperintensities seen on MRI scans of older persons (Ketonen, 1998) may account in part for the decline in white matter volume. These changes are well established to increase with advancing age (Ylikoski et al., 1995), and their bright appearance on MRI implies that myelin has been replaced by water. However, preliminary studies have found that these hyperintensities are not correlated with white matter volume (Salat et al., 1999). Alternative explanations can be derived from studies of the white matter at the molecular level. First, a decrease in subcortical myelin with aging has been demonstrated, associated with an increase in unsaturated acyl chains; this relative desaturation of myelin lipid implies an instability of the white matter in aging (Malone and Szoke, 1985). Others have shown that free radicals, believed by many to have a role in normal aging, preferentially attack myelin, in which is found abundant readily peroxidizable phospholipids (Weber,

1994). Regardless of the mechanism, there is substantial evidence that loss of brain weight and volume in aging may stem primarily from changes in the white matter.

If white matter is selectively lost in the aging brain, it is possible that this attrition has an impact on behavior. Whereas controversy exists in this area, a recent meta-analysis of computed tomography and MRI studies of normal older people concluded that cerebral white matter abnormalities are associated specifically with attenuated performance on tasks of processing speed, immediate and delayed memory, executive functions, and indices of global cognitive function (Gunning-Dixon and Raz, 2000). It should be emphasized that these behavioral changes in the elderly are not disabling and should not be considered abnormal. On the contrary, they represent normal developmental phenomena that can be distiguished from the effects of neuropathologic conditions such as AD. Seen in this light, it becomes important to characterize the cognitive changes of normal aging as specifically as possible so that this profile can be clearly contrasted with disease states. The relative abundance of white matter in the frontal lobes and the right hemisphere offers a basis for developing a hypothesis for normal aging changes in that white matter loss might be expected to reflect specific dysfunction in these areas (Filley, 1998). Evidence for this prediction is indeed available.

Many of the cognitive features of normal aging closely resemble changes classically associated with frontal lobe involvement seen in clinical settings (Filley, 1995). Aging confers many cognitive advantages, such as the broad experience and expansive knowledge commonly known as wisdom, but it is also true that the mental slowing and rambling garrulousness of some older people is reminiscent of younger patients with frontal lobe dysfunction who are inattentive, distractible, and poorly organized. Three familiar and well-documented examples of aging changes are cognitive slowing (Salthouse, 1996), impaired vigilance or concentration (Filley and Cullum, 1994), and executive dysfunction (Keys and White, 2000), all of which are widely regarded as reflecting prefrontal dysfunction. Several large studies of elderly populations have found robust correlations between cognitive changes and white matter changes on MRI (Longstreth et al., 1996; de Groot et al., 2000; Swan et al., 2000), with cognitive speed being the most affected domain (de Groot et al., 2000). These considerations have led to a concept known as the "frontal aging hypothesis," in which it is postulated that cognitive functions dependent on the frontal lobes are selectively vulnerable in aging (West, 1996). Despite the appeal of this idea, it has been pointed out that evidence for selective frontal lobe atrophy in aging is not convincing, and that other, nonfrontal cognitive skills are also affected in aging (Greenwood, 2000). Resolution of this issue may be provided by considering the role of white matter. Because white matter tracts course throughout the brain, alterations in myelinated systems in aging would be expected to impact all cognitive functions to some extent, but because the frontal lobes have the largest concentration of white matter, this effect would be most apparent in the performance of frontally mediated tasks. This explanation is consistent with the notion of a myelin-based theory of aging (Greenwood, 2000), which necessarily includes the concept of distributed neural networks as proposed by Mesulam (2000). Stated alternatively, this idea posits that normal aging involves widespread structural changes in cerebral white matter that alter the function of neural networks in which the frontal lobes play a prominent but not exclusive role.

Evidence also exists for a selective decline in right hemisphere function in aging that may in part reflect loss of cerebral white matter. The classical aging pattern has long been recognized by neuropsychologists as the relative stability of the verbal intelligence quotient (IQ) on the Wechsler Adult Intelligence Scale with a decline in the performance IQ (PIQ; Weintraub, 2000). Whereas the PIQ is only roughly a measure of right hemisphere function, it is reflective of so-called "fluid" abilities that are largely nonverbal in nature (Weintraub, 2000). In this light, it is of interest that a recent study of healthy octogenarians found a selective decline in the PIQ that correlated with increasing severity of white matter hyperintensities on MRI (Garde et al., 2000). More data are clearly needed, but existing information is consistent with the conclusion that some aspects of normal aging changes may result from a selective loss of right hemisphere white matter.

To summarize, the recent emphasis on white matter loss in aging is an important development in neuroscience that is sure to stimulate much useful investigation. However, it must be acknowledged that simultaneous loss of white *and* gray matter may occur, so that a more appropriate question may be the relative importance of each process. The late development of the human brain probably includes a number of structural changes that interact to produce the complex behavioral profile of normal aging. Considering the role of the white matter in this process is an increasingly more plausible notion. Further investigation of this issue will likely produce important insights into both the origin of age-related cognitive changes and strategies aimed at their prevention and treatment.

References

Albert M. Neuropsychological and neurophysiological changes in healthy adult humans across the age range. Neurobiol Aging 1993; 14: 623–625.

Aston-Jones G, Rogers J, Shaver RD, et al. Age-impaired impulse flow from nucleus basalis to cortex. Nature 1985; 318: 462–464.

Barkovich AJ, Kjos BO, Jackson DE, Norman D. Normal maturation of the neonatal and infant brain: MR imaging at 1.5 T. Radiology 1988; 166: 173–180.

Benes FM, Turtle M, Khan Y, Farol P. Myelination of a key relay zone in the hippocampal formation occurs in the human brain during childhood, adolescence, and adulthood. Arch Gen Psychiatry 1994; 51: 477–484.

Bird CR, Hedberg M, Drayer BP, et al. MR assessment of myelination in infants and children: usefulness of marker sites. AJNR 1989; 10: 731–740.

Brody H. Organization of the cerebral cortex: III. A study of aging in the human cerebral cortex. J Comp Neurol 1955; 102: 511–556.

Byrd SE, Darling CF, Wilczynski MA. White matter of the brain: maturation and myelination on magnetic resonance in infants and children. Neuroimaging Clin N Am 1993: 3: 247–266.

Chun T, Filippi CG, Zimmerman RD, Ulug AM. Diffusion changes in the aging human brain. AJNR 2000; 21: 1078–1083.

Coleman PD, Flood DG. Neuron numbers and dendritic extent in normal aging and Alzheimer's disease. Neurobiol Aging 1987; 8: 521–545.

Creasey H, Rapoport SI. The aging human brain. Ann Neurol 1985; 17: 2–10.

de Groot JC, de Leeuw F-E, Oudkerk M, et al. Cerebral white matter lesions and cognitive function: the Rotterdam Scan Study. Ann Neurol 2000; 47: 145–151.

Double KL, Halliday GM, Kril JJ, et al. Topography of brain atrophy during normal aging and Alzheimer's disease. Neurobiol Aging 1996; 17: 513–521.

Engelter ST, Provenzale JM, Petrella JR, et al. The effect of aging on the apparent diffusion coefficient of normal-appearing white matter. AJR 2000; 175: 425–430.

Filley CM. Neurobehavioral anatomy. Niwot, CO: University Press of Colorado, 1995.

Filley CM. The behavioral neurology of cerebral white matter. Neurology 1998; 50: 1535–1540.

Filley CM, Cullum CM. Attention and vigilance functions in normal aging. Appl Neuropsychol 1994; 1: 29–32.

Flechsig P. Developmental (myelogenetic) localisation of the cerebral cortex in the human subject. Lancet 1901; 2: 1027–1029.

Fletcher JM, Bohan TP, Brandt ME, et al. Cerebral white matter and cognition in hydrocephalic children. Arch Neurol 1992; 49: 818–824.

Garde E, Mortensen EL, Krabbe K, et al. Relation between age-related decline in intelligence and cerebral white-matter hyperintensities in healthy octogenarians: a longitudinal study. Lancet 2000; 356: 628–634.

Greenwood PM. The frontal aging hypothesis evaluated. J Int Neuropsychol Soc 2000; 6: 705–726.

Gunning-Dixon FM, Raz N. The cognitive correlates of white matter abnormalities in normal aging: a quantitative review. Neuropsychology 2000; 14: 224–232.

Guttmann CRG, Jolesz FA, Kikinis R, et al. White matter changes with normal aging. Neurology 1998; 50: 972–978.

Kandel ER, Schwartz JH, Jessell TM, eds. Principles of neural science. 4th ed. New York: McGraw-Hill, 2000.

Ketonen LM. Neuroimaging of the aging brain. Neurol Clin 1998; 16: 581–598.

Keys BA, White DA. Exploring the relationship between age, executive abilities, and psychomotor speed. J Int Neuropsychol Soc 2000; 6: 76–82.

Klingberg T, Vaidya CJ, Gabrieli JDE, et al. Myelination and organization of the frontal white matter in children: a diffusion tensor MRI study. Neuroreport 1999; 10: 2817–2821.

Longstreth WT, Manolio TA, Arnold A, et al. Clinical correlates of white matter findings on cranial magnetic resonance imaging of 3301 people. The Cardiovascular Health Study. Stroke 1996; 27: 1274–1282.

Malone MJ, Szoke MC. Neurochemical changes in white matter. Aged human brain and Alzheimer's Disease. Arch Neurol 1985; 42: 1063–1066.

Meier-Ruge W, Ulrich J, Bruhlmann M, Meier E. Age-related white matter atrophy in the human brain. Ann NY Acad Sci 1992; 673: 260–269.

Mesulam M-M. Behavioral neuroanatomy. Large-scale neural networks, association cortex, frontal systems, the limbic system, and hemispheric specializations. In: Mesulam M-M. Principles of behavioral and cognitive neurology. 2nd ed. New York: Oxford University Press, 2000: 1–120.

Miller AKH, Alston RL, Corsellis JAN. Variation with age in the volumes of grey and white matter in the cerebral hemispheres of man: measurements with an image analyser. Neuropathol Appl Neurobiol 1980; 6: 119–132.

Morrison JH, Hof PR. Life and death of neurons in the aging brain. Science 1997; 278: 412–419.

Nolte J. The human brain. 4rd ed. St Louis: Mosby, 1999.

Nomura Y, Sakuma H, Takeda K, et al. Diffusional anisotropy af the human brain assessed with diffusion-weighted MR: relation with normal brain development and aging. AJNR 1994; 15: 231–238.

Pakkenberg B, Gundersen HJG. Neocortical neuron number in humans: effect of sex and age. J Comp Neurol 1997; 384: 312–320.

Pfefferbaum A, Sullivan EV, Hedehus M, et al. Age-related decline in brain white matter anisotropy measured with spatially corrected echo-planar diffusion tensor imaging. Magn Res Med 2000; 44: 259–268.

Salat DH, Kaye JA, Janowsky JS. Prefrontal gray and white matter volumes in healthy aging and Alzheimer Disease. Arch Neurol 1999; 56: 338–344.

Salthouse TA. The processing-speed theory of adult age differences in cognition. Psychol Rev 1996; 103: 403–428.

Swan GE, DeCarli C, Miller BL, et al. Biobehavioral characteristics of nondemented older adults with subclinical brain atrophy. Neurology 2000; 54: 2108–2114.

Symonds LL, Archibald SL, Grant I, et al. Does an increase in sulcal or ventricular fluid predict where brain tissue is lost? J Neuroimaging 1999; 9: 201–209.

Tang Y, Nyengaard JR, Pakkenberg B, Gundersen HJ. Age-induced white matter changes in the human brain: a stereological investigation. Neurobiol Aging 1997; 18: 609–615.

Uylings HBM, West MJ, Coleman PD, et al. Neuronal and cellular changes in the aging brain. In: Clark CM, Trojanowski JQ, eds. Neurodegenerative dementias. New York: McGraw-Hill, 2000: 61–76.

van der Knaap MS, Valk J, Bakker CJ, et al. Myelination as an expression of the functional maturity of the brain. Dev Med Child Neurol 1991; 33: 849–857.

Weber GF. The pathophysiology of reactive oxygen intermediates in the central nervous system. Med Hypotheses 1994; 43: 223–230.

Weintraub S. Neuropsychological assessment of mental state. In: Mesulam M-M, ed. Principles of behavioral and cognitive neurology. 2nd ed. New York: Oxford Univeristy Press, 2000: 121–173.

West RL. An application of prefrontal cortex function theory to cognitive aging. Psychol Bull 1996; 120: 272–292.

Yakovlev PI, Lecours AR. The myelogenetic cycles of regional maturation of the brain. In: Minkowski A, ed. Regional development of the brain in early life. Oxford: Blackwell Scientific Publications, 1967: 3–79.

Ylikoski A, Erkinjuntti T, Raininko R, et al. White matter hyperintensities on MRI in the neurologically nondiseased elderly. Analysis of cohorts of consecutive subjects aged 55 to 85 years living at home. Stroke 1995; 26: 1171–1177.

4

Neuroimaging

Since the emergence of neurology as a clinical discipline in the nineteenth century, no more revolutionary development has occurred than the advance of neuroimaging in the past three decades. The classic clinical techniques of neurology have been greatly augmented by the capacity to view the brain directly during life with the use of noninvasive, safe, and readily available instruments. In addition, a host of new techniques currently evolving promise to enhance research on the structure and function of the brain in health and disease (Mazziotta, 2000). One of the areas that has been particularly advanced is the understanding of white matter, as modern techniques have allowed for increasingly detailed and precise imaging of this component of the brain (Grossman, 1998; Barkovich, 2000). In this chapter, the contemporary status of white matter neuroimaging is reviewed, as well as new directions in which this fast moving field is proceeding.

Computed Tomography

Computed tomography (CT) was first introduced in the 1970s and immediately altered the practice of neurology. Based on a three-dimensional reconstruction of thousands of x-ray images, the typical CT scan is able to show clear distinctions between brain tissue, cerebrospinal fluid (CSF), and bone (Fig. 4-1). The white matter, however, is not well demarcated from the gray matter, and only a rough es-

41

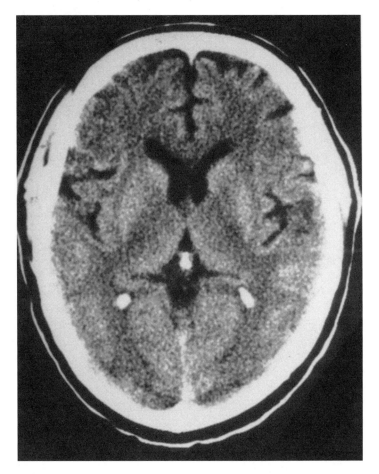

Figure 4-1. Computed tomography scan of a normal 65-year-old man. The scan shows appropriate age-related cerebral volume loss, but the white matter is not well seen.

timate of its integrity is possible with CT. Moreover, the detection of white matter lesions, while possible in many cases, is not ideal. In multiple sclerosis (MS), for example, CT is clearly inferior to magnetic resonance imaging (MRI) in detecting demyelinative plaques (Simon, 1993). The value of CT is somewhat improved with the use of iodinated contrast material, which discloses more lesions than plain CT (Simon, 1993). However, the CT scan cannot be considered particularly sensitive to either normal or abnormal white matter (Bradley, 1986). Computed to-mography may be normal in patients with substantial white matter pathology, and if the clinical setting suggests the presence of lesions of this type, MRI is usually the more useful neuroimaging procedure.

Magnetic Resonance Imaging

The appearance of MRI in the early 1980s radically changed the field of neuroimaging (Grossman, 1998). Although CT scanning remains useful for such purposes as detecting acute intracranial hemorrhage and the imaging of calcified structures (Bradley, 1986), MRI has become the preferred method for the imaging of most brain lesions because of the absence of patient exposure to ionizing radiation, and the much improved sensitivity to most neuropathologic conditions. Widely used in general neurology because of its safety and efficacy, MRI has also had a major impact on behavioral neurology by proving to be superior for the detection and localization of focal cerebral lesions affecting behavior (Tanridag and Kirshner, 1987).

One of the most impressive aspects of MRI is its capacity to demonstrate the cerebral white matter, which can now be viewed with unprecedented detail. Both the understanding of known white matter disorders and the discovery of new ones were rapidly propelled by this technology, and new insights into the development and aging of normal white matter were made possible (Chapter 3). Most of the neuroimaging scans to be shown in later chapters are conventional MRI scans, which are in routine clinical use and provide a continuing source of insight into the cerebral white matter in health and disease.

The extraordinary growth of neuroradiology continues to produce new techniques that improve the visualization of white matter. An often bewildering array of MRI methods is available at some stage of development, as is expected with the torrid pace of advances in the technology of neuroimaging. These advances will have a major impact on both the differential diagnosis (Grossman et al., 2000) and neurobehavioral impact of white matter disorders (Comi et al., 2000). For clinicians dealing with cognitive and emotional aspects of these disorders, some familiarity with emerging new techniques is indispensible.

A complete account of the physical basis of MRI is beyond the scope of this book, but a brief review of elementary principles will be helpful (Jackson et al., 1997). Magnetic resonance imaging is based on the fact that protons—the nuclei of hydrogen atoms—can be induced to emit electrical signals giving information about the structure and function of the living brain. Protons normally rotate around their axes in a random fashion. When individuals to be scanned are placed in a powerful magnetic field, the protons in the brain are aligned so as to create a net vertical magnetic field. A second magnetic field is then formed by the application of a radiofrequency pulse, which causes the protons to begin "wobbling" around their axes, a process called precession. When this radiofrequency pulse is turned off, the protons "relax," precession decreases, and the axes of the protons become realigned with the original magnetic field. Magnetic resonance imaging measures the rates of two relaxation processes that are characterized by time constants known as T1 and T2; these changes occur as the excited protons return to their lower energy state after the removal of the radiofrequency pulse. From this point, axial, sagittal, or coronal brain images are generated that provide detailed information about normal and abnormal brain tissue. In addition, the use of contrast enhancement with ga-dolinium enables the visualization of regions where the neuropathologic process involves breakdown of the blood–brain barrier. Even blood vessels can be imaged with the use of magnetic resonance angiography (Jackson et al., 1997).

Magnetic resonance imaging images generated for routine clinical purposes are determined by the selection of several pulse sequences, depending on the neuro-logic setting (Jackson et al., 1997). Most often used is the spin echo (SE) sequence, which is characterized by two parameters: the repetition time (TR) and the echo time (TE). The choice of TR and TE determines the degree of T1-weighting, T2-weighting, or proton density-weighting in the images produced. T1-weighted im-ages have a short TR (500–700 ms) and a short TE (15–25 ms), T2-weighted im-ages have a long TR (2500–3500) and long TE (80–100 ms), and proton density images have a long TR (2500–3500 ms) but a short TE (15–25 ms; Jackson et al., 1997). These various images reveal aspects of normal and pathologic neuroanatomy by providing unmatched tissue contrast; T1-weighted images (Fig. 4-2) are espe-

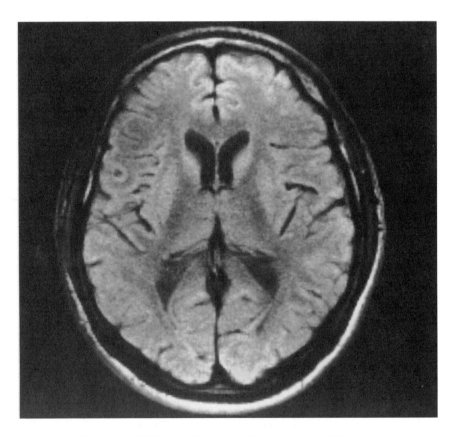

Figure 4-2. T1-weighted MRI scan of a normal 60-year-old man. Mild age-related volume loss is apparent, and there is good resolution of neuroanatomic detail.

cially useful for study of neuroanatomic detail, whereas T2-weighted images are usually superior for visualizing neuropathologic conditions (Jackson et al., 1997).

White matter disorders of the hemispheres, brainstem, and cerebellum are best seen on moderately to heavily T2-weighted images, which provide good discrimination between gray and white matter areas because of their long TR (Fig. 4-3). This degree of T2-weighting, however, causes the CSF to appear as bright, and in some patients with periventricular white matter disease, the high signal in the adjacent CSF obscures the visualization of hyperintense lesions. Thus proton density images, also known as mildly T2-weighted images (Fig. 4-4), are often useful because their short TE assures that the CSF is dark (Jackson et al., 1997).

Another approach to the problem of high CSF signal within the ventricular system is the development of fluid attenuated inversion recovery (FLAIR) imaging. These images allow for improved imaging of the periventricular white matter by suppressing the signal from the ventricular CSF while preserving the T2-weighting of the brain parenchyma (De Coene et al., 1992). With this technique, white matter lesions can be seen with still more clarity, and FLAIR imaging is routinely performed with this objective in mind (Fig. 4-5).

In the two decades since the advent of MRI, enormous strides have been taken in the understanding of white matter and its disorders. The best example of this phenomenon can be seen with MS, in which MRI has fundamentally altered the clinical approach to the disease. Magnetic resonance imaging has now become the

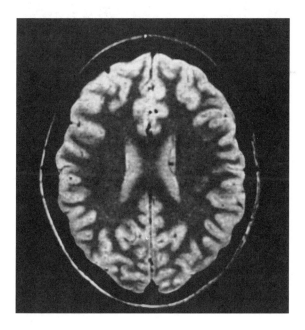

Figure 4-3. T2-weighted MRI scan of a normal 30-year-old man. The brain has no volume loss, and the white matter is well demarcated from the gray matter.

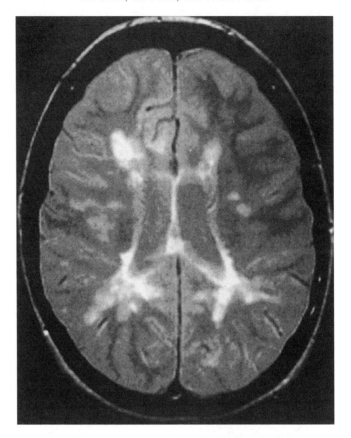

Figure 4-4. Proton density MRI scan of patient with MS, demonstrating good visualization of periventricular white matter lesions because the CSF appears dark. (Reprinted with permission from Miller DH, Kesselring J, McDonald WI, et al. Magnetic resonance in multiple sclerosis. Cambridge: Cambridge University Press, 1997.)

most important diagnostic test for MS, usually obviating the need for lumbar puncture and evoked potentials, and it plays an increasingly prominent role in the treatment and follow-up of affected individuals (Simon, 1993). Moreover, the clinical assessment of other white matter disorders is becoming equally dependent on MRI scanning.

In the 1990s, additional MRI techniques were developed that have further refined the detection of white matter damage. One of these is magnetic resonance spectroscopy (MRS), which identifies and quantifies chemicals in living tissue (Rudkin and Arnold, 1999). Magnetic resonance spectroscopy findings are displayed in spectra of peaks that represent the chemical structure and concentration of metabolites in the tissue of interest (Fig. 4-6). This technique has been used to detect axonal damage by identifying a decrease in N-acetyl aspartate (NAA), an

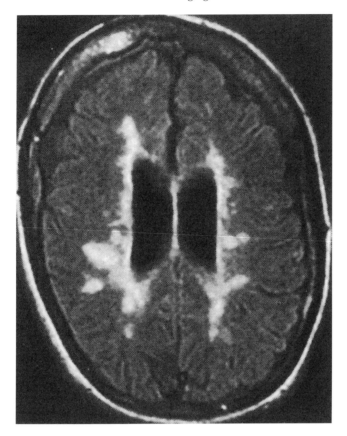

Figure 4-5. FLAIR MRI scan of a patient with MS, showing excellent visualization of periventricular plaques as a result of suppression of the ventricular CSF signal. (Reprinted with permission from Miller DH, Kesselring J, McDonald WI, et al. Magnetic resonance in multiple sclerosis. Cambridge: Cambridge University Press, 1997.)

amino acid regarded as a marker of neuronal integrity (Simmons et al., 1991). Magnetic resonance spectroscopy may be particularly useful in white matter disorders; in MS, for example, reductions in NAA are found not only within demyelinative plaques, but in white matter areas that appear normal on conventional MRI (Grossman et al., 2000). Thus, MRS may enable more sensitive detection of early abnormalities in white matter disorders that can be correlated with clinical variables.

Neuroradiologists have also begun using the technique of magnetization transfer imaging (MTI), which is based on interactions between protons in water and macromolecules in the brain. When a radiofrequency saturation pulse is combined with an imaging sequence, it is possible to derive a magnetization transfer ratio (MTR; van Buchem, 1999), the most popular MTI parameter. In white matter, a

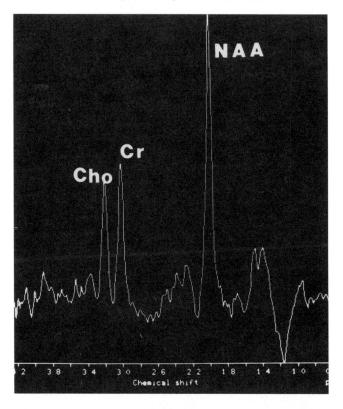

Figure 4-6. Normal MRS spectrum. Reduction of the NAA peak in white matter would be an index of axonal damage. (Reprinted with permission from Fogel BS, Schiffer RB, Rao SM, eds. Neuropsychiatry. Baltimore: Williams and Wilkins, 1996.)

low MTR reflects damage to myelin and axons from a wide variety of disorders, including MS (Cercignani et al., 2000) and white matter ischemia (Tanabe et al., 1997), and as with MRS abnormalities, a low MTR may be seen in the normal appearing white matter before conventional MRI shows any change (Loevner et al., 1995). The MTR also correlates with the degree of normal myelination, rendering MTI applicable to the study of development and aging (Rademacher et al., 1999). In addition to the use of the MTR in specific regions of interest, which has enabled study of the evolution of individual white matter lesions, whole brain histograms also permit quantification of total disease burden (van Buchem, 1999). Magnetizatoin transfer imaging thus has promise for measuring the entire range of white matter neuropathology, macroscopic and microscopic, and for providing a basis for improved correlations with neurobehavioral data (van Buchem, 1999).

Another new development in MRI that assists in the study of cerebral white matter is the technique of diffusion-weighting (Rowley et al., 1999). Diffusion-weighted MRI (DWMRI) enables the measurement of the diffusional motion of water molecules in the brain, which is quantified by a parameter known as the apparent diffusion coefficient (ADC; Neumann-Haftelin et al., 2000). When water diffusion is restricted by a neuropathologic process, the ADC declines, and a hyperintense area appears on the reconstructed image (Fig. 4-7). At present, DWMRI is most used in the setting of acute stroke, where it appears to be able to identify ischemic tissue sooner after the onset than conventional MRI or CT (Neumann-Haefelin et al. 2000).

Most recently, the arrival of the technique of diffusion tensor MRI (DTI) promises to offer particularly relevant information to the study of higher function (Peled et al., 1998; Jones et al., 1999b; Shimony et al., 1999). The chief advantage of this method over DWMRI is that it is capable of measuring the directionality as well as the magnitude of water diffusion (Neumann-Haefelin et al., 2000). Diffusion in

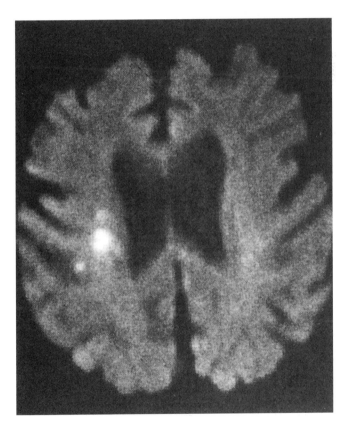

Figure 4-7. Diffusion-weighted MRI scan showing a small right centrum semiovale infarct; after onset, this lesion is typically seen earlier with DWMRI than with conventional MRI. (Reprinted with permission from Baird et al. Enlargement of human cerebral ischemic lesion volumes measured by diffusion-weighted magnetic resonance imaging. Ann Neurol 1997; 41: 581–589.)

white matter is anisotropic or directional, meaning that diffusion of water molecules normally occurs in parallel with the direction of a given tract; isotropic diffusion, in contrast, takes place in a random manner. The property of anisotropic diffusion permits the visualization of fiber tracts on a DTI image (Fig. 4-8). Reduced anisotropy as evaluated by DTI has been interpreted as the common denominator of structural white matter lesions due to a variety of disorders, including stroke, leukoaraiosis, trauma, neoplasms, and MS (Weishmann et al., 1999; Mukherjee et al., 2000; Jones et al., 1999a). Like other techniques discussed above, DTI can also detect abnormalities in areas that appear normal on conventional MRI, and, in addition, can do so within specific white matter tracts (Neumann-Haefelin et al., 2000). Thus, DTI enables the imaging of specific white matter tracts in a unique fashion,

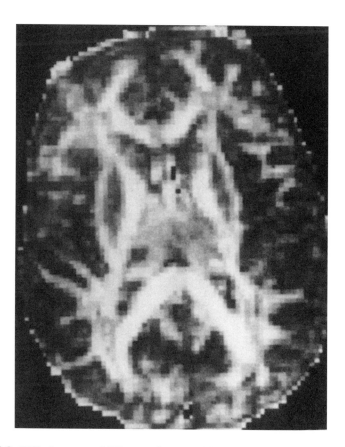

Figure 4-8. Diffusion tensor MRI scan of a normal individual showing numerous white matter tracts in the brain. (Reprinted with permission from Werring et al. The structural and functional mechanisms of motor recovery: complementary use of diffusion tensor and functional magnetic resonance imaging in a traumatic injury of the internal capsule. J Neurol Neurosurg Psychiatry 1998; 65: 863–869.)

permitting analysis of normal and disrupted cerebral connectivity (Makris, et al., 1997; Fig. 4-8). Diffusion tensor MRI appears poised to facilitate the in vivo identification of all the white matter tracts in the brain, and in so doing address a major deficiency of neuroanatomy, which has to date been unable to provide a detailed map of the origin, course, and termination of cerebral white matter tracts (Chapter 2). On the basis of this information, lesion analysis can then proceed in a more precise fashion.

Functional Neuroimaging

Conventional CT and MRI both provide static information about the structure of the brain. As such, they are unable to illuminate its function other than by indirect means. Functional neuroimaging techniques provide the opportunity to observe the metabolic activity of the brain as it is engaged in the performance of elemental or higher neurologic functions. Whereas these techniques are more relevant to gray matter areas where metabolic activity is higher than in white matter, they are complimentary in the investigation of distributed neural networks in which white matter tracts play a vital role.

Functional neuroimaging techniques can be divided into those that involve radioisotopes as labels for metabolic activity and those that utilize MRI principles. Radioisotopes are used to tag molecules of biologic interest, and after these molecules are injected into the bloodstream, emissions can be measured outside the body to reflect metabolism in the brain. The most readily obtainable of this group is single photon emission computed tomography (SPECT), which makes use of radioisotopes that emit single photon radiation, typically in the form of gamma rays (Alavi and Hirsch, 1991). Single photon emission computed tomography is widely available and inexpensive, and can often identify areas of cortical dysfunction. However, this technique is compromised to some extent by low spatial resolution.

More elegant than SPECT is positron emission tomography (PET), which uses short-lived radioisotopes attached to a variety of compounds involved in brain metabolism (Roland, 1993; Fig. 4-9). These isotopes decay by emitting a positron, and this property allows the localization of metabolically active regions within gray matter. Positron emission tomography scans reveal greater detail about brain activity than does SPECT, and the procedure has made possible the collection of impressive data on the localization of higher functions in the cerebral cortex (Nadeau and Crosson, 1995; Cabeza and Nyberg, 1997). However, the routine access to PET scanning for clinical purposes is limited in some centers by its high cost and reduced availability.

Functional MRI (FMRI) presents an immediately attractive alternative to PET scanning because it provides excellent spatial resolution and can be performed using standard MRI scanners found in medical centers and hospitals (Prichard and Cummings, 1997; Fig. 4-10). Functional MRI is founded on the idea that brain activity can be indexed by means of a method known as blood oxygen level detection (BOLD). In metabolically active regions of the brain, neuronal activity is as-

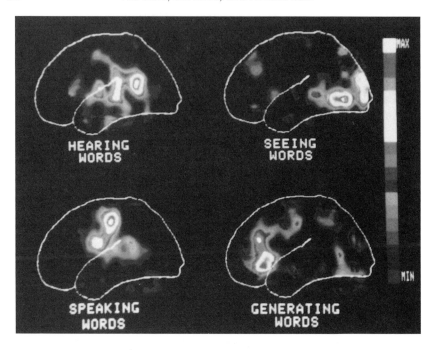

Figure 4-9. PET images of a normal individual showing activation of left hemisphere cortical regions with various mental tasks. (Reprinted with permission from Pechura CM, Martin JB, eds. Mapping the brain and its functions. Integrating enabling technologies into neuroscience research. Washington, D.C.: National Academy Press, 1991.)

sociated with a greater supply of oxygenated blood than is required, resulting in a higher than normal ratio of oxygenated to deoxygenated blood. The BOLD technique exploits this phenomenon, and provides a measure of cerebral cortical activity that has spatial resolution considered to be better than that of PET scanning. The field of FMRI is rapidly evolving, and from this work steady advances are occurring in the understanding of brain–behavior relationships at the level of the cerebral cortex (Nadeau and Crosson, 1995; Cabeza and Nyberg, 2000).

Mapping Neural Networks

According to contemporary neurologic thinking, neurobehavioral functions are represented in the brain by a collection of distributed neural networks (Mesulam, 2000). These networks are comprised of multiple cortical and subcortical structures linked into coherent assemblies that are dedicated to specific aspects of cognition and emotion. White matter tracts are essential components of these networks, connecting the gray matter areas into functional ensembles; indeed, without the white matter, neural networks could not exist. Reference to neural networks will be made

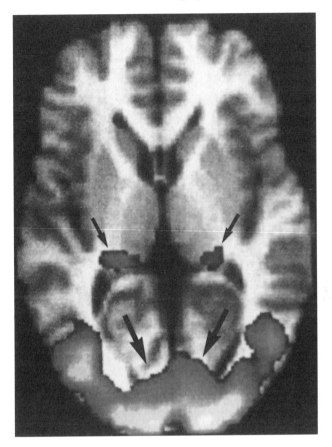

Figure 4-10. FMRI scan of a normal individual using the BOLD technique to demonstrate activation of the lateral geniculate nuclei (*small arrows*) and the visual cortices (*large arrows*) during a visual task. (Reprinted with permission from Kandel ER, Schwartz JH, Jessell TM, eds. Principles of neural science. 4th ed. New York: McGraw-Hill, 2000.)

throughout this book, and a detailed discussion of their structure, function, and disruption appears in Chapter 18.

The neuroradiologic methods discussed above will permit an integrative synthesis of both the structure of white matter tracts and the functions of the cortical areas they interconnect. A combination of functional and connectional assessment is now being applied to the study of the brain; DTI and functional MRI presently seem to offer the most exciting combination of techniques (Conturo et al., 1999; Werring et al., 1999). As is clear from a review of the history of behavioral neurology (Chapter 1), a given neurobehavioral function cannot strictly be assigned to a single cerebral area, and a consideration of the complex circuitry underlying the behavior is more appropriate.

The role of white matter connectivity of the brain in neurobehavioral function thus becomes as important as understanding gray matter function. The joint use of structural and functional MRI to identify both white matter and gray matter components of these distributed neural networks is becoming feasible. Despite perhaps formidable methodological obstacles, the integrated combination of these techniques promises to yield unique insights into the structure and function of white matter in the living brain.

References

Alavi A, Hirsch LJ. Studies of central nervous system disorders with single photon emission computed tomography and positron emission tomography. Semin Nucl Med 1991; 21: 58–81.

Barkovich AJ. Concepts of myelin and myelination in neuroradiology. AJNR 2000; 21: 1099–1109.

Bradley WG. Magnetic resonance imaging in the central nervous system: comparison with computed tomography. Magn Reson Annu 1986; 81–122.

Cabeza R, Nyberg L. Imaging cognition: an empirical review of PET studies with normal subjects. J Cogn Neurosci 1997; 9: 1–26.

Cabeza R, Nyberg L. Imaging cognition II: an empirical review of 275 PET and MRI studies. J Cogn Neurosci 2000; 12: 1–47.

Cercignani M, Iannucci G, Rocca MA, et al. Pathologic damage in MS assessed by diffusion-weighted and magnetization transfer MRI. Neurology 2000; 54: 1139–1144.

Comi G, Rovaris M, Leocani L, et al. Assessment of damage of the cerebral hemispheres in MS using neuroimaging techniques. J Neurol Sci 2000; 172: S63–S66.

Conturo TE, Lori NF, Cull TS, et al. Tracking neuronal fiber pathways in the living human brain. Proc Natl Acad Sci 1999; 96: 10422–10427.

De Coene B, Hajnal JV, Gatehouse P, et al. MR of the brain using fluid-attenuated inversion recovery (FLAIR) pulse sequences. AJNR 1992; 13: 1555–1564.

Grossman R. Brain imaging. AJNR 1998; 21: 9–18.

Grossman RI, Kappos L, Wolinsky JS. The contribution of magnetic resonance imaging in the differential diagnosis of the damage of the cerebral hemispheres. J Neurol Sci 2000; 172: S57–S62.

Jackson EF, Ginsberg LE, Schomer DF, Leeds NE. A review of MRI pulse sequences and techniques in neuroimaging. Surg Neurol 1997; 47: 185–199.

Jones DK, Lythgoe D, Horsfield MA, et al. Charaterization of white matter damage in ischemic leukoaraiosis with diffusion tensor MRI. Stroke 1999a; 30: 393–397.

Jones DK, Simmons A, Williams SCR, Horsfield MA. Non-invasive assessment of axonal fiber connectivity in the human brain via diffusion tensor imaging. Magn Res Med 1999b; 42: 37–41.

Loevner LA, Grossman RI, Cohen JA, et al. Microscopic disease in normal-appearing white matter on conventional MR imaging in patients with multiple sclerosis: assessment with magnetization-transfer measurements. Radiology 1995; 196: 511–515.

Makris N, Worth AJ, Sorensen AG, et al. Morphometry of in vivo human white matter association pathways with diffusion-weighted magnetic resonance imaging. Ann Neurol 1997; 42: 951–962.

Mazziotta JC. Imaging. Window on the brain. Arch Neurol 2000; 57: 1413–1421.

Mesulam M-M. Behavioral neuroanatomy. Large-scale neural networks, association cortex, frontal systems, the limbic system, and hemispheric specializations. In: Mesulam M-M. Principles of behavioral and cognitive neurology. 2nd ed. New York: Oxford University Press, 2000: 1–120.

Mukherjee P, Bahn MM, McKinstry RC, et al. Differences between gray and white matter water diffusion in stroke: diffusion-tensor MR imaging in 12 patients. Radiology 2000; 215: 211–220.

Nadeau SE, Crosson B. A guide to the functional imaging of cognitive processes. Neuropsychiatry Neuropsychol Behav Neurol 1995; 8: 143–162.

Neumann-Haefelin T, Moseley ME, Albers GW. New magnetic resonance imaging methods for cerebrovascular disease: emerging clinical applications. Ann Neurol 2000; 47: 559–570.

Peled S, Gudbjartsson H, Westin C-F, et al. Magnetic resonance imaging shows orientation and asymmetry of white matter fiber tracts. Brain Res 1998; 780: 27–33.

Prichard JW, Cummings JL. The insistent call from functional MRI. Neurology 1997; 48: 797–800.

Rademacher J, Engelbrecht V, Burgel U, et al. Measuring in vivo myelination of human white matter fiber tracts with magnetization transfer MR. Neuroimage 1999; 9: 393–406.

Roland P. Brain activation. New York: Wiley-Liss, 1993.

Rowley HA, Grant PE, Roberts TP. Diffusion MR imaging. Theory and applications. Neuroimaging Clin N Am 1999; 9: 343–361.

Rudkin TM, Arnold DL. Proton magnetic resonance spectroscopy for the diagnosis and management of cerebral disorders. Arch Neurol 1999; 56: 919–926.

Shimony JS, McKinstry RC, Akbudak E, et al. Quantitative diffusion-tensor anisotropy brain MR imaging: normative human data and anatomic analysis. Radiology 1999; 212: 770–784.

Simmons M, Frondoza C, Coyle J. Immunocytochemical localization of N-acetyl-aspartate with monoclonal antibodies. Neuroscience 1991; 45: 37–45.

Simon JH. Neuroimaging of multiple sclerosis. Neuroimaging Clin N Am 1993; 3: 229–246.

Tanabe JL, Ezekiel F, Jagust WJ, et al. Volumetric method for evaluating magnetization transfer ratio of tissue categories: application to areas of white matter signal hyperintensity in the elderly. Radiology 1997; 204: 570–575.

Tanridag O, Kirshner HS. Magnetic resonance imaging and CT scanning in neurobehavioral syndromes. Psychosomatics 1987; 28: 517–528.

van Buchem MA. Magnetization transfer: applications in neuroradiology. J Comp Assist Tomogr 1999; 23 (suppl 1): S9–S18.

Weishmann UC, Clark CA, Symms MR, et al. Reduced anisotropy of water diffusion in structural cerebral abnormalities demonstrated with diffusion tensor imaging. Magn Res Imaging 1999; 17: 1269–1274.

Werring DJ, Clark CA, Parker GJ, et al. A direct demonstration of both structure and function in the visual system: combining diffusion tensor imaging with functional magnetic resonance imaging. Neuroimage 1999; 9: 352–361.

II

DISORDERS OF
WHITE MATTER

5

Genetic Disorders

To begin a survey of white matter disorders of the brain, the category of genetic disorders serves as an appropriate departure. These disorders fall largely within the province of child neurology, but in some cases they come to the attention of the adult neurologist as well. At any age, however, neurobehavioral manifestations are prominent. Genetic white matter disorders highlight the importance of myelinated tracts in the ontogeny of behavior because they demonstrate how defective white matter can profoundly disrupt the development of cognition and emotion. This group of disorders is now considered with special attention to the neurobehavioral syndromes that are regularly encountered.

The understanding of inherited neurologic disorders continues to evolve, and many unanswered questions remain about their classification. Among the white matter disorders, a number of leukoencephalopathies are defined by their genetic origin, whereas many others have an unknown etiology. It is becoming commonplace for reports of newly described disorders to appear, both in children—as in leukoencephalopathy with vanishing white matter (van der Knaap et al., 1997a), and in adults—as in autosomal dominant leukoencephalopathy with neuroaxonal spheroids (van der Knaap et al., 2000). Although a genetic cause can often be assumed in these diseases, it is estimated that at least half of the childhood leukoencephalopathies seen clinically remain idiopathic and unclassified (van der Knaap et al., 1999). The diseases discussed in this chapter are those leukoencephalopathies caused by a known or presumed genetic abnormality that are relatively well characterized. The primary goal is to consider the impact of genetic white matter disease on behavior, and in so doing provide a framework for neurobehavioral analysis of new entities that will doubtless be better understood in the near future (van der Knaap et al., 1999).

Leukodystrophies

Traditional neurologic teaching has emphasized a distinction between the two neuropathologic categories of dysmyelination and demyelination. As reviewed in Chapter 3, myelin is laid down in an orderly sequence that begins in utero and continues for several decades. Dysmyelination implies the abnormal development of myelin because of a metabolic error preventing the normal sequence of events that participate in the establishment and maintenance of the myelin sheath. The leukodystrophies provide the most familiar examples of the category of dysmyelination. Although some abnormalities of white matter can also be observed in primary neuronal diseases such as Tay-Sachs disease and Niemann-Pick disease, these effects occur secondarily because of neuronal dysfunction and metabolic effects on oligodendrocytes (Folkerth, 2000). In contrast, the dysmyelinative diseases represent valuable opportunities to examine altered brain function in white matter disorders resulting from a primary deficiency of myelin formation. Demyelination, alternatively known as myelinoclasis, refers to the loss of previously acquired normal myelin through some superimposed neuropathologic process. Multiple sclerosis (MS) remains the prototype example of demyelination, as is discussed in Chapter 6. The contrast between dysmyelination and demyelination still provides a useful framework in which to consider genetic disorders of white matter.

The leukodystrophies typically begin in early life and are caused by an autosomal recessive gene defect. In these diseases, significant neurologic dysfunction occurs because of interference with normal myelination caused by an inborn error of metabolism. These single gene defects, while at present clinically devastating, offer to improve the understanding of the events leading to normal myelination, and eventually leading to effective therapies. As will be apparent, such therapies are beginning to appear. Promising therapeutic interventions for the leukodystrophies now provide hope for improved treatment for these severe neurologic diseases, and also suggest how diseases of white matter may exhibit substantial reversibility.

Metachromatic Leukodystrophy

Metachromatic leukodystrophy (MLD) is the most common of the leukodystrophies. The usual age of onset is in the second or third year of life, but the disease may present at any time throughout adulthood. Common initial manifestations include developmental delay, intellectual deterioration, gait disorder, strabismus, and spasticity, and dysmyelination in peripheral nerves also produces neuropathy with hyporeflexia. Steady deterioration progresses inexorably toward a vegetative state and death within a few years. Cases with a later age of onset cases have a somewhat less severe course.

Metachromatic leukodystrophy is caused by a deficiency of the enzyme arylsulfatase A, which converts sulfatide to cerebroside, a major component of myelin (Austin et al., 1968). The resulting sulfatide accumulation in myelin and the lysosomes of oligodendrocytes is visible microscopically as metachromatically staining granules, the characteristic neuropathologic feature of MLD. There is also diffuse dysmyelination in the cerebrum, cerebellum, spinal cord, and peripheral nerves. In the central nervous system, the eventual death of oligodendrocytes precludes the possibility of any remyelination. The diagnosis is confirmed by the demonstration of reduced arylsulfatase A activity in leukocytes.

Neuroimaging studies are useful in demonstrating the dysmyelination associated with MLD. Computed tomography (CT) shows symmetric low density white matter lesions and ventriculomegaly (Skomer et al., 1983). Magnetic resonance imaging (MRI), particularly with the use of T2-weighted images, provides a more detailed view of diffuse and symmetric cerebral white matter involvement (Filley and Gross, 1992; Fig. 5-1).

In older children and adults, the more protracted disease course has permitted some study of the neurobehavioral features of MLD. Dementia is the major syndrome, often dominated by features of frontal lobe dysfunction with disinhibition, impulsivity, and poor attention span; neuropsychological testing discloses a pattern of findings including inattention, poor vigilance, impaired memory, relatively intact language, impaired visuospatial function, and executive dysfunction (Shapiro et al., 1994). Consistent with these observations, a frontal predominance of dysmyelination may be apparent (Shapiro et al., 1994). In addition, a frequent tendency for psychosis to herald the onset of the disease has been noted (Filley and Gross, 1992). In a thorough review, Hyde and colleagues (1992) reported that 53% of published cases of adolescent and early-adult onset MLD had psychosis as an early clinical feature. It has been postulated that psychosis occurs because of disrupted corticocortical connections between frontal and temporal lobes (Hyde et al., 1992), and that dementia follows as more extensive dysmyelination proceeds to disrupt other connections and produce more widespread cerebral dysfunction (Filley and Gross, 1992).

Treatment of MLD has been limited to supportive therapy until recently. However, the introduction of bone marrow transplantation has raised the hope that normal arylsulfatase A activity and clinical benefit can be achieved (Krivit et al., 1990). This procedure entails the engraftment of hematopoietic stem cells from a healthy donor, which results in normal monocytes entering the brain of the recipient to correct the deficient enzymatic activity associated with the disease (Krivit et al., 1999). Treatment is desirable early in the disease course, presumably because oligodendrocytes are still viable and remyelination can proceed. Preliminary reports indicate that the procedure can indeed restore the activity of the enzyme, and also stabilize cognitive deterioration in MLD, both in children (Shapiro et al., 1992) and in adults (Navarro et al., 1996). Bone marrow transplantation seems to

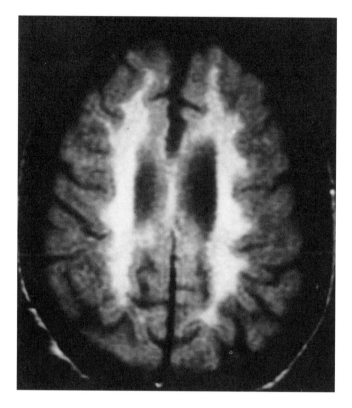

Figure 5-1. Mildly T2-weighted MRI scan of a patient with metachromatic leukodystrophy. Diffuse cerebral dysmyelination is apparent. (Reprinted with permission from Filley CM, Gross KF. Erratum. Psychosis with cerebral white matter disease. Neuropsychiatry Neuropsychol Behav Neurol 1993; 6: 142.)

exert its effects on cognition by improving the structure of cerebral white matter as shown on MRI scanning (Krivit et al., 1990). Success in treating MLD with this approach provides evidence for the neurobehavioral importance of white matter in that cognitive improvement occurs in parallel with restoration of the integrity of myelinated tracts in the brain.

Globoid Cell Leukodystrophy (Krabbe's Disease)

Globoid cell leukodystrophy (GCL) differs little from MLD in its clinical features, although it is not as common (Menkes, 1990). Globoid cell leukodystrophy is an autosomal recessive disease caused by a deficiency of the enzyme galactocerebrosidase, which can be assayed in leukocytes for diagnostic purposes. Onset is usually in early infancy, with evidence of both central and peripheral dysmyelination. Intellectual decline and dementia are the most prominent features, and as in MLD, later onset cases with a more prolonged course are known to occur. Neuropathologically, there is dysmyelination in the brain, spinal cord, and peripheral nerves, and accumulations of galactocerebroside are found in the characteristic globoid cells. Computed tomography scans show ventricular enlargement consistent with reduced white matter volume (Ieshima et al., 1983), and MRI scans reveal diffuse white matter hyperintensity that tends to involve more posterior brain regions (Kapoor et al., 1992). Neuroradiologic white matter abnormalities correlate with the absence of normal myelination throughout the cerebrum (Percy et al., 1994).

As in MLD, bone marrow transplantation has been used for selected cases of GCL, and similar favorable results have been observed (Krivit et al., 1999). Transplantation restores normal galactocerebroside activity in the brain, and reversal or prevention of neurologic dysfunction has been shown (Krivit et al., 1998). As is the case with MLD, treatment of CGL enhances neurobehavioral function at the same time that improvement is demonstrable in the MRI appearance of the cerebral white matter (Krivit et al., 1998).

Adrenoleukodystrophy

Adrenoleukodystrophy (ALD) is an X-linked disease of males characterized by neurologic dysfunction and adrenal insufficiency (Moser, 1997). The disease usually manifests between the ages of 3 and 10, with behavioral disturbances, visual loss, and intellectual decline. Gait disorder and spastic quadriparesis follow, and a rapidly progressive course is typical, with death in 2 to 3 years from neurologic deterioration. The adrenal manifestations, if treated with hormone replacement, do not significantly affect longevity.

Adrenoleukodystrophy results from defective beta-oxidation of very long chain fatty acids (VLCFAs), the accumulation of which leads to dysmyelination in the central and peripheral nervous system as well as damage to adrenocortical cells. In the brain, the effect of VLCFAs is speculated to be a destabilization of the myelin membrane, and in severe cases inflammation is also thought to contribute to white matter damage (Moser, 1997).

Computed tomography scans show low density lesions in the hemispheric white matter (Patel et al., 1995). Magnetic resonance imaging scans reveal symmetric white matter hyperintensity that tends to be most prominent in parietooccipital regions (Loes et al., 1994; Fig. 5-2). Although ALD is a disease of males, female heterozygotes may have neurologic signs and symptoms suggesting MS, and MRI findings consistent with this disease may be present (van Geel et al., 1997).

Adrenoleukodystrophy has several phenotypic variants, indicating that a later age of onset can also occur (van Geel et al., 1997). One patient with onset at the age of 57 has been reported (Weller et al., 1992). In later-onset cases, neurobehavioral implications have been more amenable to detailed study. Cognitive decline and progressive dementia occur, often heralded by neuropsychiatric dysfunction that manifests as personality change, mania, or psychosis (Rosebush et al., 1999).

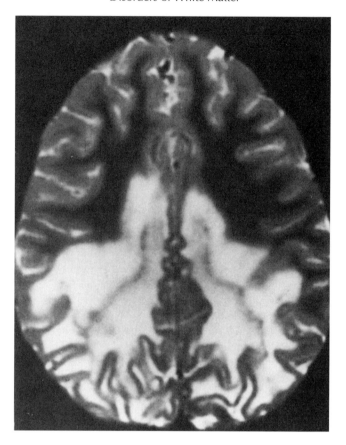

Figure 5-2. T2-weighted MRI scan of a patient with adrenoleukodystrophy. The dysmyelination has a predilection for the posterior hemispheric white matter. (Reprinted with permission from Atlas SW, ed. Magnetic resonance imaging of the brain and spine. 2nd ed.
Philadelphia: Lippincott-Raven, 1996.)

In a neuropsychological study of ALD children, Riva and colleagues (2000) found
deficits in nonverbal intelligence, memory, and executive function, with relative
sparing of language, that was closely reminiscent of cognitive impairment seen in
adults with white matter disorders (Filley, 1998). Moreover, the cognitive loss in
these children correlated significantly with posterior hemispheric dysmyelination
on MRI (Riva et al., 2000).

   Treatment of ALD has been improving in recent years. Initial attempts at dietary treatment by reducing the intake of VLCFAs was ineffective, but a formulation known as Lorenzo's oil became popular in the 1980s. Lorenzo's oil is a 4:1
combination of oleic acid and erucic acid intended to decrease the production of
VLCFAs, but despite the reduction of VLCFAs that could be demonstrated, the
treatment did not affect cerebral deterioration (Rosebush et al., 1999). Treatment

with immunosuppressive drugs has also been suggested on the basis of inflammatory mechanisms that are postulated to contribute to dysmyelination (van Geel et al.,
1997), but results of these trials are still pending (Rosebush et al., 1999). Use of intravenous immunoglobulin (IVIG) has been attempted, but clinical improvement,
if any, was temporary (Sawaya, 2000). Bone marrow transplantation appears to
have the most promise in treating ALD, as sustained clinical, biochemical, and
MRI improvement has been documented in several cases so treated (Aubourg et
al., 1990; Shapiro et al., 2000). This procedure seems to be most suitable for those
who are very young and have an early form of the disease (Shapiro et al., 2000).
Finally, gene therapy has been considered with the use of viral carriers placed
stereotactically into the brain, but is still in an experimental phase and has not been
attempted in humans (Sawaya, 2000).

Adrenomyeloneuropathy

Adrenomyeloneuropathy (AMN) was described by Griffin and colleagues (1977)
as a variant of ALD in which myelopathy and neuropathy dominate the clinical
course. Typically beginning in the third or fourth decade, AMN has a more benign
course than ALD, with near normal life expectancy despite slowly progressive
spastic quadriparesis and peripheral neuropathy (van Geel et al., 1997). Treatment
of this disease is supportive.

The brain was initially believed to be spared in AMN, but recent developments
have indicated that cognition may be affected. Magnetic resonance imaging scans
of the brain show white matter abnormalities in 45% of affected patients (Kumar et
al., 1995). Moreover, neuropsychological studies of individuals with cerebral AMN
indicate cognitive loss consistent with white matter involvement, and severe MRI
lesion burden is associated with more pronounced impairment (Edwin et al., 1996).

Canavan's Disease

Canavan's disease is an autosomal recessive disease that presents in early infancy
with intellectual decline, macrocephaly, optic atrophy, and hypotonia (Menkes,
1990). The course is rapidly progressive and a fatal outcome soon ensues. There
is a mutation in the gene coding for the enzyme aspartoacylase (ASPA), which
leads to an accumulation of the amino acid N-acetyl-aspartic acid (NAA); diagnosis is based on the demonstration of NAA in the urine. In the brain, a spongiform
leukodystrophy develops, which appears on MRI as increased signal throughout
the white matter (Brismar et al., 1990a).

Treatment of Canavan's disease has heretofore been confined to supportive
measures, but a recent report describing gene therapy in this disease was encouraging. Using a nonviral delivery system, Leone and colleagues (2000) showed that
intraventricular treatment with the ASPA gene could normalize NAA levels, improve the appearance of the white matter on MRI, and produce clinical improvement in two affected children. The investigators also demonstrated widespread
gene expression in astrocytes, neurons, and oligodendrocytes within the deep

white matter (Leone et al., 2000). This study, the first to report on gene therapy for a neurologic disease, represents an important event in neurologic therapeutics in general. In addition, it emphasizes again that white matter disorders may be particularly well suited to therapeutic interventions because of the relative sparing of gray matter elements in many cases. Futher study of this therapy as it relates to correction of leukodystrophy and neurobehavioral impairment will be of considerable interest.

Pelizaeus-Merzbacher Disease

An X-linked dysmyelinative disease of the central nervous system, Pelizaeus-Merzbacher disease usually presents in infancy with intellectual delay but may also appear in later life. This slowly progressive disorder of myelin formation has been linked to an abnormality of the gene coding for proteolipid protein, one of the major protein constituents of myelin (Koeppen et al., 1987). More than 30 different mutations in this gene have now been identified (Seitelberger, 1995), although the phenotype of the disease may also appear in individuals who do not have one of these mutations (Sasaki et al., 2000). Dementia and psychiatric dysfunction are common in adult onset cases. Neuropathologically, patchy areas of myelin loss combined with preserved myelin islets in the brain produce the so-called tigroid pattern of dysmyelination that is considered characteristic. On MRI, there is a diffusely increased signal suggesting hypomyelination (van der Knaap and Valk, 1989), and occasionally evidence of the tigroid pattern can be found (Sasaki et al., 2000). Treatment is limited to supportive measures.

Alexander's Disease

In contrast to many other leukodystrophies, Alexander's disease has no known genetic or biochemical correlates. Rather, the defining features are neuropathologic: Rosenthal fibers and diffuse myelin loss in the brain. This disease typically presents in early life with psychomotor retardation, macrocephaly, and spasticity, and pursues a rapidly fatal course. Cases appearing in adolescence and adulthood are also described, and in these individuals the clinical picture may resemble MS because of prominent motor system involvement (Russo et al., 1976). Dementia has also been noted as the core feature of a very late–onset case (Murphy et al., 1990). Computed tomography scans show low attenuation of the periventricular and centrum semiovale white matter (Hess et al., 1990), and MRI scans demonstrate diffusely increased white matter signal (Takanashi et al., 1998); these changes are most prominent in the frontal lobes. No effective treatment has been found.

Cockayne's Disease

Cockayne's disease is a clinically diverse disease of unknown etiology that has been regarded as a leukodystrophy similar to Pelizaeus-Merzbacher disease. An autosomal recessive pattern of transmission is suspected (Soffer et al., 1979), although X-linked inheritance cannot be excluded (Houston et al., 1982). The disease usually presents in late infancy and includes progressive mental retardation, microcephaly, dwarfism, deafness, retinal degeneration, and dysmorphic facial features. White matter atrophy with myelin loss has been consistently documented neuropathologically, along with variable cerebral and cerebellar cortical calcifications and cerebellar cortical atrophy (Soffer et al., 1979). Cases appearing in childhood have also been recognized, in which white matter hyperintensities on MRI scans and neuropsychological impairment have been found (Sugita et al., 1992). Treatment is confined to supportive interventions.

Cerebrotendinous Xanthomatosis

A rare autosomal recessive disease of bile acid synthesis, cerebrotendinous xanthomatosis is characterized by loss of myelinated fibers in the brain, and deposition of cholestanol xanthomas in the peripheral nerves, lungs, and tendons. White matter throughout the brain, especially the cerebellum, is severely affected (Soffer et al., 1995). The disease presents in adulthood with gait disorder and dementia, and MRI scans reveal diffuse white matter abnormality and cerebral atrophy (Swanson and Cromwell, 1986). In one series, 66% of affected individuals had cognitive impairment (Verrips et al., 2000). Diagnosis is established by the finding of elevated plasma cholestanol, and treatment to lower cholestanol with chenodeoxycholic acid can be effective (Pedley et al., 1985). However, the dementia may not respond even if the cholestanol is reduced significantly (Swanson and Cromwell, 1986).

Membranous Lipodystrophy

Membranous lipodystrophy is a very rare disease affecting the brain and the skeletal system (Tanaka, 1980). Appearing in mid-adulthood, the disease manifests with dementia and neuropsychiatric changes, accompanied at some point by parallel features of bone pain and pathologic fractures (Tanaka, 1980; Minagawa et al., 1985). The course is progressive. An inherited disorder of lipid metabolism affecting both cerebral myelin and adipose tissue is suspected, but the etiology is unknown. In the brain, there is diffuse and symmetric myelin degeneration, particularly in the frontal and temporal lobes, that spares the U fibers (Tanaka, 1980). Magnetic resonance imaging scans show increased white matter signal on T2-weighted images and dilated ventricles (Araki et al., 1991). No effective treatment is known.

Aminoacidurias

Among the many inborn errors of metabolism, several affect amino acid metabolism. Of these autosomal recessive aminoacidurias, two—phenylketonuria and maple syrup urine disease (MSUD)—are known to disturb normal myelination. These diseases highlight the potential for salutary effects of dietary treatment in genetic disorders of white matter.

Phenylketonuria

Phenylketonuria (PKU) is one of the most common disorders associated with mental retardation, and its recognition and treatment have led to significant reduction of neurologic disability. The disease appears in newborns as a result of an autosomal recessive deficiency of hepatic phenylalanine hydroxylase that prevents the conversion of phenylalanine to tyrosine (Pietz, 1998). The resulting hyperphenylalaninemia is associated with mental retardation and motor dysfunction. Neuropathologically, it has long been recognized that myelin is primarily affected by PKU (Malamud, 1966). In untreated patients, findings include delayed myelination, fibrillary gliosis, excess white matter water, and low concentrations of cerebrosides, sulfatides, and cholesterol (Martin and Schlote, 1972). These observations have suggested that dysmyelination is the most accurate model to explain the white matter changes in PKU (Hommes and Matsuo, 1987; Pietz, 1998). More recent studies have suggested that elevated phenylalanine may induce oligodendrocytes to adopt a nonmyelinating phenotype (Dyer et al., 1996). In any case, the diffuse hypomyelination of untreated PKU correlates well with MRI observations of increased signal on T2-weighted images in the periventricular white matter (Shaw et al., 1991).

Neuropsychological studies of PKU patients have documented a variety of deficits that can be interpreted as reflecting white matter involvement. These impairments are present in both treated and untreated individuals, although dietary restriction of phenylalanine clearly improves cognitive function (Ris et al., 1994). While domains including memory and language are relatively preserved (Pennington et al., 1985), a pattern of deficits in sustained attention (Schmidt et al., 1994), executive function (Welch et al., 1990), and visuospatial skills (Fishler et al., 1987) has emerged, a profile consistent with the prominence of white matter in the frontal lobes (Filley, 1998) and the right hemisphere (Gur et al., 1980). Impaired reaction time and sustained attention have been significantly correlated with MRI white matter burden (Pietz et al., 1996), although motor impairment has not generally shown this correlation (Pietz, 1998).

Further evidence for the importance of dysmyelination in the cognitive loss of PKU patients comes from observations of the reversibility of MRI findings with control of phenylalanine levels (Shaw et al., 1991; Cleary et al., 1995), and from occasional reports of clinical exacerbations being closely associated with worsening of MRI findings (Thompson et al., 1990). However, the biochemical complexity of PKU suggests that a multifactorial process may best explain the neurobehavioral manifestations of PKU (Pietz, 1998). Further correlational studies of MRI status and neuropsychological function are needed to elucidate the contribution of white matter neuropathology to the clinical phenomenology of this disease.

Maple Syrup Urine Disease

Formerly rapidly fatal in infancy, MSUD can now be treated effectively with dietary measures so that affected children can be expected to survive indefinitely. The disease is caused by a defect in the enzyme-branched chain alpha-keto acid dehydrogenase, which results in excessive urinary levels of leucine, isoleucine, and valine. In untreated cases, severe mental and motor decline is observed along with the characteristic odor of the urine. The neuropathology is confined to the brain white matter, where myelin formation is uniformly defective (Silberman et al., 1961). Computed tomography and MRI scans show variable white matter changes consistent with these observations (Brismar et al., 1990b).

Neuropsychological studies of treated MSUD children reveal that cognition and learning are typically affected, although a gratifyingly good outcome can be expected in many cases (Nord et al., 1991). Similar to PKU, the pattern of cognitive deficits in MSUD shows relative sparing of verbal functions and prominent visuospatial impairment (Nord et al., 1991). Improvement in cognition and the CT apprearance of white matter have been documented with dietary treatment (Taccone et al., 1992), supporting a role of dysmyelination in the neurobehavioral profile of MSUD.

Phakomatoses

The phakomatoses, or neurocutaneous syndromes, are diseases of known or suspected genetic etiology in which the skin and the nervous system are involved. At least 20 different phakomatoses are recognized, the three most common being neurofibromatosis, tuberous sclerosis, and Sturge-Weber syndrome (Roach, 1992). These diseases are best known for their propensity to produce benign and malignant tumors, but the range of neuropathologic lesions is broad. In recent years, MRI and neuropathologic studies of patients with these diseases have brought to light various abnormalities of the cerebral white matter (Pont and Elster, 1992; Roach, 1992). Some suggestions that white matter lesions in these diseases may contribute to neurobehavioral decline have appeared, although the presence of other abnormalities complicates this hypothesis. In this section, the phakomatoses characterized by documented cerebral white matter changes will be discussed, as well as the evidence that these changes contribute to neurobehavioral impairment.

Neurofibromatosis

The most common of the phakomatoses, neurofibromatosis has recently been established to have two main clinical varieties, both transmitted in an autosomal dominant pattern (Roach, 1992). Neurofibromatosis-1 (NF-1), the classic von Recklinghausen's disease with café-au-lait spots, axillary freckling, Lisch nodules, multiple neurofibromas, and a tendency for the development of optic glioma and other malignancies, is far more common that NF-2, which essentially features bilateral acoustic neuromas (Roach, 1992). Gene defects have been identified on chromsomes 17 and 22 for NF-1 and NF-2, respectively (Roach, 1992).

White matter changes of two varieties have emerged in NF-1. First, high signal changes have been seen on MRI in the subcortical white matter, and in the basal ganglia, cerebellum, and brainstem as well (Pont and Elster, 1992). The origin of these alterations is unknown, although it has been speculated that they represent dysmyelination, hamartomas, heterotopias, or even edema (Denckla et al., 1996). Second, increased cerebral white matter volume has been observed, both in the cerebrum as a whole (Said et al., 1996) and in the corpus callosum (Moore et al., 2000). These changes have been interpreted as reflecting insufficient growth control (Said et al., 1996), perhaps through delayed developmental apoptosis (Moore et al., 2000).

The neurobehavioral consequences of these changes are equally obscure. Some investigators have found that children with MRI hyperintensities have impaired cognition (North et al., 1994; Denckla et al., 1996), whereas others have not (Ferner et al., 1993). Moreover, studies specifically examining the role of white matter hyperintensities apart from gray matter lesions have not been conducted. Diminished visuospatial and motor function have been correlated with increased corpus callosum size (Moore et al., 2000), but few studies have examined the correlates of excessive white matter volume. However, neuropsychological studies of both children and adults with NF-1 demonstrate a general pattern of impairment in cognitive speed, attention, memory retrieval, visuospatial function, and problem solving (Zöller et al., 1997). This profile resembles that of subcortical dementia (Zöller et al., 1997), and is also similar to that of white matter dementia (Filley, 1998), suggesting that white matter changes in NF-1 may have important cognitive sequelae.

Tuberous Sclerosis

Tuberous sclerosis consists of a combination of skin lesions including facial angiofibroma (adenoma sebaceum), hypomelanotic macules (ash leaf spots), ungual fibromas, and shagreen patches, and neurologic features including seizure disorders and mental retardation (Roach, 1992). Systemic manifestations are also common in the kidney, heart, and other organs. The disease is transmitted as an autosomal dominant, and two gene loci, on chromosomes 9 and 16, have been identified recently (Hyman and Whittemore, 2000).

In the brain, a complex pattern of neuropathology is found, including cortical tubers, subependymal nodules, giant cell astrocytomas, and white matter heterotopias (Scheithauer, 1992). Despite the name of the disease deriving from the tubers in the cortex, all the other lesions are found in the white matter, as is well demonstrated by MRI (Braffman et al., 1992). Disordered migration of dysgenetic cells has been postulated as important in the pathogenesis (Braffman et al., 1992).

Patients with tuberous sclerosis may have severe mental retardation, mild cognitive impairment, neuropsychiatric abnormalities, or normal neurobehavioral function (Harrison et al., 1999). However, it is difficult to tease apart the contribution of specific white matter lesions to mental status abnormalities. In one study of tuberous sclerosis patients with normal intelligence quotients (IQs), neuropsychological deficits were found on tests reflecting frontal lobe function (Harrison et al., 1999). This result is of interest in view of the fact that white matter lesions are most commonly found in the frontal lobes (Braffman et al., 1992). However, it should be noted that cortical tubers are also most often found in the frontal lobes (Braffman et al., 1992), confounding the clinical-pathologic correlation. Further study of this question is clearly needed.

Sturge-Weber Syndrome

Although not known to be a genetic disease, Sturge-Weber syndrome is congenital and bears sufficient similarity to other disorders in this section to merit inclusion here. This is a disease of children who have a port wine nevus in the distribution of the trigeminal nerve and an ipsilateral leptomeningeal angioma (Roach, 1992). Bilateral angiomas can occur, and cause more severe neurologic morbidity. Cortical calcifications, classically in a "tram track" configuration, are also encountered. Seizure disorders, often refractory, are the most common neurologic manifestation, and cognitive impairment, which may be severe, occurs in about 50% of patients (Roach, 1992). White matter changes have recently been identified on MRI, and attributed to ischemia from the hypoperfusion associated with the angiomas or to dysmyelination (Marti-Bonmarti et al., 1992). The neurobehavioral significance of these changes has yet to be investigated.

Hypomelanosis of Ito

Also known as incontinentia pigmenti achromiens, hypomelanosis of Ito is the fourth most common phakomatosis (Ruggieri et al., 1996). The characteristic hypopigmented skin lesions are accompanied by neurologic features in more than 60% of cases, typically including cognitive deterioration and seizures (Pascual-Castroviejo et al., 1988). Magnetic resonance imaging changes including periventricular white matter hyperintensity (Ruggieri et al., 1996) and absent delineation between cortical gray and white matter (Malherbe et al., 1993) have been noted, explained alternatively by Wallerian degeneration or altered myelination. The significance of white matter changes is unclear, but in a small series of affected children, those with the most extensive changes had the most severe psychomotor delay and the lowest IQ scores (Ruggieri et al., 1996).

Fabry's Disease

Fabry's disease (angiokerotoma corporis diffusum) is an X-linked disease characterized by a deficiency of alpha-galactosidase (Mitsias and Levine, 1996). Cerebrovascular involvement is a major feature of this disease (Mitsias and Levine, 1996), with both cortical and subcortical strokes that accumulate with increasing age (Crutchfield et al., 1998). Early in the course, which typically begins in young adulthood, white matter lesions may predominate because of the initial involvement of long penetrating arterioles in the cerebrum, and later on, cortical strokes also occur (Crutchfield et al., 1998). Recent studies with magnetic resonance spectroscopy indicate that white matter damage may extend beyond the areas of damage visible with conventional MRI (Tedeschi et al., 1999). The neurobehavioral correlates of white matter involvement are not well defined, but vascular dementia has been described in Fabry's disease (Mendez et al., 1997).

Mucopolysaccharidoses

The mucopolysaccharidoses (MPS) are a group of lysosomal storage diseases in which an enzyme defect prevents the metabolic degradation of mucopolysaccharides (Walsh and Moran, 1993). Systemic morphologic abnormalities are apparent in all these diseases, and nervous system involvement occurs in most. The two most familiar of these diseases, Hurler's and Hunter's syndrome, both feature prominent white matter involvement and will be appropriate to consider at this point. In neither syndrome have precise correlations between white matter changes and cognitive loss been made, but similarities to other genetic leukoencephalopathies suggest that such a relationship may exist.

Hurler's Syndrome

Also known as MPS I, Hurler's syndrome is the prototype for this family of diseases. Developmental slowing appears in the first year of life, and dementia progresses over the few years that the child can be expected to live. Hurler's syndrome is an autosomal recessive disease caused by a deficiency of the enzyme alpha-L-iduronidase. Neuropathology shows white matter involvement from disordered myelin and from associated hydrocephalus that seems to result from mucopolysaccharide accumulations in the arachnoid villi (Walsh and Moran, 1993). Magnetic resonance imaging findings of diffusely delayed myelination have been reported (Johnson et al., 1984). Treatment with bone marrow transplantation has extended life expectancy in some affected individuals (Krivit et al., 1999).

Hunter's Syndrome

Hunter's syndrome, or MPS II, can be considered a milder form of MPS I. It is an X-linked disease that appears in young boys, and the deficient enzyme is iduronate sulfatase (Walsh and Moran, 1993). The neuropathology affecting white matter structures is similar to that of MPS I but less severe. Mental function is variably preserved. Magnetic resonance imaging scans reveal diffuse white matter abnormalities (Shinomiya et al., 1996).

Muscular Dystrophy

Until recently, the muscular dystrophies were considered strictly to be diseases of muscle. However, neurobehavioral impairment has been noted in a number of these diseases, and attention has thus been directed to the brain. Although cognitive loss has been found in the most common of this group, Duchenne muscular dystrophy (Bresolin et al., 1994), and in its milder relative, Becker muscular dystrophy (North et al., 1996), white matter lesions are not prominent, and the defect in these diseases appears to stem from a lack of dystrophin in gray matter structures (Blake and Kroger, 2000). White matter is affected, however, in two of the other muscular dystrophies, and evidence pertaining to the possible neurobehavioral importance of this feature is accumulating.

Congenital Muscular Dystrophy

This term encompasses a heterogeneous group of congenital muscle diseases that typically show an autosomal recessive pattern of inheritance. The classification of congenital muscular dystrophy (CMD) is in progress, but several types are generally accepted: "pure" CMD, Fukuyama-type CMD, Walker-Warburg syndrome, muscle-eye-brain disease, and merosin-deficient CMD (van der Knaap et al., 1997b). All of these variants may have cerebral white matter changes on MRI, including the pure form of CMD, which was formerly thought to feature no brain involvement (Mackay et al., 1998). Congenital muscular dystrophy types also include a variety of gray matter abnormalities, however, so that interpretation of the white matter changes is complex. One study did conclude that CMD children with white matter changes had more perceptuo-motor difficulties and soft neurologic signs than those who did not (Mercuri et al., 1995). For the present, it is reasonable to conclude that the clinical significance of white matter changes in CMD, as well as their origin, remains largely unknown.

Myotonic Dystrophy

Myotonic dystrophy is an autosomal dominant neuromuscular disease characterized by distal myopathy, cataracts, cardiac conduction defects, and hypogonadism. Cognitive impairment in myotonic dystrophy may take the form of mental retardation, mild cognitive loss, or progressive dementia (Huber et al., 1989; Abe et al., 1994). Neuropsychiatric impairment in the form of depression (Huber et al., 1989) and attention deficit disorder (Steyaert et al., 1997) may also be prominent. The pathogenesis of neurobehavioral dysfunction in myotonic dystrophy is not understood, but autopsy study has shown myelin pallor and an increased interfascicular space with relative sparing of axons, cortical gray matter, and subcortical gray matter (Abe et al., 1994). Conventional MRI has revealed T2 hyperintensities in the cerebral white matter of these patients, and fluid attenuated inversion recovery imaging appears to demonstrate these lesions more clearly (Abe et al., 1998).

Neuropsychological studies of myotonic dystrophy patients have documented deficits in attention, memory, visuospatial function, and cognitive speed, with relative sparing of language (Woodward et al., 1982; Huber et al., 1989; Malloy et al., 1990). One study compared myotonic dystrophy and MS patients, and concluded that white matter lesions in the former that were immediately subjacent to the cortex disrupted cognition more that the periventricular lesions found in the latter (Damian et al., 1994). Huber and colleagues (1989) observed that white matter lesions, particularly in the anterior temporal lobe, correlated with severe cognitive impairment. Abe and colleagues (1994) found that, compared to control subjects, myotonic dystrophy patients had cognitive dysfunction and depression in association with white matter lesions, and that cognitive loss worsened as white matter lesion burden increased. Despite the sparse existing knowledge of their origin, white matter lesions in myotonic dystrophy increasingly appear to be implicated in neurobehavioral impairments.

Callosal Agenesis

Incomplete development of the corpus callosum is an idiopathic developmental anomaly, but will be considered at this point because it is a congenital disorder frequently associated with a wide variety of chromosomal and single gene defects (Lassonde and Jeeves, 1994). Callosal agenesis may in fact be seen in a number of white matter disorders described elsewhere in this book, including fetal alcohol syndrome, Krabbe's disease, Hurler's syndrome, neurofibromatosis, tuberous sclerosis, cytomegalovirus encephalitis, and hydrocephalus (Lassonde and Jeeves, 1994). Complete agenesis is relatively rare, and various forms of partial agenesis are more often encountered. Magnetic resonance imaging is the neuroimaging procedure of choice for this disorder, as the optimal midsagittal view cannot be achieved on routine CT scans (Fig. 5-3). Other developmental defects frequently co-exist in these patients, including seizure disorder, Dandy-Walker cyst, and corpus callosum lipoma (Lassonde and Jeeves, 1994).

The neurobehavioral consequences of callosal agenesis are difficult to ascertain because of the frequency with which other developmental abnormalities are present. Many children with this disorder suffer with mental retardation or various degrees of learning disability, and it is generally thought that associated cerebral anomalies in large part account for these problems (Lassonde and Jeeves, 1994). Indeed, the apparent normalcy of cognition in persons whose only abnormality is a callosal defect has contributed to doubt about the neurobehavioral importance of the corpus callosum (Bogen, 1993).

As a general rule, individuals with isolated callosal agenesis are frequently free of major neurobehavioral disturbances, but they do tend to function at the lower end of the normal range intellectually (Chiarello, 1980; Lassonde and Jeeves, 1994; Sauerwein and Lassonde, 1994). No specific pattern of cognitive dysfunction has been detected (Lassonde and Jeeves, 1993). Disconnection effects have been detected (Hannay, 2000) but are also relatively subtle, as they are more prominent in those who have undergone corpus callosotomy (Chapter 12). This discrepancy has been explained as a result of compensatory mechanisms that allow for near normal interhemispheric transfer. Other intact connecting tracts between the hemispheres, most notably the anterior commissure, can probably compensate for the callosal disconnection (Fischer et al., 1992). In addition, it has been speculated that acallosal patients make use of the Probst bundles—longitudinal fibers that run along the medial aspect of each hemisphere—to convey information from the posterior hemispheres for transfer across the anterior commissure (Bogen,

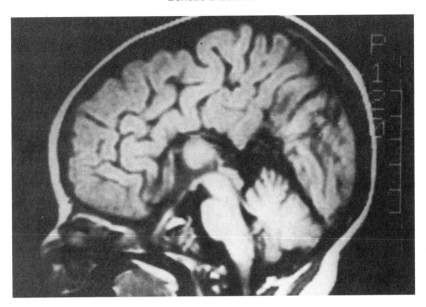

Figure 5-3. Midsagittal T1-weighted MRI scan of a patient with callosal agenesis. The corpus callosum is absent. (Reprinted with permission from Lassonde M, Jeeves MA. Collosal agenesis. A natural split brain? New York: Plenum Press, 1994.)

1993). Some suggestions exist that developmental callosal abnormalities may be associated with major psychiatric disorders, including schizophrenia, bipolar disorder, Asperger's syndrome, anxiety, and depression (David et al., 1993). These speculations are of interest in view of callosal abnormalities in schizophrenia demonstrated by advanced MRI techniques (David, 1994). The relationship of schizophrenia and white matter abnormalities is further examined in Chapter 17.

References

Abe K, Fujimura H, Soga F. The fluid-attenuated inversion-recovery pulse sequence in assessment of central nervous system involvement in myotonic dystrophy. Neuroradiology 1998; 40: 32–35.

Abe K, Fujimura H, Toyooka K, et al. Involvement of the central nervous system in myotonic dystrophy. J Neurol Sci 1994; 127: 179–185.

Araki T, Ohba H, Monzawa S, et al. Membranous lipodystrophy: MR imaging appearance of the brain. Radiology 1991; 180: 793–797.

Aubourg P, Blanche S, Jambaqué I, et al. Reversal of early neurological and neuroradiologic manifestations of X-linked adrenoleukodystrophy by bone marrow transplantation. N Engl J Med 1990; 322: 1860–1866.

Austin J, Armstrong D, Fouch S, et al. Metachromatic leukodystrophy (MLD). VIII. MLD in adults: diagnosis and pathogenesis. Arch Neurol 1968; 18: 225–240.

Blake DJ, Kroger S. The neurobiology of Duchenne muscular dystrophy: learning lessons from muscle? Trends Neurosci 2000; 23: 92–99.

Bogen JE. The callosal syndromes. In: Heilman KM, Valenstein E, eds. Clinical neuropsychology. 3rd ed. New York: Oxford University Press, 1993: 337–407.

Braffman BH, Bilaniuk LT, Naidich TP, et al. MR imaging of tuberous sclerosis: pathogenesis of this phakomatosis, use of gadopentetate dimeglumine, and literature review. Radiology 1992; 183: 227–238.

Bresolin N, Castelli E, Comi GP, et al. Cognitive impairment in Duchenne muscular dystrophy. Neuromuscul Disord 1994; 4: 359–369.

Brismar J, Aqeel A, Brismar G, et al. Maple syrup urine disease: findings on CT and MRI scans of the brain in 10 infants. AJNR 1990a; 11: 1219–1228.

Brismar J, Brismar G, Gascow G, et al. Canavan disease: CT and MR imaging of the brain AJNR 1990b; 11: 805–810.

Chiarello C. A house divided? Cognitive functioning with callosal agenesis. Brain Lang 1980; 11: 128–158.

Cleary MA, Walter JH, Wraith JE, et al. Magnetic resonance imaging in phenylketonuria: reversal of cerebral white matter change. J Pediatr 1995; 127: 251–255.

Crutchfield KE, Patronas NJ, Dambrosia JM, et al. Quantitative analysis of cerebral vasculopathy in patients with Fabry disease. Neurology 1998; 50: 1746–1749.

Damian MS, Schilling G, Bachmann G, et al. White matter lesions and cognitive deficits: relevance of lesion pattern? Acta Neurol Scand 1994; 90: 430–436.

David AS. Schizophrenia and the corpus callosum: developmental, structural and functional relationships. Behav Brain Res 1994; 20: 203–211.

David AS, Wacharasindhu A, Lishman WA. Severe psychiatric disturbance and abnormalities of the corpus callosum: review and case series. J Neurol Neurosurg Psychiatry 1993: 56: 85–93.

Denckla MB, Hofman K, Mazzocco MMM, et al. Relationship between T2-weighted hyperintensities (unidentified bright objects) and lower IQs in children with neurofibromatosis-1. Am J Med Genet 1996: 67: 98–102.

Dyer CA, Kendler A, Philibote T, et al. Evidence for central nervous system glial cell plasticity in phenylketonuria. J Neuropathol Exp Neurol 1996; 55: 795–814.

Edwin D, Speedie L, Kohler W, et al. Cognitive and brain magnetic resonance imaging findings in adrenomyeloneuropathy. Ann Neurol 1996; 40: 675–678.

Ferner RE, Chaudhuri R, Bingham J, et al. MRI in neurofibromatosis 1. The nature and evolution of increased intensity T2 weighted lesions and their relationship to intellectual impairment. J Neurol Neurosurg Psychiatry 1993; 56: 492–495.

Filley CM. The behavioral neurology of cerebral white matter. Neurology 1998; 50: 1535–1540.

Filley CM, Gross KF. Psychosis with cerebral white matter disease. Neuropsychiatry Neuropsychol Behav Neurol 1992; 5: 119–125.

Fischer M, Ryan SB, Dobyns WB. Mechanisms of interhemispheric transfer and patterns of cognitive function in acallosal patients of normal intelligence. Arch Neurol 1992; 49: 271–277.

Fishler K, Azen CG, Henderson R, et al. Psychoeducational findings among children treated for phenylketonuria. Am J Ment Defic 1987: 92: 65–73.

Folkerth RD. Abnormalities of developing white matter in lysosomal storage diseases. J Neuropathol Exp Neurol 2000; 58: 887–902.

Griffin J, Goren E, Schaumburg H, et al. Adrenomyeloneuropathy: a probable variant of adrenoleukodystrophy. Neurology 1977; 27: 1107–1113.

Gur RC, Packer IK, Hungerbuhler JP, et al. Differences in the distribution of gray and white matter in the human cerebral hemispheres. Science 1980; 207: 1226–1228.

Hannay HJ. Functioning of the corpus callosum in children with early hydrocephalus. J Int Neuropsychol Soc 2000; 6: 351–361.

Harrison JE, O'Callaghan FJ, Hancock E, et al. Cognitive deficits in normally intelligent patients with tuberous sclerosis. Am J Med Genet 1999; 88: 642–646.

Hess DC, Fischer AQ, Yaghmai F, et al. Comparative neuroimaging with pathologic correlates in Alexander's Disease. J Child Neurol 1990; 5: 248–252.

Hommes FA, Matsuo K. On a possible mechanism of abnormal brain development in experimental hyperphenylalaninemia. Neurochem Int 1987: 11: 1–10.

Houston CS, Zaleski WA, Rozdilsky B. Identical male twins and brother with Cockayne syndrome. Am J Med Genet 1982; 13: 211–223.

Huber SJ, Kissel KT, Shuttleworth EC, et al. Magnetic resonance imaging and clinical correlates of intellectual impairment in myotonic dystrophy. Arch Neurol 1989; 46: 536–540.

Hyde TM, Ziegler JC, Weinberger DR. Psychiatric disturbances in metachromatic leukodystrophy. Insights into the neurobiology of psychosis. Arch Neurol 1992; 49: 401–406.

Hyman MH, Whittemore VH. National Institutes of Health Consensus Conference: tuberous sclerosis complex. Arch Neurol 2000; 57: 662–665.

Ieshima A, Eda I, Matsui A, et al. Computed tomography in Krabbe's disease: comparison with neuropathology. Neuroradiology 1983; 25: 323–327.

Johnson MA, Desai S, Hugh-Jones K, Starer F. Magnetic resonance imaging of the brain in Hurler syndrome. AJNR 1984; 5: 816–819.

Kapoor R, McDonald WI, Crockard A, Moseley IF. Clinical and MRI features of Krabbe's disease in adolescence. J Neurol Neurosurg Psychiatry 1992; 55: 331–332.

Koeppen AH, Ronca NA, Greenfield EA, Hans MB. Defective biosynthesis of proteolipid protein in Pelizaeus-Merzbacher Disease. Ann Neurol 1987; 21: 159–170.

Krivit W, Peters C, Shapiro EG. Bone marrow transplantation as effective treatment of central nervous system disease in globoid cell leukodystrophy, metachromatic leukodystrophy, adrenoleukodystrophy, mannosidosis, fucosidosis, aspartylglucosaminuria, Hurler, Maroteaux-Lamy, and Sly syndromes, and Gaucher disease type III. Curr Opin Neurol 1999; 12: 167–176.

Krivit W, Shapiro E, Kennedy W, et al. Treatment of late infantile metachromatic leukodystrophy by bone marrow transplantation. N Engl J Med 1990; 322: 28–32.

Krivit W, Shapiro EG, Peters C, et al. Hematopoietic stem-cell transplantation in globoid-cell leukodystrophy. N Engl J Med 1998; 338: 1119–1126.

Kumar AJ, Kohler W, Kruse B, et al. MR findings in adult onset adrenoleukodystrophy. AJNR 1995; 16: 1227–1237.

Lassonde M, Jeeves MA. Callosal agenesis. A natural split brain? New York: Plenum Press, 1994.

Leone P, Janson CG, Bilianuk L, et al. Aspartoacylase gene transfer to the mammalian central nervous system with therapeutic implications for Canavan's Disease. Ann Neurol 2000; 48: 27–38.

Loes DJ, Hite S, Moser H, et al. Adrenoleukodystrophy: a scoring method for brain MR observations. AJNR 1994; 15: 1761–1766.

Mackay MT, Kornberg AJ, Shield L, et al. Congenital muscular dystrophy, white matter abnormalities, and neuronal migration disorders: the expanding concept. J Child Neurol 1998; 13: 481–487.

Malamud N. Neuropathology of phenylketonuria. J Neuropathol Exp Neurol 1966; 25: 254–268.

Malherbe V, Pariente D, Tardieu M, et al. Central nervous system lesions in hypomelanosis of Ito: an MRI and neuropathological study. J Neurol 1993; 240: 302–304.

Malloy P, Mishra SK, Adler SH. Neuropsychological deficits in myotonic muscular dystrophy. J Neurol Neurosurg Psychiatry 1990; 53: 1011–1013.

Marti-Bonmati L, Menor F, Poyatos C, Cortina H. Diagnosis of Sturge-Weber syndrome: comparison of the efficacy of CT and MR imaging in 14 cases. AJR 1992; 158: 867–871.

Martin JJ, Schlote W. Central nervous system lesions in disorders of amino-acid metabolism. A neuropathological study. J Neurol Sci 1972; 15: 49–76.

Mendez MF, Stanley TM, Medel NM, et al. The vascular dementia of Fabry's disease. Dement Geriatr Cogn Disord 1997; 8: 251–257.

Menkes JH. The leukodystrophies. N Engl J Med 1990; 322: 54–55.

Mercuri E, Dubowitz L, Berardinelli A, et al. Minor neurological and perceptuo-motor deficits in children with congenital muscular dystrophy: correlation with brain MRI changes. Neuropediatrics 1995; 26: 156–162.

Minagawa M, Maeshiro H, Shioda K, Hirano A. Membranous lipodystrophy (Nasu disease): clinical and neuropathological study of a case. Clin Neuropathol 1985: 4: 38–45.

Mitsias P, Levine SR. Cerebrovascular complications of Fabry's disease. Ann Neurol 1996; 40: 8–17.

Moore BD, Slopis JM, Jackson EF, et al. Brain volume in children with neurofibromatosis type 1: relation to neuropsychological status. Neurology 2000; 54: 914–920.

Moser HW. Adrenoleukodystrophy: phenotype, genetics, pathogenesis and therapy. Brain 1997; 120: 1485–1508.

Murphy FM, Saini N, Schwankhaus J, et al. Adult Alexander's Disease and dementia. Neurology 1990; 40 (Suppl 1): 451.

Navarro C, Fernandez JM, Dominguez C, et al. Late juvenile matechromatic leukodystrophy treated with bone marrow transplantation: a 4–year follow-up study. Neurology 1996; 46: 254–256.

Nord A, van Doorninck WJ, Greene C. Developmental profile of patients with maple syrup urine disease. J Inher Metab Dis 1991; 14: 881–889.

North K, Joy P, Yuille D, et al. Specific learning disability in children with neurofibromatosis type 1: significance of MRI abnormalities. Neurology 1994; 44: 878–883.

North KN, Miller G, Iannaccone ST, et al. Cognitive dysfunction as the major presenting feature of Becker's muscular dystrophy. Neurology 1996; 46: 461–465.

Pascual-Castroviejo I, Lopez-Rodriguez L, de la Cruz Medina M, et al. Hypomelanosis of Ito. Neurological complications in 34 cases. Can J Neurol Sci 1988; 15: 124–129.

Patel PJ, Kolawole TM, Malabarey TM, et al. Adrenoleukodystrophy: CT and MRI findings. Pediatr Neurol 1995; 25: 256–268.

Pedley TA, Emerson RG, Warner CL, et al. Treatment of cerebrotendinous xanthomatosis with chenodeoxycholic acid. Ann Neurol 1985; 18: 517–518.

Pennington BF, van Doorninck WJ, McCabe LL, McCabe ER. Neuropsychological deficits in early treated phenylketonuric children. Am J Ment Defic 1985; 89: 467–474.

Percy AK, Odrezin GT, Knowles PD, et al. Globoid cell leukodystrophy: comparison of neuropathology with magnetic resonance imaging. Acta Neuropathol 1994; 88: 26–32.

Pietz J. Neurological aspects of adult phenylketonuria. Curr Opin Neurol 1998; 11: 679–688.

Pietz J, Kreis R, Schmidt H, et al. Phenylketonuria: findings at MR imaging and localized in vivo H-1 MR spectroscopy of the brain in patients with early treatment. Radiology 1996; 201: 413–420.

Pont MS, Elster AD. Lesions of skin and brain: modern imaging of the neurocutaneous syndromes. AJR 1992; 158: 1193–1203.

Ris MD, Williams SE, Hunt MM, et al. Early-treated phenylketonuria: adult neuropsychologic outcome. J Pediatr 1994; 124: 388–392.

Riva D, Bova SM, Bruzzone MG. Neuropsychological testing may predict early progression of asymptomatic adrenoleukodysrophy. Neurology 2000; 54; 1651–1655.

Roach ES. Neurocutaneous syndromes. Pediatr Clin N Am 1992; 39: 591–620.

Rosebush PI, Garside S, Levinson AJ, Mazurek MF. The neuropsychiatry of adult-onset adrenoleukodystrophy. J Neuropsychiatry Clin Neurosci 1999; 11: 315–327.

Ruggieri M, Tigano G, Mazzone D, et al. Involvement of the white matter in hypomelanosis of Ito (incontinentia pigmenti achromiens). Neurology 1996; 46: 485–492.

Russo LS, Aron A, Anderson PJ. Alexander's disease: a report and reappraisal. Neurology 1976; 26: 607–614.

Said SMA, Yeh T-L, Greenwood RS, et al. MRI morphometric analysis and neuropsychological function in patients with neurofibromatosis. Neuroreport 1996; 7: 1941–1944.

Sasaki A, Miyanaga K, Ototsuji M, et al. Two autopsy cases with Pelizaeus-Merzbacher disease phenotype of adult onset, without mutation of proteolipid protein gene. Acta Neuropathol 2000; 99: 7–13.

Sauerwein HC, Lassonde M. Cognitive and sensori-motor functioning in the absence of corpus callosum: neuropsychological studies in callosal agenesis and callosotomized patients. Behav Brain Res 1994; 64: 229–240.

Sawaya RA. Adrenoleukodystrophy: a review. Neurologist 2000; 6: 214–219.

Scheithauer BW. The neuropathology of tuberous sclerosis. J Dermatol 1992; 19: 897–903.

Schmidt E, Rupp A, Burgard P, et al. Sustained attention in adult phenylketonuria: the influence of the concurrent phenylalanine-blood-level. J Clin Exp Neuropsychol 1994; 16: 681–688.

Seitelberger F. Neuropathology and genetics of Pelizaeus-Merzbacher disease. Brain Pathol 1995; 5: 267–273.

Shapiro E, Krivit W, Lockman L, et al. Long-term effect of bone-marrow transplantation for childhood-onset cerebral X-linked adrenoleukodystrophy. Lancet 2000; 356: 713–718.

Shapiro EG, Lipton ME, Krivit W. White matter dysfunction and its neuropsychological correlates: a longitudinal study of a case of metachromatic leukodystrophy treated with bone marrow transplant. J Clin Exp Neuropsychol 1992; 14: 610–624.

Shapiro EG, Lockman LA, Knopman D, Krivit W. Characteristics of the dementia in late-onset metachromatic leukodystrophy. Neurology 1994; 44: 662–665.

Shaw DWW, Maravilla KR, Weinberger E, et al. MR imaging of phenylketonuria. AJNR 1991; 12: 403–406.

Shinomiya N, Nagayama T, Fujiyoka Y, Aoki T. MRI in the mild type of mucopolysaccharidosis II (Hunter's syndrome). Neuroradiology 1996; 38: 483–485.

Silberman J, Dancis J, Feigin I. Neuropathological observations in maple syrup urine disease. Arch Neurol 1961; 5: 351–363.

Skomer C, Stears J, Austin J. Metachromatic leukodystrophy (MLD). XV. Adult MLD with focal lesions by computed tomography. Arch Neurol 1983; 40: 354–355.

Soffer D, Benharroch D, Berginer V. The neuropathology of cerebrotendinous xanthomatosis revisited: a case report and review of the literature. Acta Neuropathol 1995; 90: 213–220.

Soffer D, Grotsky HW, Rapin I, Suzuki K. Cockayne syndrome: unusual neuropathological findings and review of the literature. Ann Neurol 1979; 6: 340–348.

Steyaert J, Umans S, Willekens D, et al. A study of the cognitive and psychological profile in 16 children with congenital or juvenile myotonic dystrophy. Clin Genet 1997; 52: 135–141.

Sugita K, Takanashi J, Ishii M, Niimi H. Comparison of white matter changes with neuropsychologic impairment in Cockaye syndrome. Pediatr Neurol 1992; 8: 295–298.

Swanson PD, Cromwell LD. Magnetic resonance imaging in cerebrotendinous xanthomatosis. Neurology 1986; 36: 124–126.

Taccone A, Schiaffino MC, Cerone R, et al. Computed tomography in maple syrup urine disease. Eur J Radiol 1992; 14: 207–212.

Takanashi J, Sugita K, Tanabe Y, Niimi H. Adolescent case of Alexander disease: MR imaging and MR spectroscopy. Pediatr Neurol 1998; 18: 67–70.

Tanaka J. Leukoencephalopathic alteration in membranous lipodystrophy. Acta Neuropathol 1980; 50: 193–197.

Tedeschi G, Bonavita S, Banerjee TK, et al. Diffuse central neuronal involvement in Fabry disease: a proton MRS imaging study. Neurology 1999; 52: 1663–1667.

Thompson AJ, Smith I, Brenton D, et al. Neurological deterioration in young adults with phenylketonuria. Lancet 1990; 336: 602–605.

van der Knaap MS, Barth PG, Gabreels FJ, et al. A new leukoencephalopathy with vanishing white matter. Neurology 1997a; 48: 845–855.

van der Knaap MS, Breiter SN, Naidu S, et al. Defining and categorizing leukoencephalopathies of unknown origin: MR imaging approach. Radiology 1999; 213: 121–133.

van der Knaap MS, Kleinschmidt-DeMasters BK, Kamphorst W, Weinstein HC. Autosomal dominant leukoencephalopathy with neuroaxonal spheroids. Neurology 2000; 54: 463–468.

van der Knaap MS, Smit LME, Barth PG, et al. Magnetic resonance imaging in classification of congenital muscular dystrophies with brain abnormalities. Ann Neurol 1997b; 42: 50–59.

van der Knaap MS, Valk J. The reflection of histology in MR imaging of Pelizaeus-Merzbacher disease. AJNR 1989; 10: 99–103.

van Geel BM, Assies J, Wanders RJA, Barth PG. X linked adrenoleukodystrophy: clinical presentation, diagnosis, and therapy. J Neurol Neurosurg Psychiatry 1997; 63: 4–14.

Verrips A, van Engelen BG, Wevers RA, et al. Presence of diarrhea and absence of tendon xanthomas in patients with cerebrotendinous xanthomatosis. Arch Neurol 2000; 57: 520–524.

Walsh LE, Moran CC. The mucopolysaccharidoses. Clinical and neuroradiographic features. Neuroimaging Clin N Am 1993; 3: 291–303.

Welch MC, Pennington BF, Ozonoff S, et al. Neuropsychology of early-treated phenylketonuria: specific executive function deficits. Child Dev 1990; 61: 1697–1713.

Weller M, Liedtke W, Petersen D, et al. Very-late-onset adrenoleukodystrophy: possible precipitation of demyelination by cerebral contusion. Neurology 1992: 42: 367–370.

Woodward JB, Heaton RK, Simon DB, Ringel SP. Neuropsychological findings in myotonic dystrophy. J Clin Neuropsychol 1982; 4: 335–342.

Zöller MET, Rembeck B, Bäckman L. Neuropsychological deficits in adults with neurofibromatosis type 1. Acta Neurol Scand 1997; 95: 225–232.

6

Demyelinative Diseases

In contrast to dysmyelination, demyelination refers to a stripping away of myelin from the axon. The demyelinative diseases target the normal myelin only after it is fully formed, and these diseases are characterized by an inflammatory attack on the myelin sheath. The most familiar demyelinative disease is multiple sclerosis (MS), and several related disorders with similar clinical and neuropathologic features are also recognized. This category is undoubtedly the most intensely investigated group of white matter disorders. Multiple sclerosis is the most common nontraumatic disabling neurologic disease of young adults, and the processes of inflammatory demyelination have generated much interest as a key to understanding basic pathophysiologic mechanisms that could apply to many other neurologic disorders. The demyelinative diseases are discussed with an emphasis on their many neurobehavioral manifestations.

Multiple Sclerosis

Despite more than a century of study, MS remains a perplexing disease whose clinical variability, etiology, and therapy continue to preoccupy neurologists (Noseworthy, 1999). Among the many issues with MS that require further elucidation is the characterization, significance, and treatment of neurobehavioral dysfunction. As recognized by Charcot in the nineteenth century (Charcot, 1877), the occurrence of both cognitive and emotional disturbances is acknowledged, but many details of these aspects of the disease remain to be more fully understood. The wide range of neurobehavioral disturbances that afflict individuals with MS (Filley, 1996) presents a challenge to clinicians and an opportunity for researchers.

Cognitive impairment is an important problem affecting many patients with MS (Rao, 1986; Feinstein, 1999). This syndrome may range from subtle cognitive loss that may easily escape clinical detection to severe dementia that mandates total care. For much of the history of MS, however, the high prevalence of cognitive impairment was not fully appreciated. As late as 1970, for example, the prevalence of cognitive dysfunction of any degree in MS was estimated to be in the vicinity of 5% (Kurtzke, 1970). Using more sensitive neuropsychological tests and improved research design, subsequent studies put this figure much higher. Peyser and colleagues, for example, found a prevalence of 55% in their series of hospitalized MS patients (Peyser et al., 1980). Heaton and colleagues considered the two major subtypes of relapsing-remitting and chronic-progressive MS, and found that 46% and 72%, respectively, were cognitively impaired (Heaton et al., 1985). Moreover, cognitive disturbances are not confined to MS patients referred to university hospital clinics, as Rao and colleagues found a prevalence of 43% in a community-based population (Rao et al., 1991). Given the variability in patient selection and methods of quantitating cognitive impairment, an overall prevalance figure of 40%–70% thus seems reasonable, and it is generally thought that more severe forms of the disease predict more significant degrees of cognitive loss.

A crucial point is that cognitive dysfunction in MS may not be associated with more obvious features of neurologic disease. Whereas it is true that memory and other disturbances often appear in parallel with elemental neurologic dysfunction in MS, cognitive loss may by itself constitute the major source of disability. Clinicians working with MS patients should be aware of this possibility, as it is often overlooked in patients who appear intact because of the absence of major motor and sensory findings on examination. Franklin and colleagues presented 12 patients in whom cognitive dysfunction was limiting, but physical disability, as measured by the Extended Disability Status Scale (EDSS; Kurtzke, 1983), was minimal (Franklin et al., 1989). This report highlights the important point that the EDSS, which remains the most widely used clinical measure of overall disability in MS, is generally insensitive to neurobehavioral dysfunction in this disease (Franklin et al., 1990). Another way clinicians can be misled by the disease is that the cognitive impairment of MS may be subtle in comparison to that of more familiar dementia syndromes such as that caused by Alzheimer's disease (AD). The typical pattern of cognitive deficits in AD, for example, is one of prominent amnesia and aphasia, whereas MS patients are likely to manifest greater impairment in sustained attention (Filley et al., 1989). These distinctions mean that the use of routine cognitive screening instruments may be inadequate. For example, because the dementia of MS (similar to many other white matter disorders) does not significantly disrupt language function, heavily language-weighted tests such as the Mini-Mental State Examination (MMSE; Folstein et al., 1976) are not well suited to detecting any cognitive loss that may be present (Franklin et al., 1988; Beatty and Goodkin, 1990; Swirsky-Sacchetti et al., 1992). In view of the inadequacy of both the EDSS and the MMSE for identifying cognitive dysfunction, detailed mental status testing and often neuropsychological evaluation may be required to confirm a clinical suspicion of cognitive dysfunction.

Understanding the origin of cognitive impairment in MS begins with the neuropathology of the disease. Whereas some patients have predominantly spinal cord disease, most individuals experience some degree of demyelinative plaque burden in the brain. Even the variant of MS known as neuromyelitis optica or Devic's syndrome, considered by many a demyelinative process confined to the optic nerves and spinal cord, may produce cerebral white matter lesions on MRI scans (Arnold and Myers, 1987; O'Riordan et al., 1996; Wingerchuk et al., 1999) and at autopsy (Filley et al., 1984), raising the possibility that subtle neurobehavioral dysfunction may also attend this disorder. The distribution of cerebral plaques in patients with MS was studied by Brownell and Hughes (1962), who found that periventricular sites were the most common, that left and right hemispheres were equally affected, and that plaques were distributed proportionately throughout the white matter. These findings are familiar to neurologists, and MRI studies of MS patients typically show a pattern of hyperintensities on T2–weighted images consistent with these observations (Fig. 6-1).

Further observations using MRI have clarified the neuropathologic significance of white matter lesions in MS (Simon, 1999). T2 hyperintensities generally reflect an increase in the water content of the white matter region affected, and are therefore nonspecific. T2 lesions may thus range in severity from simple interstitial edema, to demyelination with astrogliosis, and finally to axonal destruction. The acute lesion of MS is an inflammatory process revealed by contrast enhancement that transiently increases the T2 signal until the inflammation subsides, and then variable degrees of tissue loss remain. With time, these lesions conspire to produce brain atrophy, which is most prominent around the third ventricle (Simon, 1999). That is, atrophy results from widespread lesions that collectively reduce brain volume by destroying white matter (Simon, 1999). This process is not limited to more severe forms of the disease. In relapsing MS, for example, the lesion load of T2 hyperintensities increases by about 0.6 cm^3 per year (Simon, 1999). Multiple sclerosis is thus increasingly understood today as a progressive brain disease even in those with a presumably more benign course.

Brain atrophy in MS has important neurobehavioral implications in itself, but more specific white matter involvement is also important. Atrophy implies only diffuse white matter loss, and in attempting to define the specific cognitive profile of MS, the regional distribution of lesions assumes significance. In the study of Brownell and Hughes (1962), the subfrontal white matter had the heaviest plaque burden in the brain. This predilection presumably reflects the fact that the frontal lobe is the largest of the brain, and because demyelinative lesions occur randomly in the cerebral white matter, the subfrontal white matter stands to be the most heavily targeted of all the four lobes. Using the same logic, the possibility that more white matter is present in the right hemisphere than the left (Gur et al., 1980) implies that the disease may have disproportionate cognitive effects on right hemisphere function. These observations suggest that whereas MS is usually a diffuse

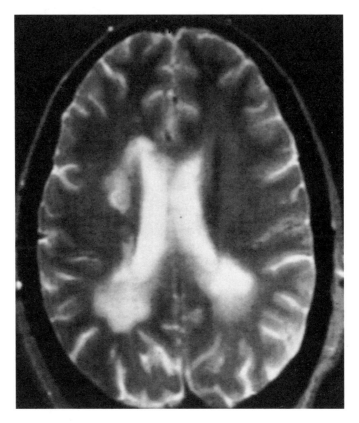

Figure 6-1. T2-weighted MRI scan of a patient with MS showing typical periventricular demyelinative plaques. (Reprinted with permission from Atlas SW, ed. Magnetic resonance imaging of the brain and spine. 2nd ed. Philadelphia: Lippincott-Raven, 1996.)

brain disease, its neurobehavioral effects may still reflect selective interference with frontal and right hemisphere systems.

The neuroanatomic basis of cognitive dysfunction has been actively investigated with neuroimaging, and there is overwhelming evidence that the burden of white matter disease correlates with cognitive dysfunction. At least 20 studies have found that total lesion burden on MRI predicts cognitive impairment as assessed neuropsychologically (Medaer et al., 1987; Franklin et al., 1988; Reisches et al., 1988; Rao et al., 1989b; Callanan et al., 1989; Anzola et al., 1990; Pozzilli et al., 1991; Swirsky-Sacchetti et al., 1992; Maurelli et al., 1992; Huber et al., 1992; Feinstein et al., 1992; Comi et al., 1993; Pugnetti et al., 1993; Feinstein et al., 1993; Arnett et al., 1994; Möller et al., 1994; Tsolaki et al., 1994; Patti et al., 1995; Ryan et al., 1996; Hohol et al., 1997). As a general rule, cognitive loss becomes more severe as plaques assume a more confluent appearance in the periventricular white matter and cerebral atrophy develops (Fig. 6-2). A threshold disease

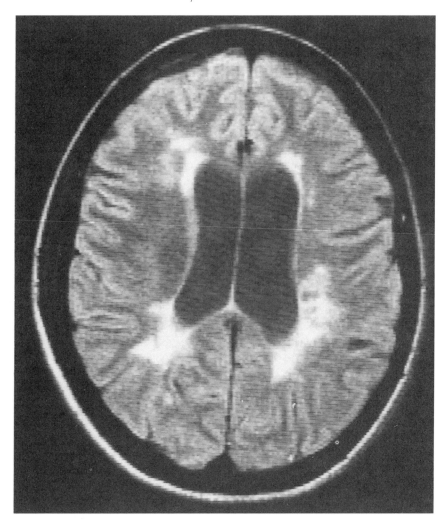

Figure 6-2. Proton density MRI scan of a patient with long-standing MS showing widespread periventricular white matter disease and ventricular enlargement. (Reprinted with permission from Filley CM, Gross KF. Psychosis with white matter disease. Neuropsychiatry Neuropsychol Behav Neurol 1992; 5:119–125, 1992.)

burden of approximately 30 cm^2 has been suggested as the cutoff area above which cognitive impairment is likely (Rao et al., 1989b; Swirsky-Sacchetti et al., 1992). Multiple sclerosis plaques that occur in the cortex, judged to be 5% of the total by neuropathologic study (Brownell and Hughes, 1962) do not appear to cause cognitive decline, as Catalaa and colleagues (1999) found that cortical plaques as revealed by MRI accounted for only 6% of the total lesion volume and did not correlate with neurocognitive test results. Moreover, white matter lesions and atrophy on MRI are associated with significantly reduced quality of life among MS patients (Janardhan and Bakshi, 2000). Taken together, these findings leave little doubt that cerebral white matter lesions in MS have important neurobehavioral implications.

Recently, more advanced MRI techniques have added additional information. Both magnetic resonance spectroscopy (MRS; Sarchielli et al., 1999) and magnetization transfer imaging (MTI; Filippi et al., 2000) studies of MS have shown abnormalities in normal appearing white matter that correlate with clinical dysfunction. These observations have been confirmed by postmortem studies of MS brains that have detected axonal loss in areas of white matter that are normal on conventional MRI (Evangelou et al., 2000). These findings suggest that subtle white matter neuropathology can be detected with advanced neuroimaging techniques, and that MTI and MRS findings may add to the clinical assessment and treatment of cognitively impaired MS patients.

Some interest has also developed in the use of event-related potentials (ERPs) to assess cognitive function in MS (Comi et al., 1999). Studies of the auditory and visual P300 in patients with MS have found that an increase in P300 latency correlates with both the degree of cognitive impairment and the MRI white matter disease burden (Newton et al., 1989; Honig et al., 1992; Giesser et al., 1992). As it is generally accepted that ERPs measure information processing speed (Comi et al., 1999), these data are consistent with the propensity of MS to produce slowed cognition (Litvan et al., 1988). However, even though delayed a P300 latency probably reflects the disconnection of inter- and intrahemispheric areas concerned with cognitive efficiency, ERPs in general do not offer good neuroanatomic localization. Nevertheless, these techniques may contribute to monitoring clinical trials in MS, as one study reported that high-dose methylprednisolone significantly shortened the P300 latency in MS patients (Filipović et al., 1997).

Attempts to characterize the cognitive deficits in MS have been made, and Rao (1986) concluded that MS has neuropsychological features that qualify it as one of the subcortical dementias. In his view, the prominence of deficits in attention, concentration, memory, executive function, and neuropsychiatric status combined with the absence of significant language disturbance and other cortical deficits compels this conclusion (Rao, 1986). Soon thereafter, others concurred with this opinion (Cummings, 1990). Subsequently, however, additional data appeared that invited the possibility that MS might have unique neuropsychological features that separate it not only from cortical diseases but also from subcortical gray matter diseases. First, the memory disturbance in MS was reported to involve a retrieval rather than an encoding deficit (Rao et al., 1989a), and despite some evidence suggesting that memory encoding may be primarily affected (DeLuca et al., 1994; DeLuca et al., 1998), most studies have supported this claim (Brassington and Marsh, 1998). Later, another feature that seemed to characterize MS was the sparing of procedural memory, known to be affected in subcortical gray matter diseases (Rao et al., 1993). These characteristics were thus postulated to distinguish MS from both the cortical dementias, which involve an encoding deficit, and the traditional subcortical dementias, in which procedural memory is affected; moreover, they suggest that MS may be a prototype for all the white matter dementias (Rao, 1996; Filley, 1998). A further analysis of these considerations appears in Chapter 15, where it will be seen that other white matter disorders also manifest this pattern.

Treatment of cognitive dysfunction in MS is only beginning to be explored. For the present, corticosteroid treatment of acute exacerbations remains the mainstay of conventional treatment, and it is plausible, although unproven, that cognitive decline in the context of an acute exacerbation might respond to this intervention. More pertinent is the use of immunomodulatory drugs, three of which—interferon β-1–b, glatiramer, and interferon β-1–a—have appeared for routine use in the United States within the last decade. The rationale for the use of these drugs in relapsing MS is persuasive: this form of the disease, if untreated, is associated with progressive brain atrophy (Simon et al., 1999), and all three drugs appear to reduce relapse rate and improve white matter disease burden on MRI (Rudick et al., 1997). Therapy of this kind could therefore in theory improve or stabilize cognitive function. A preliminary study of interferon β-1–b in MS did in fact find improvement in a visual reproduction test after 4 years of therapy (Pliskin et al., 1996). In contrast, the use of glatiramer in patients with MS did not affect cognitive function compared to those treated with a placebo (Weinstein et al., 1999). The most comprehensive study of this kind to date was a prospective placebo-controlled trial of interferon β-1–a in MS that showed significant benefit in information processing, memory, visuospatial ability, and executive function (Fischer et al., 2000). One important implication of these studies is that they may justify the use of immunomodulatory drugs in MS for cognitive dysfunction alone. Trials of the cholinergic agent donepezil, now approved only for AD, are also in progress and have been encouraging thus far (Krupp et al., 1999).

As reviewed above, MS is a diffuse demyelinative disease that typically disturbs the function of multiple cerebral regions simultaneously. For this reason, the most common neurobehavioral syndrome thus far identified is dementia. In relatively few situations can a single plaque or region of white matter involvement be securely correlated with a focal neurobehavioral syndrome. However, a growing number of case reports demonstrate that isolated cognitive syndromes may also occur in MS (Table 6-1).

These syndromes include amnesia (Pozzilli et al., 1991), Broca's aphasia (Achiron et al., 1992), transcortical motor aphasia (Devere et al., 2000), conduction aphasia (Arnett et al., 1996), Wernicke's aphasia (Day et al., 1987), global aphasia (Friedman et al., 1983), mixed transcortical aphasia (Devere et al., 2000), pure alexia (Doğulu et al., 1996), alexia with agraphia (Day et al., 1987), left hemineglect (Graff-Radford and Rizzo, 1987), visual agnosia (Okuda et al., 1996), left tactile anomia, agraphia, and apraxia (Schnider et al., 1993), and executive dysfunction (Arnett et al., 1994). From Table 6-1, it is apparent that the site(s) of the lesions responsible for the appearance of these familiar neurobehavioral syndromes are consistent with what would be expected on the basis of classic teachings on localization in behavioral neurology. Therapy of these syndromes should be individualized, although the comments made above concerning immunomodu-

Table 6-1. Focal Neurobehavioral Syndromes in Multiple Sclerosis

Syndrome	White Matter Lesion(s)
Verbal memory deficit	Left temporal
Broca's aphasia	Left frontal
Transcortical motor aphasia	Left frontal
Conduction aphasia	Left arcuate fasciculus
Wernicke's aphasia	Left temporoparietal
Global aphasia	Left periventricular
Mixed transcortical aphasia	Left frontal and diffuse
Pure alexia	Left occipital, Splenium of corpus callosum
Alexia with agraphia	Left temporoparietal
Left hemineglect	Right hemispheric
Visual agnosia	Bilateral occipitotemporal
Left tactile anomia, agraphia, and apraxia	Corpus callosum and bihemispheric
Executive dysfunction	Bifrontal

latory agents may equally apply to the prevention and treatment of these focal disturbances. Further discussion of focal syndromes in MS and other white matter disorders can be found in Chapter 16.

Finally, a number of neuropsychiatric syndromes have been described in patients with MS. This broad category includes a variety of emotional disorders that may come to the attention of psychiatrists and neurologists alike. These include depression, mania, psychosis, personality changes, and fatigue. As might be expected, the site(s) of white matter involvement to produce these syndromes are usually unknown, and other factors in addition to structural brain disease are likely to play a role in their pathogenesis (Feinstein, 1999). Multiple sclerosis, like other chronic neurologic diseases, frequently produces disturbances that can be ascribed to psychological distress. However, white matter lesions probably also contribute to the development of neuropsychiatric syndromes.

Depression is the most significant neuropsychiatric syndrome, arising in 50% of MS patients at some point (Feinstein, 1999). A sobering statistic for clinicians to keep in mind is that MS patients have been found to be seven times as likely to commit suicide than age-matched control subjects (Sadovnick et al., 1991). Assiduous follow-up to ensure the recognition and treatment of this problem is crucial. Mania is much less common than depression in MS, but more so than would be expected as compared to the normal population (Schiffer et al., 1986). A small case series suggested that temporal lobe demyelination could be pathogenetic in bipolar disorder (Honer et al., 1987), but little formal study of its etiology in MS has been conducted. Standard treatment as indicated for bipolar disorder in a psychiatric setting is appropriate. Psychosis is rarer still, but may occur in 5% of MS cases at some point in the disease course (Filley and Gross, 1992). The pathogenesis of psychosis may involve frontal-limbic disconnection or temporal lobe demyelination (Filley and Gross, 1992), but data to address this question are not yet available. Neuroleptic drugs are often used for these patients, although it is intriguing to consider that corticosteroids—in doses low enough to prevent mania—may be more appropriate if psychosis is related to acute demyelination. Personality changes include emotional incontinence and euphoria. Emotional incontinence, also known as pathologic laughter and crying or pseudobulbar affect, may occur in up to 10% of MS patients (Minden and Schiffer, 1990). This syndrome has traditionally been associated with disease of the corticobulbar tracts originating in the frontal lobes, but evidence for this assertion is not compelling (Feinstein, 1999). Amitriptyline has proven to be a useful treatment in this setting (Schiffer et al., 1985). A state of sustained and undue cheerfulness called euphoria has often been described, a recent estimate suggesting that it may occur in 25% of MS patients (Rabins, 1990). Computed tomography studies have found enlarged ventricles and brain atrophy implying bifrontal demyelination as the cause of euphoria (Rabins et al., 1986), but MRI studies have yet to be carried out. Treatment of euphoria is usually unnecessary, as euphoria in this setting, while inappropriate, may be a desirable state to maintain on compassionate grounds. Lastly, fatigue is a problem for many patients with MS (Krupp et al., 1988), and may relate to motor, cognitive, or emotional factors. Treatment with amantadine has been effective in some cases (Rosenberg and Appenzeller, 1988). These syndromes are discussed in more detail in Chapter 17.

Acute Disseminated Encephalomyelitis

Acute disseminated encephalomyelitis (ADEM) is a rapidly evolving, monophasic demyelinative disease of the brain and spinal cord that classically follows an antecedent infection or vaccination. The disease has long interested neurologists because of its similarity to experimental allergic encephalomyelitis (EAE), a model animal disease extensively studied because of its relevance to some aspects of demyelinative disease (Tselis and Lisak, 1995), but the neurobehavioral features of ADEM have also recently attracted attention. In contrast to MS, ADEM may often present as a fulminant leukoencephalopathy characterized by a prominent acute confusional state. A wide range of associated neurobehavioral and neurologic features may occur as well, as would be expected with this multifocal cerebral disease (Kesselring et al., 1990). Common neurobehavioral features include confusion, irritability, and frontal lobe dysfunction (Patel and Friedman, 1997). Acute psychosis has also been observed as the presenting syndrome of ADEM (Nasr et al., 2000). Magnetic resonance imaging shows multifocal white matter lesions, often with gadolinium enhancement consistent with acute demyelination and breakdown of the blood–brain barrier. Brain biopsy may be necessary for definitive diagnosis (Paskavitz et al., 1995). Treatment with corticosteroids is commonly attempted, but no controlled trials are available to assess the value of these agents; anticonvulsants and neuroleptics may also be of use during the acute phase and perhaps thereafter (Patel and Friedman, 1997). The outcome is variable, ranging from full recovery to death; many individuals experience lasting cognitive and emotional deficits (Patel and Friedman, 1997).

Acute Hemorrhagic Leukoencephalitis

This disease is a very rare and severe demyelinative disorder with many clinical and neuropathologic features in common with ADEM. First described 60 years ago (Hurst, 1941), acute hemorrhagic leukoencephalitis is a fulminant cerebral demyelinative disease that typically follows an upper respiratory or other minor infection. Initial confusion and focal signs rapidly give way to coma, and a progressive course and fatal outcome ensue. Neuropathogically, there is severe bilateral hemispheric demyelination with perivascular hemorrhage and necrosis (Vartanian and de la Monte, 1999). Although the disease is nearly always fatal, a remarkable case has been reported in which vigorous treatment with immunosuppression and reduction of increased intracranial pressure led to complete recovery (Seales and Greer, 1991).

Schilder's Disease

Schilder's disease has caused considerable confusion in the neurologic literature. In 1912, the Austrian neuropathologist Paul Schilder described a cerebral demyelinative disease in a 14-year-old girl that bore a close resemblance to MS (Schilder, 1912). Over the next few decades, he reported other similar cases under the name encephalitis periaxialis diffusa (Schilder, 1913, 1924), and the term Schilder's disease came to be applied to all of these diseases. In retrospect, however, these cases were probably not all the same disease; it is likely the 1913 case was an instance of adrenoleukodystrophy, and the 1924 case one of subacute sclerosing panencephalitis (Poser et al., 1986). Nevertheless, Schilder's initial case does appear to represent a distinct entity, and Schilder's disease is now best considered a rare variant of MS that occurs mainly in children (Poser et al., 1986). A variety of neurobehavioral deficits can be seen, in keeping with the presence of large demyelinative lesions in the centrum semiovale of both hemispheres, and corticosteroids may be helpful in treatment (Poser et al., 1986). Schilder's disease differs from ADEM in that there is typically no antecedent infection or vaccination, and because of the absence of spinal cord involvement.

Marburg's Disease

This disease was first described as a fulminant, monophasic demyelinative disease leading to death in a few weeks (Marburg, 1906). Other similar cases have been reported since then, and Marburg's disease is now considered an acute and severe variant of MS. Although resembling Schilder's disease, Marburg's disease affects adults rather than children, involves the brainstem in addition to the cerebral hemispheres, and has a more rapid and lethal course (Mendez and Pogacar, 1988; Johnson et al., 1990; Poser et al., 1992). Severe demyelination with variable axonal loss and necrosis is seen at autopsy, and has been attributed to brainstem involvement affecting bulbar function. A confusional state can be seen admixed with many other neurologic and neurobehavioral features (Mendez and Pogacar, 1988).

Balò's Concentric Sclerosis

Balò's concentric sclerosis is probably another rare variant of MS. First described by Balò in 1928, (Balò, 1928) the defining feature of this disease is concentric rings in the cerebral white matter that represent alternating areas of demyelinated and relatively normal tissue (Yao et al., 1994). In addition to elemental neurologic findings, cognitive deficits including confusion and memory loss have been noted (Chen et al., 1999). Only about 50 cases have been reported, most of them with autopsy verification (Chen et al., 1996). The disease can now be identified in life with conventional MRI, which may show the concentric rings of demyelination developing in a centrifugal direction (Chen et al., 1999). Magnetic resonance spectroscopy has shown changes in the affected white matter similar to those seen in MS (Kim et al., 1997).

References

Achiron A, Ziv I, Djaldetti R, et al. Aphasia in multiple sclerosis: clinical and radiologic correlations. Neurology 1992; 42: 2195–2197.

Anzola GP, Bevilacqua L, Cappa SF, et al. Neuropsychological assessment in patients with relapsing-remitting multiple sclerosis and mild functional impairment: correlation with magnetic resonance imaging. J Neurol Neurosurg Psychiatry 1990; 53: 142–145.

Arnett PA, Rao SM, Bernardin L, et al. Relationship between frontal lobe lesions and Wisconsin Card Sorting Test performance in patients with multiple sclerosis. Neurology 1994; 44: 420–425.

Arnett PA, Rao SM, Hussain M, et al. Conduction aphasia in multiple sclerosis: a case report with MRI findings. Neurology 1996; 47: 576–578.

Arnold TW, Myers GJ. Neuromyelitis optica (Devic syndrome) in a 12–year-old male with complete recovery following steroids. Pediatr Neurol 1987; 3: 313–315.

Balò J. Encephalitis periaxialis concentrica. Arch Neurol Psychiatry 1928; 19: 242–264.

Beatty WE, Goodkin DE. Screening for cognitive impairment in multiple sclerosis. Arch Neurol 1990; 47: 297–301.

Brassington JC, Marsh NV. Neuropsychological aspects of multiple sclerosis. Neuropsychol Rev 1998; 8: 43–77.

Brownell B, Hughes JT. The distribution of plaques in the cerebrum in multiple sclerosis. J Neurol Neurosurg Psychiatry 1962; 25: 315–320.

Callanan MM, Logsdail SJ, Ron MA, Warrington EK. Cognitive impairment in patients with clinically isolated lesions of the type seen in multiple sclerosis. A psychometric and MRI study. Brain 1989; 112: 361–374.

Catalaa I, Fulton JC, Zhang X, et al. MR imaging quantitation of gray matter involvement in multiple sclerosis and its correlation with disability measures and neurocognitive testing. AJNR 1999; 20: 1613–1618.

Charcot JM. Lectures on the diseases of the nervous system delivered at La Salpêtrière. London: New Sydenham Society, 1877.

Chen C-J, Chu N-S, Lu C-S, Sung C-Y. Serial magnetic resonance imaging in patients with Balò's concentric sclerosis: natural history of lesion development. Ann Neurol 1999; 46: 651–656.

Chen C-J, Ro L-S, Chang C-N, et al. Serial MRI studies in pathologically verified Balò's concentric sclerosis. J Comp Assist Tomogr 1996; 20: 732–735.

Comi G, Filippi M, Martinelli V, et al. Brain magnetic resonance imaging correlates of cognitive impairment in multiple sclerosis. J Neurol Sci 1993; 115 (Suppl): S66–73.

Comi G, Leocani L, Locatelli T, et al. Electrophysiological investigations in multiple sclerosis dementia. In: Comi G, Lücking CH, Kimura J, Rossini PM, eds. Clinical neurophysiology : from receptors to perception (EEG Suppl 50). Amsterdam: Elsevier Science, 1999: 480–485.

Cummings JL, ed. Subcortical dementia. New York: Oxford University Press, 1990.

Day TJ, Fisher AG, Mastaglia FL. Alexia with agraphia in multiple sclerosis. J Neurol Sci 1987; 78: 343–348.

DeLuca J, Barbieri-Berger S, Johnson SK. The nature of memory acquisition in multiple sclerosis: acquisition versus retrieval. J Clin Exp Neuropsychol 1994; 16: 183–189.

DeLuca J, Gaudino EA, Diamond BJ, et al. Acquisition and storage deficits in multiple sclerosis. J Clin Exp Neuropsychol 1998; 20: 376–390.

Devere TR, Trotter JL, Cross AH. Acute aphasia in multiple sclerosis. Arch Neurol 2000; 57: 1207–1209.

Doğulu CF, Kansu T, Karabudak R. Alexia without agraphia in multiple sclerosis. J Neurol Neurosurg Psychiatry 1996; 61: 528.

Evangelou N, Esiri MM, Smith S, et al. Quantitative pathological evidence for axonal loss in normal appearing white matter in multiple sclerosis. Ann Neurol 2000; 47: 392–395.

Feinstein A. The clinical neuropsychiatry of multiple sclerosis. Cambridge: Cambridge University Press, 1999.

Feinstein A, Kartsounis LD, Miller DH, et al. Clinically isolated lesions of the type seen in multiple sclerosis: a cognitive, psychiatric, and MRI follow up study. J Neurol Neurosurg Psychiatry 1992; 55: 869–876.

Feinstein A, Ron MA, Thompson A. A serial study of psychometric and magnetic resonance imaging changes in multiple sclerosis. Brain 1993; 116: 569–602.

Filipović SR, Drulović J, Stojsavljević N, Lević Z. The effects of high-dose intravenous methylprednisolone on event-related potentials in patients with multiple sclerosis. J Neurol Sci 1997; 152: 147–153.

Filley CM. Behavioural manifestations of multiple sclerosis. Int MSJ 1996; 2: 91–97.

Filley CM. The behavioral neurology of cerebral white matter. Neurology 1998; 50: 1535–1540.

Filley CM, Gross KF. Psychosis with cerebral white matter disease. Neuropsychiatry Neuropsychol Behav Neurol 1992; 5: 119–125.

Filley CM, Heaton RK, Nelson LM, et al. A comparison of dementia in Alzheimer's Disease and multiple sclerosis. Arch Neurol 1989; 46: 157–161.

Filley CM, Sternberg PE, Norenberg MD. Neuromyelitis optica in the elderly. Arch Neurol 1984; 41: 670–673.

Fillippi M, Tortorella C, Rovaris M, et al. Changes in the normal appearing brain tissue and cognitive impairment in multiple sclerosis. J Neurol Neurosurg Psychiatry 2000; 68: 157–161.

Fischer JS, Priore RL, Jacobs LD, et al. Neuropsychological effects of interferon β-1–a in relapsing multiple sclerosis. Ann Neurol 2000; 48: 885–892.

Folstein MF, Folstein SE, McHugh PR. "Mini-Mental State": A practical method for grading the cognitive state of patients for the clinician. J Psychiat Res 1976; 12: 189–198.

Franklin GM, Heaton RK, Nelson LM, et al. Correlation of neuropsychological and magnetic resonance imaging findings in chronic/progressive multiple sclerosis. Neurology 1988; 38: 1826–1829.

Franklin GM, Nelson LM, Filley CM, Heaton RK. Cognitive loss in multiple sclerosis. Case reports and review of the literature. Arch Neurol 1989; 46: 162–167.

Franklin GM, Nelson LM, Heaton RK, Filley CM. Clinical perspectives in the identification of cognitive impairment. In: Rao SM, ed. Neurobehavioral aspects of multiple sclerosis. New York: Oxford University Press, 1990: 161–174.

Friedman JH, Brem H, Mayeux R. Global aphasia in multiple sclerosis. Ann Neurol 1983; 222–223.

Giesser BS, Schroeder MM, LaRocca NG, et al. Endogenous event-related potentials as indices of dementia in multiple sclerosis patients. Electroenceph Clin Neurophysiol 1992; 82: 320–329.

Graff-Radford NR, Rizzo M. Neglect in a patient with multiple sclerosis. Eur Neurol 1987; 26: 100–103.

Gur RC, Packer IK, Hungerbuhler JP, Reivich M, et al. Differences in the distribution of gray and white matter in the human cerebral hemispheres. Science 1980; 207: 1226–1228.

Heaton RK, Nelson LM, Thompson DS, et al. Neuropsychological findings in relapsing-remitting and chronic-progressive multiple sclerosis. J Consul Clin Psychol 1985; 53: 103–110.

Hohol MJ, Guttmann CRG, Orav J, et al. Serial neuropsychological assessment and magnetic resonance imaging analysis in multiple sclerosis. Arch Neurol 1997; 54: 1018–1025.

Honer WG, Hurwitz T, Li DKB, et al. Temporal lobe involvement in multiple sclerosis patients with psychiatric disorders. Arch Neurol 1987; 44: 187–190.

Honig LS, Ramsay RE, Sheremata WA. Event-related potential P300 in multiple sclerosis. Relation to magnetic resonance imaging and cognitive impairment. Arch Neurol 1992; 49: 44–50.

Huber SJ, Bornstein RA, Rammohan KW, et al. Magnetic resonance imaging correlates of neuropsychological impairment in multiple sclerosis. J Neuropsychiatry Clin Neurosci 1992; 4: 152–158.

Hurst EW. Acute hemorrhagic leukoencephalitis: a previously undefined entity. Med J Aust 1941; 2: 1–6.

Janardhan V, Bakshi R. Quality of life and its relationship to brain lesions and atrophy on magnetic resonance images in 60 patients with multiple sclerosis. Arch Neurol 2000; 57: 1485–1491.

Johnson MD, Lavin P, Whetsell WO. Fulminant monophasic multiple sclerosis, Marburg's type. J Neurol Neurosurg Psychiatry 1990; 53: 918–921.

Kesselring J, Miller DH, Robb SA, et al. Acute disseminated encephalomyelitis: MRI findings and the distinction from multiple sclerosis. Brain 1990; 113: 291–302.

Kim MO, Lee SA, Choi CG, et al. Balò's concentric sclerosis: a clinical case study of brain MRI, biopsy, and proton magnetic resonance spectroscopic findings. J Neurol Neurosurg Psychiatry 1997; 62: 655–658.

Krupp LB, Alvarez LA, LaRocca NG, Scheinberg LC. Fatigue in multiple sclerosis. Arch Neurol 1988; 45: 435–437.

Krupp LB, Elkins LE, Scheffer RS, et al. Donepezil for the treatment of memory impairments in multiple sclerosis. Neurology 1999 (suppl 2); 52: A137.

Kurtzke JF. Neurologic impairment in multiple sclerosis and the Disability Status Scale. Acta Neurol Scand 1970; 46: 493–512.

Kurtzke JF. Rating neurologic impairment in multiple sclerosis: an expanded disability scale. Neurology 1983; 33: 1444–1452.

Litvan I, Grafman J, Vendrell P, Martinez JM. Slowed information processing in multiple sclerosis. Arch Neurol 1988; 45: 281–285.

Marburg O. Die sogenannte "akute multiple Sklerose." Jhrb Psychiatr Neurol 1906; 27: 211–312.

Maurelli M, Marchioni E, Cerretano R, et al. Neuropsychological assessment in MS: clinical, neurophysiological and neuroradiological relationships. Acta Neurol Scand 1992; 86: 124–128.

Medaer R, Nelissen E, Appel B, et al. Magnetic resonance imaging and cognitive functioning in multiple sclerosis. J Neurol 1987; 235: 86–89.

Mendez MF, Pogacar S. Malignant monophasic multiple sclerosis or "Marburg's disease." Neurology 1988; 38: 1153–1155.

Minden SL, Schiffer RB. Affective disorders in multiple sclerosis. Review and recommendations for clinical research. Arch Neurol 1990; 47: 98–104.

Möller A, Wiedemann G, Rhode U, et al. Correlates of cognitive impairment and depressive mood disorder in multiple sclerosis. Acta Psychiatr Scand 1994; 89: 117–121.

Nasr JT, Andriola MR, Coyle PK. ADEM: literature review and case report of acute psychosis presentation. Pediatr Neurol 2000; 22: 8–18.

Newton MR, Barrett G, Callanan MM, Towell AD. Cognitive event-related potentials in multiple sclerosis. Brain 1989; 112: 1637–1660.

Noseworthy JH. Progress in determining the causes and treatment of multiple sclerosis. Nature 1999; 399 (Suppl): A40–A47.

Okuda B, Tanaka H, Tachibana H, et al. Visual form agnosia in multiple sclerosis. Acta Neurol Scand 1996; 94: 38–44.

O'Riordan JI, Gallagher HL, Thompson AJ, et al. Clinical, CSF and MRI findings in Devic's neuromyelitis optica. J Neurol Neurosurg Psychiatry 1996; 60: 382–387.

Paskavitz JF, Anderson CA, Filley CM, et al. Acute arcuate fiber demyelinative encephalopathy following Epstein-Barr virus infection. Ann Neurol 1995; 38:127–131.

Patel SP, Friedman RS. Neuropsychiatric features of acute disseminated encephalomyelitis. J Neuropsychiatry Clin Neurosci 1997; 9: 534–540.

Patti F, Di Stefano M, De Pascalis D, et al. May there exist specific MRI findings predictive of dementia in multiple sclerosis patients? Funct Neurol 1995; 10: 83–90.

Peyser JM, Edwards KR, Poser CM, Filskov SB. Cognitive function in patients with multiple sclerosis. Arch Neurol 1980; 37: 577–579.

Pliskin NH, Hamer DP, Goldstein DS, et al. Improved delayed visual reproduction test performance in multiple sclerosis patients receiving interferon β-1–b. Neurology 1996; 47: 1463–1468.

Poser CM, Goutières F, Carpentier M-A, Aicardi J. Schilder's myelinoclastic diffuse sclerosis. Pediatrics 1986; 77: 107–112.

Poser S, Luer W, Bruhn H, et al. Acute demyelinating disease. Classification and noninvasive diagnosis. Acta Neurol Scand 1992; 86: 579–585.

Pozzilli C, Passfiume D, Bernardi S, et al. SPECT, MRI and cognitive functions in multiple sclerosis. J Neurol Neurosurg Psychiatry 1991; 54: 110–115.

Pugnetti L, Mendozzi L, Motta A, et al. MRI and cognitive patterns in relapsing-remitting multiple sclerosis. J Neurol Sci 1993; 115 (Suppl): S59–65.

Rabins PV. Euphoria in multiple sclerosis. In: Rao SM, ed. Neurobehavioral aspects of multiple sclerosis. New York: Oxford University Press, 1990: 180–185.

Rabins PV, Brooks BR, O'Donnell P, et al. Structural brain correlates of emotional disorder in multiple sclerosis. Brain 1986; 109: 585–597.

Rao SM. Neuropsychology of multiple sclerosis: a critical review. J Clin Exp Neuropsychol 1986; 8; 503–542.

Rao SM. White matter disease and dementia. Brain Cogn 1996; 31: 250–268.

Rao SM, Grafman J, DiGiulio D, et al. Memory dysfunction in multiple sclerosis: its relation to working memory, semantic encoding, and implicit learning. Neuropsychology 1993; 7: 364–374.

Rao SM, Leo GJ, Aubin-Faubert P. On the nature of memory disturbance in multiple sclerosis. J Clin Exp Neuropsycyhol 1989a; 11: 699–712.

Rao SM, Leo GJ, Bernardin L, Unverzagt F. Cognitive dysfunction in multiple sclerosis. I. Frequency, patterns, and prediction. Neurology 1991; 41: 685–691.

Rao SM, Leo GJ, Haughton VM, et al. Correlation of magnetic resonance imaging with neuropsychological testing in multiple sclerosis. Neurology 1989b; 39: 161–166.

Reischies FM, Baum K, Brau H, et al. Cerebral magnetic resonance imaging findings in multiple sclerosis. Relation to disturbance of affect, drive and cognition. Arch Neurol 1988; 45: 1114–1116.

Rosenberg GA, Appenzeller O. Amantadine, fatigue, and multiple sclerosis. Arch Neurol 1988; 45: 1104–1106.

Rudick RA, Cohen JA, Weinstock-Guttman B, et al. Management of multiple sclerosis. N Engl J Med 1997; 337: 1604–1611.

Ryan L, Clark CM, Klonoff H, et al. Patterns of cognitive impairment in relapsing-remitting multiple sclerosis and their relationship to neuropathology on magnetic resonance images. Neuropsychology 1996; 10: 176–193.

Sadovnick AD, Eisen K, Ebers CG, Paty DW. Cause of death in patients attending multiple sclerosis clinics. Neurology 1991; 412: 1193–1196.

Sarchielli P, Presciutti O, Pellicioli G, et al. Absolute quantification of brain metabolites by proton magnetic spectroscopy in normal-appearing white matter of multiple sclerosis patients. Brain 1999; 122: 513–521.

Schiffer RB, Herndon RM, Rudick RA. Treatment of pathologic laughing and weeping with amitriptyline. N Engl J Med 1985; 312: 1480–1482.

Schiffer RB, Wineman NM, Weitkamp LR. Association between bipolar affective disorder and multiple sclerosis. Am J Psychiatry 1986; 143: 94–95.

Schilder P. Zur Kenntnis der sogannanten diffusen Sklerose. Z Gesamte Neurol Psychiat 1912; 10: 1–60.

Schilder P. Zur Frage der Encephalitis periaxialis diffusa. Z Gesamte Neurol Psychiatr 1913; 15: 359–376.

Schilder P. Die Encephalitis periaxialis diffusa. Arch Psychiatr Nervenkr 1924; 71: 327–356.

Schnider A, Benson DF, Rosner LJ. Callosal disconnection in multiple sclerosis. Neurology 1993; 43: 1243–1245.

Seales D, Greer M. Acute hemorrhagic leukencephalitis. A successful recovery. Arch Neurol 1991; 48: 1086–1088.

Simon JH. From enhancing lesions to brain atrophy in relapsing MS. J Neuroimmunol 1999; 98: 7–15.

Simon JH, Jacobs LD, Campion MK, et al. A longitudinal study of brain atrophy in relapsing multiple sclerosis. Neurology 1999; 53: 139–148.

Swirsky-Sacchetti T, Field HL, Mitchell DR, et al. The sensitivity of the mini-mental state
exam in the white matter dementia of multiple sclerosis. J Clin Psychol 1992; 48: 779–
786.

Swirsky-Sacchetti T, Mitchell DR, Seward J, et al. Neuropsychological and structural brain
lesions in multiple sclerosis: a regional analysis. Neurology 1992; 42: 1291–1295.

Tselis AC, Lisak RP. Acute disseminated encephalomyelitis and isolated central nervous
system demyelinative syndromes. Curr Opin Neurol 1995; 8: 227–229.

Tsolaki M, Drevelegas A, Karachristianou S, et al. Correlation of dementia, neuropsychological and MRI findings in multiple scerosis. Dementia 1994; 5: 48–52.

Vartanian TK, de la Monte S. Case 1–1999. N Engl J Med 1999; 327; 127–135.

Weinstein A, Schwid SI, Schiffer RB, et al. Neuropsychologic status in multiple sclerosis
after treatment with glatiramer. Arch Neurol 1999; 56: 319–324.

Wingerchuk DM, Hogancamp WF, O'Brien PC, Weinshenker BG. The clinical course of
neuromyelitis optica (Devic's syndrome). Neurology 1999; 53: 1107–1114.

Yao DL, Webster HD, Hudson LD, et al. Concentric sclerosis (Balò): morphometric and in
situ hybridization study of lesions in six patients. Ann Neurol 1994; 35: 18–30.

7

Infectious Diseases

The white matter of the brain can be affected by a number of infectious diseases. The majority of these infections are caused by viruses, and many clinical and immunopathologic similarities to demyelinative diseases have invited comparison with multiple sclerosis (MS) and related diseases. As is often the case with white matter disorders, infectious diseases may also involve gray matter regions, and the selectivity for white matter may only be relative. Nevertheless, consideration of these diseases will serve to point out that infection prominently affecting the white matter can have important neurobehavioral consequences.

Acquired Immunodeficiency Syndrome Dementia Complex

Infection with the human immunodeficiency virus type 1 (HIV-1), commonly known as HIV, has come to be one of the most publicized medical problems of the last 2 decades. Since its recognition in 1981, the acquired immunodeficiency syndrome (AIDS) has become a major public health problem worldwide. Despite rapid progress on determining its etiology, prevention, and treatment, AIDS continues to be an incurable disease.

One of the more ominous manifestations of this systemic retroviral infection is involvement of the brain, which was recognized soon after the epidemic was identified (Price et al., 1988). The most commonly used name for this disorder is the AIDS dementia complex (ADC), which emphasizes the constellation of cognitive, motor, and behavioral changes that occur (Navia et al., 1986b); other names include subacute HIV encephalitis, AIDS-related dementia, and AIDS encephalopathy. A consensus group also introduced the term HIV-1-associated cognitive/motor complex (HIV-CMC), and distinguished between mild (HIV-1-associated minor cognitive/motor disorder) and severe (HIV-1-associated dementia complex) forms of the disorder (Report of a Working Group of the American Academy of Neurology AIDS Task Force, 1991). This terminology signals a growing tendency in the characterization of neurologic disorders to recognize an early and mild form of cognitive dysfunction that contrasts with the more severe syndrome of dementia.

The ADC affects approximately 30% of patients with AIDS at some point in the disease course (McArthur et al., 1998), and may even be its presenting or sole manifestation (Navia and Price, 1987). In approximately half of those affected, the disorder takes the form of frank dementia (Navia et al., 1986b), and in the other half a milder cognitive impairment can be detected neuropsychologically (Wilkie et al., 1990). The severity of ADC generally parallels the degree to which AIDS itself has advanced (McArthur et al., 1998). At any stage, the neurobehavioral effects of HIV infection contribute importantly to the overall impact of the disease (Heaton et al., 1995), but the onset of dementia in AIDS is particularly serious, as the median survival time after this development is only 6 months (Brew, 1999).

Since its identification in the 1980s, the most common neuropathologic feature of the ADC has been diffuse myelin pallor in the cerebral white matter (Navia et al., 1986a). White matter may be severely and selectively involved, as documented by a case in which fulminant fatal leukoencephalopathy was the only manifestation of HIV infection (Jones et al., 1988). Human immunodeficiency virus enters the central nervous system from the bloodstream via infected monocytes and does not infect neurons; the virus is in fact concentrated more in the white matter and basal ganglia than in the cortex (McArthur et al., 1999). In typical cases of ADC, pallor of the white matter is accompanied by gliosis, multinucleated giant cells, microglial nodules, and increased numbers of perivascular macrophages (Sharer, 1992). Demyelination is not seen, and it has been suggested that white matter pallor is caused by a breakdown of the blood–brain barrier and development of vasogenic edema, which appear to be early pathogenic events in brain infection with HIV (Power et al., 1993). Investigations of the cortex in HIV infection have found either no cortical neuronal loss in patients with ADC (Seilhean et al., 1993), or that the loss of cortical neurons is not correlated with the severity of dementia (Weis et al., 1993; Everall et al., 1994). Cortical cell loss may be a late event in the course of the disease, but white matter pallor and gliosis are more prominent initial events (Gray et al., 1996).

White matter changes are also visible on conventional computed tomography (CT) and especially magnetic resonance imaging (MRI), where there may be patchy or diffuse hyperintensity on T2–weighted images (Fig. 7-1) combined with cerebral atrophy (Bencherif and Rottenberg, 1998). The subcortical and cortical gray matter are not affected as early or as significantly as the white matter on neuroimaging scans. Subcortical gray matter involvement has been recognized along with white matter changes (Navia et al., 1986b), but recent studies with magnetic

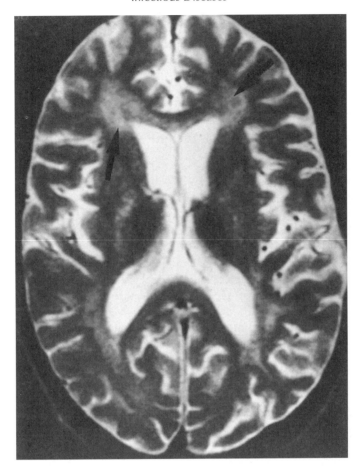

Figure 7-1. T2-weighted MRI scan of a patient with AIDS dementia complex. White matter hyperintensities are most apparent in the frontal lobes (*arrows*). (Reprinted with permission from Osborn AG. Diagnostic neuroradiology. St. Louis: Mosby-Year Book, 1994.)

resonance spectroscopy (MRS) of patients with ADC patients have suggested that the white matter is affected earliest, followed by the basal ganglia and lastly the cortical gray matter (Chang et al., 1999).

The ADC has been characterized as a subcortical dementia (Navia et al., 1986b; Tross et al., 1988). Patients typically present with impairments in attention, concentration, memory, and personality, and the loss of cognitive speed and mental flexibility may be striking (Grant et al., 1987). Tests of choice reaction time have shown marked impairment in studies of AIDS patients (Perdices and Cooper, 1989). Language is usually normal (McArthur et al., 1999), but visuospatial function is impaired (Tross et al., 1988). Memory is uniformly affected, and the pattern of memory dysfunction renders ADC a close fit with the hypothesized profile of white matter dementia (Filley, 1998) in that there appears to be a retrieval deficit in declarative memory (White et al., 1997) and a sparing of procedural memory (Jones and Tranel, 1991). Psychomotor slowing, apathy, and withdrawal are common in this disease (Navia et al., 1986b).

In clinical terms, a good overall correlation between white matter pallor and degree of cognitive impairment has been observed (Navia et al., 1986a; Grant et al., 1987; Price et al., 1988; Bencherif and Rottenberg, 1998). This correlation is most apparent in ADC with severe dementia, but there is a suggestion that milder cognitive impairment is also associated with white matter changes (Post et al., 1991). This observation exemplifies a general trend for white matter disorders to present with subtle neurobehavioral features that precede more obvious signs but which are still identifiable with careful evaluation. Early and selective involvement of frontal white matter has been suggested by a pattern of neuropsychological deficits implicating prominent attentional impairment and executive dysfunction in mildly affected ADC patients (Krikorian and Wrobel, 1991).

However, the neuropathology of the ADC also includes the subcortical gray matter to some extent (Navia et al., 1986a), and some have regarded changes in the gray matter of the thalamus, basal ganglia, and brainstem as equal to or more prominent than those in the white matter (McArthur et al., 1998; Brew, 1999). In light of this dilemma, it is difficult to determine what proportion of the neurobehavioral syndrome of ADC can be attributed to white matter versus subcortical gray matter involvement. This confusion is illustrated by neuropsychological studies of HIV infected individuals finding prominent deficits suggesting subcortical dysfunction that have been attributed to frontodiencephalic (Perdices and Cooper, 1990) and frontostriatal dysfunction (Sahakian et al., 1995). In view of the neuropathologic heterogeneity of HIV infection, there is a need for careful studies correlating clinical features with neuroimaging and neuropathologic data to define with greater precision the origin of neurobehavioral dysfunction in these patients. This principle applies to most other white matter disorders as well, in which there is also some degree of neuropathologic overlap with gray matter structures.

Despite the uncertainty of clinical–pathologic correlation in the ADC, further indirect evidence of white matter dysfunction comes from studies of AIDS treatment. A gratifying development in the 1990s has been the marked reduction in the incidence of ADC that has accompanied the widespread use of antiretroviral therapy of AIDS (Clifford, 2000), possibly through its prevention of initial cerebral white matter involvement. In addition, the more effective treatment of established ADC made possible by new drug therapy may also imply a beneficial effect on the white matter. Zidovudine (AZT), an antiretroviral drug that is a mainstay of AIDS pharmacotherapy, has been shown to improve cognitive function in ADC (Sidtis et al., 1993), and this improvement is accompanied by reduction in white matter lesion burden on MRI (Tozzi et al., 1993). Similarly, the use of the protease inhibitors in the ADC may also be associated with improvement in both cognitive function and extent of white matter involvement on MRI (Filippi et al., 1998; Thurnher et al., 2000).

In summary, these observations support the hypothesis that the neurobehavioral features of ADC are related in part to primary involvement of cerebral white matter. This notion does not preclude a contribution of changes in gray matter to the clinical picture. In addition, the impact of diffuse metabolic dysfunction in ADC, most likely involving a variety of neurotoxic cytokines (Merrill and Chen, 1991; McArthur et al., 1998), should also be considered. In determining the relative importance of the many factors involved in the pathogenesis of cognitive loss in ADC, white matter dysfunction deserves inclusion.

Progressive Multifocal Leukoencephalopathy

Acquired immunodeficiency syndrome is a disease of the immune system, and the vulnerability of the nervous system to a variety of opportunistic infections and neoplasms in AIDS patients was recognized early in the course of the epidemic (Snider et al., 1983). These disorders are frequently superimposed on ADC and often complicate the diagnosis and treatment of AIDS patients. In general, these diseases add to the neurobehavioral disability of HIV infection and significantly worsen overall prognosis.

Progressive multifocal leukoencephalopathy (PML) is an infection of the white matter caused by a member of the papavovirus family called the JC virus. The specific target of the virus is the oligodendrocyte, a feature that results in disrupted myelin synthesis (Gilden, 1983). This disease is confined to patients who are immunocompromised by AIDS or other disorders, and it is now thought to occur in 5% of HIV-infected individuals (Berger and Concha, 1995). Progressive multifocal leukoencephalopathy manifests clinically with focal neurologic signs including paresis and visual loss, and subtle neurobehavioral signs may also be presenting features. The course is rapidly progressive, and no pharmacologic treatment has been effective (Berger and Concha, 1995). In contrast to the ADC, the hallmark neuropathologic feature of PML is demyelination, which may occur anywhere in the central nervous system (CNS) but has a predilection for the parietooccipital white matter (Berger and Concha, 1995). Computed tomography scanning reveals nonenhancing focal white matter lesions, and these are particularly well visualized on MRI (Berger and Concha, 1995; Fig. 7-2). These lesions differ from those seen in ADC because they tend to be less diffuse and more rapidly progressive.

Although there have been no studies correlating white matter disease burden and cognitive impairment in PML, it is likely that the leukoencephalopathy produces the clinical picture. Neurobehavioral features of PML include personality and behavioral changes, inattention, and memory loss, with relatively little language impairment (Berger and Concha, 1995), all consistent with the pattern of white matter dementia (Filley, 1998). Parietooccipital involvement has produced higher visual dysfunction in the form of visual agnosia, pure alexia, and Balint's syndrome (Berger and Concha, 1995).

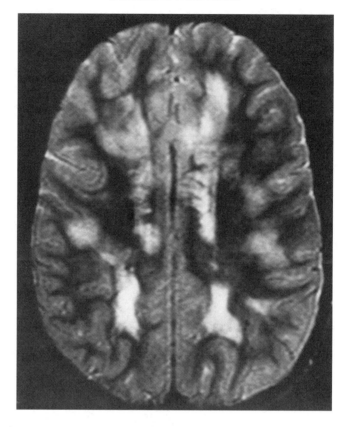

Figure 7-2. T2-weighted MRI scan of a patient with PML. There are multifocal white matter lesions scatted throughout the cerebral hemispheres. (Reprinted with permission from Atlas SW, ed. Magnetic resonance imaging of the brain and spine. 2nd ed. Philadelphia: Lippincott-Raven, 1996.)

Subacute Sclerosing Panencephalitis

Subacute sclerosing panencephalitis (SSPE) is a demyelinative disease caused by persistence and reactivation of the measles (rubeola) virus in the brain. It affects mainly children and adolescents, usually presenting between the ages of 14 and 20 (Gilden, 1983). An initial personality change with irritability and apathy evolves to progressive dementia, and then myoclonus, seizures, corticospinal dysfunction, coma, and death follow over a period of months to years. Although the name SSPE implies diffuse cerebral involvement, the disease may involve the white matter selectively and produce fulminant demyelination as a predominant feature (Poser, 1990). A predilection for white matter is also suggested by MRI studies in which high signal lesions on T2–weighted images in the periventricular or subcortical white matter are the most common findings (Anlar et al., 1996). Treatment for this disease has been supportive only.

Progressive Rubella Panencephalitis

In a manner reminiscent of SSPE, persistent rubella infection of the brain can involve the cerebral white matter. Progressive rubella panencephalitis (PRP) usually occurs in the second decade of life, about 10 years after primary rubella infection (Gilden, 1983). The disease is characterized by dementia, spasticity, and ataxia that culminates in coma and death. Widespread demyelination with vasculitis has been observed neuropathologically (Townsend et al., 1982). Recent MRI studies have disclosed that children with congenital rubella also have white matter lesions (Lane et al., 1996), implying that the later development of PRP involves an exacerbation of preexisting white matter neuropathology. As with SSPE, the prognosis of PRP is very poor, and no effective treatment has been found.

Varicella Zoster Encephalitis

Varicella zoster virus (VZV) is a human herpesvirus that typically causes chickenpox in childhood, remains latent in cranial and dorsal root ganglia, and may reactivate many years later to cause shingles and postherpetic neuralgia (Gilden et al., 2000). Varicella zoster virus can also affect the CNS, and the most common manifestation in the brain is a small vessel encephalitis (Gilden et al., 2000). Varicella zoster virus encephalitis typically follows a premonitory herpes zoster skin rash, and then presents with mental status changes, headache, fever, seizures, and focal neurologic signs (Amlie-Lefond et al., 1995). The neuropathology consists mainly of vasculopathy involving both gray and white matter, but white matter lesions predominate; a combination of ischemic and demyelinative lesions is encountered in this multifocal leukoencephalopathy (Amlie-Lefond et al., 1995). Consistent with this picture are MRI studies showing multiple subcortical white matter lesions that may enhance with contrast administration (Lentz et al., 1993). Neuropsychological studies of affected patients have found a pattern of cognitive slowing, mild memory dysfunction, and emotional changes that is consistent with a subcortical process (Hokkanen et al., 1997). The outcome is variable, and treatment with antiviral agents such as acyclovir may be effective (Amlie-Lefond et al., 1995).

Cytomegalovirus Encephalitis

The AIDS era has also witnessed an increase in the incidence of infection with CMV. This pathogen rarely infects immunocompetent individuals, but CMV encephalitis has been diagnosed retrospectively in up to 40% of individuals with AIDS (Holland et al., 1994). Clinical features of CMV encephalitis are predominantly neurobehavioral, as a subacute encephalopathy with confusion, disorientation, apathy, withdrawal, and impaired memory dominates the presentation (Holland et al., 1994). Cytomegalovirus can induce inflammatory demyelination throughout the CNS (Moskowitz et al., 1984), but it has a predilection for the subependymal white matter (Holland et al., 1994). An autopsy study of AIDS patients showed that CMV encephalitis manifests as a leukoencephalopathy that can be detected during life with MRI scanning (Miller et al., 1997). Treatment has been supportive only, but the incidence of CMV encephalitis has declined considerably in recent years because of the use of more effective drug treatments for patients with AIDS (McArthur et al., 1999).

Lyme Encephalopathy

Some patients with Lyme disease, an infection of the skin, heart, joints, and nervous system caused by a recently recognized tick-borne spirochete known as *Borrelia burgdorferi* (Burgdorfer et al., 1982), experience a syndrome of cognitive and emotional dysfunction in the chronic phase of the disease following the initial infection. After injection by the tick, the spirochete produces the characteristic rash erythema migrans, which resolves within 3 to 4 weeks (Steere, 1989). Neurologic manifestations may then be seen, and the meninges, spinal nerve roots, and cranial nerves are commonly involved (Oksi et al., 1996). Encephalopathy can also appear within weeks of the initial inoculation, or months to years later (Reik et al., 1986; Ackermann et al., 1988; Halperin et al., 1989). This syndrome has engendered considerable controversy because some patients manifest no evidence of active infection yet still have symptoms. Because of the high rate of seropositivity for *Borrelia burgdorferi* among the healthy population living in endemic areas and the wide variety of neurologic and psychiatric syndromes that have been reported, caution in diagnosis has been advised (Kristoferitsch, 1991). Lyme disease may in fact be overdiagnosed in patients whose symptoms actually reflect chronic fatigue syndrome, fibromyalgia, or depression (Steere et al., 1993).

Of the individuals with late Lyme disease who have symptoms of cognitive impairment, a small number have an unequivocal infectious leukoencephalopathy with focal inflammatory white matter lesions on MRI in association with lymphocytic pleocytosis in the cerebrospinal fluid (CSF) and intrathecal production of antibody against *Borrelia burgdorferi* (Halperin, 1997). A larger number, however, have a less severe encephalopathy, characterized primarily by a confusional state, in which CSF findings are not always found (Halperin, 1997). This group is probably heterogeneous; whereas some probably have subtle CNS infection, others may have toxic-metabolic encephalopathy associated with systemic infection, and others likely have unrelated psychiatric disorders (Halperin, 1997).

Despite the ambiguity in defining Lyme encephalopathy, considerable evidence points to a prominent role of white matter involvement in many late Lyme disease patients with both mild and severe cognitive impairment. Neuropsychological studies of mildly affected individuals have reported a pattern of deficits involving memory, attention, psychomotor speed, and executive function; depression, although often present, cannot be invoked to explain these deficits (Kaplan and Jones-Woodward, 1997). These studies have been consistent in finding a memory retrieval deficit because of the sparing of recognition memory, a pattern similar to that found in MS patients (Kaplan and Jones-Woodward, 1997). Moreover, dementia with prominent memory loss and mood disorder has been observed as a late complication of Lyme disease in association with white matter changes on MRI (Reik et al., 1986; Logigian et al., 1990). In addition, when MRI scans are performed in patients with parenchymal Lyme disease, focal abnormalities of the cerebral white matter are the most common findings (Garcia-Monco and Benach, 1995). Neuropathologic studies are limited because few individuals succumb to the illness, but diffuse demyelination has been documented that may be caused by vasculitis, oligodendroglial damage, or an autoimmune attack on myelin (Oksi et al., 1996). Both cognitive dysfunction and MRI white matter changes have been noted to improve after prompt antibiotic therapy (Garcia-Monco and Benach, 1995). In summary, therefore, while Lyme encephalopathy is a nonspecific syndrome that may include a variety of diverse patients, some individuals within this category appear to have neurobehavioral dysfunction related to cerebral white matter lesions.

References

Ackermann R, Rehse-Kupper B, Gollmer E, Schmidt R. Chronic neurologic manifestations of erythema migrans borreliosis. Ann NY Acad Sci 1988; 539: 16–23.

Amlie-Lefond C, Kleinschmidt-DeMasters BK, Mahalingam R, et al. The vasculopathy of varicella-zoster encephalitis. Ann Neurol 1995; 37: 784–790.

Anlar B, Saatci I, Kose G, Yalaz K. MRI findings in subacute sclerosing panencephalitis. Neurology 1996; 47: 1278–1283.

Bencherif B, Rottenberg DA. Neuroimaging of the AIDS dementia complex. AIDS 1998; 12: 233–244.

Berger JR, Concha M. Progressive multifocal leukoencephalopathy: the evolution of a disease once considered rare. J Neurovirol 1995; 1: 5–18.

Brew BJ. AIDS dementia complex. Neurol Clin 1999; 17: 861–881.

Burgdorfer W, Barbour AG, Hayes SF, et al. Lyme disease—a tick-borne spirochetosis? Science 1982; 216: 1317–1319.

Chang L, Ernst T, Leonido-Yee M, et al. Cerebral metabolic abnormalities correlate with clinical severity of HIV-1 cognitive motor complex. Neurology 1999; 52: 100–108.

Clifford DB. Human immunodeficiency virus-associated dementia. Arch Neurol 2000; 57: 321–324.

Everall IP, Glass JD, McArthur J, et al. Neuronal density in the superior frontal and temporal gyri does not correlate with the degree of hman immunodeficiency virus-associated dementia. Acta Neuropathol 1994; 88: 538–544.

Filley CM. The behavioral neurology of cerebral white matter. Neurology 1998; 50: 1535–1540.

Filippi CG, Sze G, Farber SJ, et al. Regression of HIV encephalopathy and basal ganglia signal intensity abnormality at MR imaging in patients with AIDS after the initiation of protease inhibitor therapy. Radiology 1998; 206: 491–498.

Garcia-Monco JC, Benach JL. Lyme neuroborreliosis. Ann Neurol 1995; 37: 691–702.

Gilden DH. Slow virus diseases of the CNS. 1. Subacute sclerosing panencephalitis, progressive rubella panencephalitis, and progressive multifocal leukoencephalopathy. Postgrad Med 1983; 73: 99–101.

Gilden DH, Kleinschmidt-DeMasters BK, LaGuardia JJ, et al. Neurologic complications of the reactivation of varicella-zoster virus. N Engl J Med 2000; 342: 635–645.

Grant I, Atkinson JH, Hesselink JR, et al. Evidence for early central nervous system involvement in the acquired immunodeficiency syndrome (AIDS) and other human immunodeficiency virus (HIV) infections. Ann Int Med 1987; 107: 828–836.

Gray F, Scaravelli F, Everall I, et al. Neuropathology of early HIV-1 infection. Brain Pathol 1996; 6: 1–15.

Halperin JJ. Neuroborreliosis: central nervous system involvement. Semin Neurol 1997; 17: 19–24.

Halperin JJ, Luft BJ, Anand AK, et al. Lyme neuroborreliosis: central nervous system manifestations. Neurology 1989; 39: 753–759.

Heaton RK, Grant I, Butters N, et al. THE HRNC 500-Neuropsychology of HIV infection at different disease stages. HIV Neurobehavioral Research Center. J Int Neuropsychol Soc 1995; 1: 231–251.

Hokkanen L, Launes J, Poutiainen E, et al. Subcortical type cognitive impairment in herpes zoster encephalitis. J Neurol 1997; 244: 239–245.

Holland NR, Power C, Mathews VP, et al. Cytomegalovirus encephalitis in acquired immunodeficiency sydrome (AIDS). Neurology 1994; 44: 507–514.

Jones HR, Ho DD, Forgacs P, et al. Acute fulminating fatal leukoencephalopathy as the only manifestation of human immunodeficiency virus infection. Ann Neurol 1988; 23: 519–522.

Jones RD, Tranel D. Preservation of procedural memory in HIV-positive patients with subcortical dementia. J Clin Exp Neuropsychol 1991; 13: 74.

Kaplan RF, Jones-Woodward L. Lyme encephalopathy: a neuropsychological perspective. Semin Neurol 1997; 17: 31–37.

Krikorian R, Wrobel AJ. Cognitive impairment in HIV infection. AIDS 1991; 5: 1501–1507.

Kristoferitsch W. Neurological manifestations of Lyme borreliosis. Infection 1991; 19: 268–272.

Lane B, Sullivan EV, Lim KO, et al. White matter MR hyperintensities in adult patients with congenital rubella. AJNR 1996; 17: 99–103.

Lentz D, Jordan JE, Pike GB, Enzmann DR. MRI in varicella-zoster virus leukoencephalitis in the immunocompromised host. J Comput Assist Tomogr 1993; 17: 313–316.

Logigian EL, Kaplan RF, Steere AC. Chronic neurologic mainfestations of Lyme disease. N Engl J Med 1990; 323: 1438–1444.

McArthur JC, Sacktor N, Selnes O. Human immunodeficiency virus-associated dementia. Semin Neurol 1999; 19: 129–150.

Merrill JE, Chen ISY. HIV-1, macrophages, glial cells, and cytokines in AIDS nervous system disease. FASEB J 1991; 5: 2391–2397.

Miller RF, Lucas SB, Hall-Craggs MA, et al. Comparison of magnetic resonance imaging with neuropathological findings in the diagnosis of HIV and CMV associated CNS disease in AIDS. J Neurol Neurosurg Psychiatry 1997; 62: 346–351.

Moskowitz LB, Gregorios JB, Hensley GT, Berger JR. Cytomegalovirus. Induced demyelination associated with acquired immune deficiency syndrome. Arch Pathol Lab Med 1984; 108: 873–877.

Navia BA, Cho E-S, Petito CK, Price RW. The AIDS dementia complex: II. Neuropathology. Ann Neurol 1986a; 19: 525–535.

Navia BA, Jordan BD, Price RW. The AIDS dementia complex: I. Clinical features. Ann Neurol 1986b; 19: 517–524.

Navia BA, Price RW. The acquired immunodeficiency syndrome dementia complex as the presenting or sole manifestation of human immunodeficiency virus infection. Arch Neurol 1987; 44: 65–69.

Oksi J, Kalimo H, Marttila RJ, et al. Inflammatory brain changes in Lyme borreliosis. A report on three patients and review of literature. Brain 1996; 119: 2143–2154.

Perdices M, Cooper DA. Simple and choice reaction time in patients with human immunodeficiency virus infection. Ann Neurol 1989; 25: 460–467.

Perdices M, Cooper DA. Neuropsychological investigation of patients with AIDS and ARC. J AIDS 1990; 3: 555–564.

Poser CM. Notes on the pathogenesis of subacute sclerosing panencephalitis. J Neurol Sci 1990; 95: 219–224.

Post MJ, Berger JR, Quencer RM. Asymptomatic and neurologically symptomatic HIV-seropositive individuals: prospective evaluation with cranial MR imaging. Radiology 1991; 178: 131–139.

Power C, Kong P-A, Crawford TO, et al. Cerebral white matter changes in acquired immunodeficiency syndrome dementia: alterations of the blood-brain barrier. Ann Neurol 1993; 34: 339–350.

Price RW, Brew B, Sidtis J, et al. The brain in AIDS: central nervous system HIV-1 infection and AIDS dementia complex. Science 1988; 239: 586–592.

Reik L, Burgdorfer W, Donaldson JO. Neurologic abormalities in Lyme disease without erythema chronicum migrans. Am J Med 1986; 81: 73–78.

Report of a Working Group of the American Academy of Neurology AIDS Task Force. Nomenclature and research case definitions for neurologic manifestations of human immunodeficiency virus-type 1 (HIV-1) infection. Neurology 1991; 41: 778–785.

Sahakian BJ, Elliott R, Low N, et al. Neuropsychological deficits in tests of executive function in asymptomatic and symptomatic HIV-1 seropositive men. Psychol Med 1995; 25: 1233–1246.

Seilhean D, Duyckaerts C, Vazeux R, et al. HIV-1–associated cognitive/motor complex: absence of neuronal loss in the cerebral neocortex. Neurology 1993; 43: 1492–1499.

Sharer L. Pathology of HIV-1 infection of the central nervous system. A review. J Neuropathol Exp Neurol 1992; 51: 3–11.

Sidtis JJ, Gatsonis C, Price RW, et al. Zidovudine treatment of the AIDS dementia complex: results of a placebo-controlled trial. Ann Neurol 1993; 33: 343–349.

Snider WD, Simpson DM, Nielsen S, et al. Neurological complications of acquired immune deficiency syndrome: analysis of 50 cases. Ann Neurol 1983; 14: 403–418.

Steere AC. Lyme disease. N Engl J Med 1989; 321: 586–596.

Steere AC, Taylor E, McHugh GL, Logigian EL. The overdiagnosis of Lyme disease. JAMA 1993; 269: 1812–1816.

Thurnher MM, Schindler EG, Thurnher SA, et al. Highly active antiretroviral therapy for patients with AIDS dementia complex: effect on MR imaging findings and clinical course. AJNR 2000; 21: 670–678.

Townsend JJ, Stroop WG, Baringer JR, et al. Neuropathology of progressive rubella panencephalitis after childhood rubella. Neurology 1982; 32: 185–190.

Tozzi V, Narciso P, Galgani S, et al. Effects of zidovudine in 30 patients with mild to endstage AIDS dementia complex. AIDS 1993; 7: 683–692.

Tross S, Price RW, Navia B, et al. Neuropsychological characterization of the AIDS dementia complex: a preliminary report. AIDS 1988; 2: 81–88.

Weis S, Haug H, Budka H. Neuronal damage in the cerebral cortex of AIDS brains: a mor-
    phometric study. Acta Neuropathol 1993; 85: 185–189.
White DA, Taylor MJ, Butters N, et al. Memory for verbal information in individuals with
    HIV-associated dementia complex. HNRC Group. J Clin Exp Neuropsychol 1997; 19:
    357–366.
Wilkie FL, Eisdorfer C, Morgan R, et al. Cognition in early human immunodeficiency virus
    infection. Arch Neurol 1990; 47: 433–440.

8

Inflammatory Diseases

A diverse group of noninfectious inflammatory diseases can affect the white matter of the brain. These disorders, some of which are referred to as connective tissue or collagen vascular diseases, share the common feature of being autoimmune in nature, by which is meant that the immune system is induced to mount an assault on various tissues of the body. Thus, most of these diseases produce systemic manifestations in addition to those in the nervous system. In the brain, widespread lesions are typical, usually related to a vasculitic process, but careful perusal of the clinical and neuropathologic features of these diseases reveals that prominent damage to white matter occurs and may have significant consequences. The neurobehavioral implications of white matter involvement from inflammatory diseases are largely unknown, but some preliminary data are emerging. The limited available information on this question is reviewed in this chapter.

Systemic Lupus Erythematosus

Systemic lupus erythematosus (SLE) is the best known connective tissue disease that affects the nervous system. It is an idiopathic autoimmune disease in which the central nervous system (CNS) is affected in up to two-thirds of patients (West, 1994). When the brain is involved, the term lupus cerebritis is often used, or, more commonly, neuropsychiatric lupus (West, 1994). This latter designation is intended to include the entire range of elemental and higher neurologic deficits, but suffers from being too general to capture the individual mental status alterations to which SLE patients are susceptible. In response to this problem, more specific nomenclature has recently been proposed to clarify the neurobehavioral features of neuropsychiatric lupus: acute confusional state, cognitive dysfunction, anxiety disorder, mood disorder, psychosis, and, interestingly, a demyelinating syndrome (ACR Ad Hoc Committee on Neuropsychiatric Lupus Nomenclature, 1999). The majority of neuropsychiatric syndromes develop when patients are on little or no corticosteroid therapy (Feinglass et al., 1976), thus pointing to cerebral involvement rather than iatrogenesis in their causation.

The neuropathology of SLE is dominated by a vasculopathy with hyalinization of vessel walls and perivascular inflammation; a true vasculitis is uncommon (Johnson and Richardson, 1968). Multiple ischemic and hemorrhagic lesions in both gray and white matter are thought to result from this process. Neuroradiologic findings in SLE include cerebral atrophy, seen on both computed tomography (CT) and magnetic resonance imaging (MRI) scans, the presence of which is confounded by the fact the treatment with corticosteroids may produce this finding (Jacobs et al., 1988). White matter abnormalities are also seen, especially on MRI (Fig. 8-1), and these may be the most prominent neuroradiologic finding (Jacobs et al., 1988). These lesions can be distinguished from those of multiple sclerosis (MS) in that they display no periventricular predilection and they enhance less often with gadolinium (Miller et al., 1987).

The origin of neuropsychiatric disturbances in SLE, however, remains incompletely understood. A number of neuropathologic processes appear to be involved, and it is plausible that a combination of structural injury from vascular occlusion and neuronal damage from antineuronal antibodies and cytokines may all contribute (West, 1994). Cognitive deficits have been well documented in SLE patients, including both those with and those without features of neuropsychiatric lupus (Carbotte et al., 1986). Clinical observations indicate that leukoencephalopathy seen on MRI can be associated with dementia, and a causal relationship has been suggested (Kirk et al., 1991). Neuropsychological reports of the profile of cognitive dysfunction in SLE generally suggest that, despite considerable clinical heterogeneity, deficits in attention, concentration, visuospatial skills, and cognitive speed without major language involvement are typical (Ginsburg et al., 1992; Kozora et al., 1996; Denburg et al., 1997a). These deficits can be seen in those with and without other neurologic signs (Kozora et al., 1996). A study of SLE patients with the lupus anticoagulant noted a profile of impairment consistent with subcortical dementia, with the most robust deficit emerging in processing speed (Denburg et al., 1997b). Not surprisingly, language-based screening measures such as the Mini-Mental State Examination (MMSE; Folstein et al., 1975) are often insensitive to the cognitive impairments of SLE patients (ACR Ad Hoc Committee on Neuropsychiatric Lupus Nomenclature, 1999). Whereas these findings are consistent with subcortical neuropathology (Denburg et al., 1997), the pattern is also reminiscent of that produced by other white matter disorders (Filley, 1998).

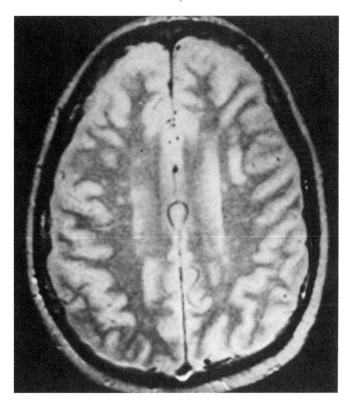

Figure 8-1. T2-weighted MRI scan of a patient with SLE and cognitive impairment. Multiple white matter hyperintensities are present in the cerebrum. (Reprinted with permission from Atlas SW, ed. Magnetic resonance imaging of the brain and spine. 2nd ed. Philadelphia: Lippincott-Raven, 1996.)

Thus, there exists considerable evidence for white matter involvement in SLE producing neurobehavioral dysfunction. However, a mild degree of MRI white matter hyperintensity does not appear to produce neuropsychological deficits (Kozora et al., 1998). One explanation for this finding may be that cognitive impairment may only be demonstrable when a certain threshold burden of disease is present on MRI (Kozora et al., 1998). Additionally, there may be damage in the white matter that is undetectable by conventional MRI. In their series of SLE patients, Brooks and colleagues (1999) found that magnetic resonance spectroscopy (MRS) measures of neuronal dysfunction in normal appearing white matter had the strongest correlation with cognitive impairment. From the available information, it can be tentatively concluded that white matter involvement contributes to neuropsychiatric dysfunction in SLE. Further work is needed to assess the relative contributions of both white and gray matter lesions, and their vascular and immunologic origin, to the pathogenesis of these disturbances.

Behçet's Disease

First described as a dermatologic condition with characteristic oral and genital ulcers and intraocular inflammation, Behçet's disease also features multisystem involvement that may include the CNS. This disease is an idiopathic inflammatory disorder of presumed autoimmune pathogenesis. Neurologic features are common, and may include corticospinal tract dysfunction, headache, and venous thrombosis in addition to neurobehavioral changes (Akman-Demir et al., 1999). In the brain, inflammatory lesions are found in both white matter and subcortical gray matter regions, and the cortex is typically spared (Akman-Demir et al., 1999). White matter hyperintensities are frequently seen on MRI (Gerber et al., 1996) and may be indistinguishable from those of MS (Coban et al., 1999). Neuropsychological deficits have been most commonly found in memory, attention, and frontal lobe function (Oktem-Tanor et al., 1999; Akman-Demir et al., 1999). Additional cognitive features include a suggestion of memory retrieval deficits and sparing of language ability (Akman-Demir et al., 1999), both of which are consistent with primary involvement of cerebral white matter (Filley, 1998). One autopsied case of Behçet's Disease revealed demyelination and gliosis of the frontal white matter in a patient who displayed indifference, euphoria, disinhibition, dementia, and finally akinetic mutism (Yamamori et al., 1994). Another clinically studied case had mutism from bilateral thalamo-capsular lesions that were thought to disconnect the thalamus from the frontal cortex (Park-Matsumoto et al., 1995). Although correlations between neurobehavioral manifestations and white matter neuropathology can only be made cautiously, evidence exists for this possibility in some cases of Behçet's disease.

Sjögren's Syndrome

Sjögren's syndrome is an autoimmune disease of the salivary and lacrimal glands that may also affect the nervous system. Mood disorder, psychosis, and dementia have been noted, elements of which may be present in 80% of patients with CNS Sjögren's syndrome (Cox and Hales, 1999). The most common brain MRI finding in patients with neuropsychiatric syndromes is the presence of multiple hyperintensities in the periventricular white matter, which appear to be caused by a small vessel vasculopathy resulting in microinfarcts and microhemorrhages (Alexander et al., 1988). Less pronounced degrees of white matter change on MRI can be seen in patients who are neurologically asymptomatic (Pierot et al., 1993), implying that mild involvement may not surpass the threshold necessary for the development of neurobehavioral features. In those who are cognitively affected, a subcortical pattern of neuropsychological impairment is found, featuring prominent attention and concentration deficits, personality change, dysphoria, and depression (Malinow et al., 1985). These observations suggest a role of white matter neuropathology in Sjögren's syndrome affecting the brain.

Wegener's Granulomatosis

Wegener's granulomatosis is a granulomatous vasculitis of unknown etiology that primarily affects the upper and lower respiratory tract and kidneys. The disease also involves the CNS in about 50% of cases (Drachman, 1963). In the brain, there is a vasculitis of small arteries and veins that produces vascular occlusion and stroke, and direct or contiguous granuloma invasion may also produce structural damage (Drachman, 1963). Magnetic resonance imaging white matter hyperintensities reflecting ischemia and infarction may be seen in 20%–30% of patients (Asmus et al., 1993; Hurst and Grossman, 1994). Neuropsychiatric features have been noted (McKeith, 1985; Nordmark et al., 1997), for which white matter lesions may be in part responsible.

Temporal Arteritis

Also known as giant cell or cranial arteritis, temporal arteritis is an inflammatory disease of the aortic arch and external carotid artery system that may also involve intracranial arteries (Caselli et al., 1988; Hurst and Grossman, 1994). Polymyalgia rheumatica is often associated with temporal arteritis, and both are seen mainly in older persons. Ischemic lesions may occur in the brain, and because prompt treatment with corticosteroids is effective in preventing stroke, early diagnosis is of paramount importance. Occipital infarcts with corresponding visual deficits and release hallucinations have been described. Cognitive deficits and depression have been noted and may relate in part to white matter ischemic disease (Caselli et al., 1988).

Polyarteritis Nodosa

Also known as periarteritis nodosa, polyarteritis nodosa is an idiopathic systemic vasculitis with a predilection for small and medium sized arteries. Peripheral neuropathy is the most common neurologic manifestation of this disease, but brain involvement occurs in a substantial percentage of patients and can produce a confusional state or psychosis (Ford and Siekert, 1965). Infarcts in the gray and white matter are likely to produce this clinical picture (Ford and Siekert, 1965). Reichhart and colleagues recently reported that lacunes were the most common strokes observed in polyarteritis nodosa; these lesions often affect the cerebral white matter and can be associated with dementia (Reichhart et al., 2000).

Scleroderma

Neurologic involvement is uncommon in scleroderma (systemic sclerosis), a disease characterized by progressive deposition of collagen in the skin, peripheral blood vessels, and visceral organs. However, corticosteroid-responsive subacute encephalopathy has been reported with angiographic evidence of focal arteritis, indicating that cerebral vasculitis can occur (Estey et al., 1979). The contribution of white matter disease to the neurobehavioral picture is difficult to assess with the limited information available, but cerebral white matter changes have been observed with both MRI and CT scanning (Liu et al., 1994). In a study of 27 consecutive scleroderma patients (Nobili et al., 1997), 30% had focal or diffuse hemispheric white matter changes that were more apparent with increasing disease severity, and in 7 patients cognitive impairment or mild dementia was found with the use of the MMSE (Folstein et al., 1975). Although many patients with scleroderma remain neurologically intact, white matter involvement may be relatively common, and in some cases cognitive loss may result.

Isolated Angiitis of the Central Nervous System

In contrast to the other diseases considered in this chapter, isolated CNS angiitis (primary CNS vasculitis, granulomatous angiitis) has no systemic manifestations. The disease thus manifests with diffuse or focal neurologic dysfunction, reflecting the location of infarcts in both cerebral gray and white matter, and because there are no other physical signs, the diagnosis is often challenging (Vollmer et al., 1993). For example, in one patient primary angiitis was initially suspected, but was found to be a case of cerebral autosomal dominant arteriopathy with subcortical infarcts and leukoencephalopathy (CADASIL; Chapter 11) after brain and skin biopsies were performed (Williamson et al., 1999). The neuropathology consists of a granulomatous angiitis that affects the vessel wall and produces vascular occlusion and infarction (Kolodny et al., 1968). Because the disease tends to favor small blood vessels (Moore, 1989), white matter involvement may occur (Hurst and Grossman, 1994), and contributes to cognitive dysfunction that is a prominent part of the clinical picture. In the cases reviewed by Younger and colleagues (1997), mental change was the most common feature, and on MRI, high signal lesions in the subcortical white matter were the most commonly seen abnormality. Although the outcome may be poor, vigorous treatment with corticosteroids and immunosuppressive agents (cyclophosphamide and azathioprine) has improved survival in patients with this disease (Rajjoub et al., 1977; Younger et al., 1997).

Sarcoidosis

Sarcoidosis is a systemic inflammatory disease featuring the characteristic pathologic finding of noncaseating granulomata. The nervous system is involved in approximately 5% of cases, and common manifestations include cranial neuropathy, aseptic meningitis, hydrocephalus, parenchymal brain disease, peripheral neuropathy, and myopathy (Stern et al., 1985). Neurosarcoidosis may develop in patients with previously known systemic disease, or as an initial presentation (Nikhar et al.,

2000). At least 35 patients with dementia caused by cerebral sarcoidosis have been reported (Cordingley et al., 1981), and white matter involvement related to ependymal disease seems to be a likely contributing factor. The neuropathology of cerebral sarcoidosis frequently involves the periventricular white matter, either from subependymal granulomatous disease or from infarction secondary to granulomatous angiitis in these areas (Miller et al., 1988). Correspondingly, MRI studies have identified the most common pattern of disease to be high signal periventricular and multifocal white matter lesions that may be indistinguishable from the lesions of MS (Miller et al., 1988; Zajicek et al., 1999). The outcome after treatment of neurosarcoidosis is usually favorable (Stern et al., 1985), suggesting that a component of the neuropathology does indeed reflect reversible white matter dysfunction.

References

ACR Ad Hoc Committee on Neuropsychiatric Lupus Nomenclature. The American College of Rheumatology Nomenclature and Case Definitions for Neuropsychiatric Lupus Syndromes. Arthritis Rheum 1999; 42: 599–608.

Akman-Demir G, Serdaroglu P, Tasçi, et al. Clinical patterns of neurological involvement in Behçet's disease: evaluation of 200 patients. Brain 1999; 122: 2171–2181.

Alexander EL, Beall SS, Gordon B, et al. Magnetic resonance imaging of cerebral lesions in Sjögren's syndrome. Ann Int Med 1988; 108: 815–823.

Asmus R, Koltza H, Muhle C, et al. MRI of the head in Wegener's granulomatosis. Adv Exp Med Biol 1993; 336: 319–321.

Brooks WM, Jung RE, Ford CC, et al. Relationship between neurometabolite derangement and neurocognitive dysfunction in systemic lupus erythematosus. J Rheumatol 1999; 26: 81–85.

Carbotte RM, Denburg SD, Denburg JA. Prevalence of cognitive impairment in systemic lupus erythematosus. J Nerv Ment Dis 1986; 174: 357–364.

Caselli RJ, Hunder GG, Whisnant JP. Neurologic disease in biopsy-proven giant cell (temporal) arteritis. Neurology 1988; 38: 352–359.

Coban O, Bahar S, Akman-Demir G, et al. Masked assessment of MR findings: is it possible to differentiate neuro-Behçet's disease from other central nervous system diseases? Neuroradiology 1999; 41: 255–260.

Cordingley G, Navarro C, Brust JCM, Healton EB. Sarcoidosis presenting as senile dementia. Neurology 1981; 31: 1148–1151.

Cox PD, Hales RE. CNS Sjögren's syndrome: an underrecognized and under appreciated neuropsychiatric disorder. J Neuropsychiatry Clin Neurosci 1999; 11: 241–247.

Denburg SD, Carbotte RM, Denburg JA. Cognition and mood in systemic lupus eythematosus. Evaluation and pathogenesis. Ann NY Acad Sci 1997; 823: 44–59.

Denburg SD, Carbotte RM, Ginsberg JS, Denburg JA. The relationship of antiphospholipid antibodies to cognitive function in patients with systemic lupus erythematosus. J Int Neuropsychol Soc 1997; 3: 377–386.

Drachman D. Neurological complications of Wegener's granulomatosis. Arch Neurol 1963; 8: 145–155.

Estey E, Lieberman A, Pinto R, et al. Cerebral arteritis in scleroderma. Stroke 1979; 10: 595–597.

Feinglass EJ, Arnett FC, Dorsch CA, et al. Neuropsychiatric manifestations of systemic lupus erythematosus: diagnosis, clinical spectrum, and relationship to other features of the disease. Medicine 1976; 55: 323–339.

Filley CM. The behavioral neurology of cerebral white matter. Neurology 1998; 50: 1535–1540.

Folstein MF, Folstein SE, McHugh PR. "Mini-mental state": a practical method for grading the cognitive state of patients for the clinician. J Psychiat Res 1975; 12: 189–198.

Ford RG, Siekert RG. Central nervous system manifestations of periarteritis nodosa. Neurology 1965; 15: 114–129.

Gerber S, Biondi A, Dormont D, et al. Long-term MR follow-up of cerebral lesions in neuro-Behçet's disease. Neuroradiology 1996; 38: 761–768.

Ginsburg KS, Wright EA, Larsen MG, et al. A controlled study of the prevalence of cognitive impairment in randomly selected patients with systemic lupus erythematosus. Arthritis Rheum 1992; 35: 776–782.

Hurst RW, Grossman RI. Neuroradiology of central nervous system vasculitis. Semin Neurol 1994; 14: 320–340.

Jacobs L, Kinkel PR, Costello PB, et al. Central nervous system lupus erythematosus: the value of magnetic resonance imaging. J Rheumatol 1988; 15: 601–606.

Johnson RT, Richardson EP. The neurological manifestations of systemic lupus erythematosus. Medicine 1968; 47: 337–369.

Kirk A, Kertesz A, Polk MJ. Dementia with leukoencephalopathy in systemic lupus erythematosus. Can J Neurol Sci 1991; 18: 344–348.

Kolodny EH, Rebeiz JJ, Caviness VS, Richardson EP. Granulomatous angiitis of the central nervous system. Arch Neurol 1968; 19: 510–524.

Kozora E, Thompson LL, West SG, Kotzin BL. Analysis of cognitive and psychological deficits in systemic lupus erythematosus patients without overt central nervous system disease. Arthritis Rheum 1996; 39: 2035–2045.

Kozora E, West SG, Kotzin BL, et al. Magnetic resonance imaging abnormalities and cognitive deficits in systemic lupus erythematosus patients without overt central nervous system disease. Arthritis Rheum 1998; 41: 41–47.

Liu P, Uziel Y, Chuang S, et al. Localized scleroderma: imaging features. Pediatr Radiol 1994: 24: 207–209.

Malinow KL, Molina R, Gordon B, et al. Neuropsychiatric dysfunction in primary Sjögren's syndrome. Ann Int Med 1985; 103: 344–350.

McKeith IG. Neuropsychiatric symptoms in the course of Wegener's granulomatosis. J Neurol Neurosurg Psychiatry 1985; 48: 713–714.

Miller BH, Kendall BE, Barter S, et al. Magnetic resonance imaging in central nervous system sarcoidosis. Neurology 1988; 38: 378–383.

Miller DH, Ormerod IEC, Gibson A, et al. MR brain scanning in patients with vasculitis: differentiation from multiple sclerosis. Neuroradiology 1987; 29: 226–231.

Moore PM. Diagnosis and management of isolated angiitis of the central nervous system. Neurology 1989; 39: 167–173.

Nikhar NK, Shah JR, Tselis AC, Lewis RA. Primary neurosarcoidosis: a diagnostic and therapeutic challenge. Neurologist 2000; 6: 126–133.

Nobili F, Cutolo M, Sulli A, et al. Impaired quantitative cerebral blood flow in scleroderma patients. J Neurol Sci 1997; 152: 63–71.

Nordmark G, Boquist L, Ronnblum L. Limited Wegener's granulomatosis with central nervous system involvement and fatal outcome. J Intern Med 1997; 242: 433–436.

Oktem-Tanor O, Baykan-Kurt B, Gurvit IH, et al. Neuropsychological follow-up of 12 patients with neuro-Behçet disease. J Neurol 1999; 246: 113–119.

Park-Matsumoto YC, Ogawa K, Tazawa T, et al. Mutism developing after bilateral thalamo-capsular lesions by neuro-Behçet disease. Acta Neurol Scand 1995; 91: 297–301.

Pierot L, Sauve C, Leger JM, et al. Asymptomatic cerebral involvement in Sjögren's syndrome: MRI findings of 15 cases. Neuroradiology 1993; 35: 378–380.

Rajjoub RK, Wood JH, Ommaya AK. Granulomatous angiitis of the brain: a successfully treated case. Neurology 1977; 27: 588–591.

Reichhart MD, Bogousslavsky J, Janzer RC. Early lacunar strokes complicating polyarteritis nodosa. Thrombotic microangiopathy. Neurology 2000; 54: 883–889.

Stern BJ, Krumholz A, Johns C, et al. Sarcoidosis and its neurological manifestations. Arch Neurol 1985; 42: 909–917.

Vollmer TL, Guarnaccia J, Harrington W, et al. Idiopathic granulomatous angiitis of the central nervous system. Diagnostic challenges. Arch Neurol 1993; 50: 925–930.

West SG. Neuropsychiatric lupus. Rheum Dis Clin N Am 1994; 20: 129–158.

Williamson EE, Chukwudelenzu FE, Meschi JF, et al. Distinguishing primary angiitis of the central nervous system from cerebral autosomal dominant arteriopathy with subcortical infarcts and leukoencephalopathy: the importance of family history. Arthritis Rheum 1999; 42: 2243–2248.

Yamamori C, Ishino H, Inagaki T, et al. Neuro-Behçet disease with demyelination and gliosis of the frontal white matter. Clin Neuropathol 1994; 13: 208–215.

Younger DS, Calabrese LH, Hays AP. Granulomatous angiitis of the nervous system. Neurol Clin 1997; 15: 821–834.

Zajicek JP, Scolding NJ, Foster O, et al. Central nervous system sarcoidosis—diagnosis and management. Quart J Med 1999; 92: 103–117.

9

Toxic Leukoencephalopathies

The nervous system can be damaged by a wide range of toxins, the study of which delimits the scope of neurotoxicology. Many physical and chemical toxins penetrate the brain and cause adverse effects, and the selective vulnerability of the white matter allows the delineation of a subset of neurotoxicology called toxic leukoencephalopathy (Filley, 1999). Many of these intoxications have been discovered and characterized by the use of magnetic resonance imaging (MRI), which has the capacity to detect subtle white matter involvement that was previously unappreciated. With the advent of new therapeutic agents for cancer and other diseases, as well as the appearance of new drugs of abuse, toxic leukoencephalopathies are being increasingly recognized.

•

Cranial Irradiation

Radiation is delivered to the brain as a therapeutic modality for neoplasia, and its benefits for the treatment of many primary and metastatic tumors has been well documented. However, like other means of treating cancer, radiation has a substantial potential for toxicity. In recent years, the problem of radiation leukoencephalopathy has been recognized as one of the major limitations of cranial irradiation.

The seminal work of Sheline and colleagues 2 decades ago established that three types of radiation injury can occur in the brain, all of which primarily affect the cerebral white matter (Sheline et al., 1980). The first is an acute reaction that occurs during treatment and is characterized by a confusional state or a worsening of preexisting neurologic signs. Typically self-limited, this mild syndrome is thought to result from cerebral white matter edema. Next in temporal order and degree of severity comes the early delayed reaction, which manifests as a so-called "somnolence syndrome" weeks to a few months after irradiation. This syndrome is ascribed to cerebral demyelination, and slow recovery usually takes place. Finally, the most ominous injury is the late delayed reaction, which develops 6 months to 2 years after therapy and presents as a progressive dementia with an often fatal outcome from widespread demyelination with necrosis. Much of the information on radiation leukoencephalopathy comes from study of these late delayed effects.

The most prominent clinical effects of any degree of radiation leukoencephalopathy are neurobehavioral. In adults, alterations including confusion, personality change, memory loss, and dementia have been repeatedly noted (Filley, 1999), and focal neurobehavioral signs may develop in association with focal neuroradiologic abnormalities (Valk and Dillon, 1991). Learning disabilities have been described in children (Constine et al., 1988), and those under 5 years of age may fare worse cognitively than older individuals (Fletcher and Copeland, 1988). Reviewing 29 studies of therapeutic cranial irradiation and 18 studies of prophylactic cranial irradiation, Crossen and colleagues found that 28% of patients seen in follow-up had encephalopathy caused by radiation (Crossen et al., 1994). DeAngelis and colleagues described 12 patients who had radiation-induced dementia and prominent white matter neuropathology on neuroimaging, cerebral biopsy, or autopsy; qualitatively, the dementia was similar to that seen with subcortical diseases (De Angelis et al., 1989). In patients irradiated for tumors at the base of the skull, neurocognitive deficits were correlated with total radiation dose, and the pattern of impairments in cognitive speed, visuospatial skills, and executive function was consistent with injury to the subcortical white matter (Meyers et al., 2000).

The dose of irradiation that induces radiation leukoencephalopathy has generally been in excess of 50 Gy in adults and 35 Gy in children (Schulthiess et al., 1995). However, much individual variability is apparent in dose-response relationships, and concomitant chemotherapy renders leukoencephalopathy more likely and more severe (Schultheiss et al., 1995). The safe lower limit of brain irradiation is not known, although a recent study of healthy adults demonstrated that no decrement in attentional functions, which are quite sensitive to radiation effects, could be detected after a dose of 1.2 Gy was delivered (Wenz et al., 1999). It also appears that focal irradiation has a less severe neurobehavioral impact than whole brain irradiation (Taphoorn et al., 1994). Significant damage may nevertheless occur with focal irradiation, as demonstrated in patients who received focal radiation therapy for nasopharyngeal carcinoma, and prominent memory and language deficits in association with bilateral temporal lobe white matter necrosis (Cheung et al., 2000).

Neuropathologic findings in radiation leukoencephalopathy may be either diffuse or focal, depending on the site(s) of irradiation. In general, a spectrum of changes from edema to demyelination and ultimately necrosis reflects the severity that can occur (Filley, 1999). Radiation does not produce significant damage to the cortex, and the often diagnosed "cortical atrophy" in irradiated patients more likely reflects loss of white matter volume (Valk and Dillon, 1991). Hypothesized causes of radiation leukoencephalopathy include *(1)* direct injury to oligodendrocytes and a secondary disturbance in myelin metabolism, and *(2)* damage to vascular endothelium that results in a breakdown of the blood–brain barrier and subsequent edema and demyelination (Sheline et al., 1980).

Neuroimaging scans reflect the spectrum of neuropathologic injury from radiation, and the most striking findings are seen on MRI in late delayed injury. Figure 9-1 shows the white matter effects of radiation in a patient with a glioblastoma multiforme. This individual also received chemotherapy (see below), which has similar neuroradiologic effects on white matter. Studies using MRI have generally supported an association between greater cognitive impairment and more extensive radiation-induced white matter disease (Corn et al., 1994). A recent study of medulloblastoma survivors provided a direct correlation between decreased white matter volume caused by radiation and cognitive loss (Mulhern et al., 1999). In children with white matter damage from brain irradiation, a correlation between abnormal P300 results and neuropsychological deficits has been found, further supporting the hypothesis that white matter damage underlies cognitive dysfunction in this syndrome (Moore et al., 1992). Armstrong and colleagues studied the effects of radiotherapy longitudinally, and reported a decline in cognitive function between 1.5 and 4.5 months after radiation followed first by improvement and then later by a decline again at 2 years; the results were interpreted as consistent with the time course of early delayed and late delayed radiation leukoencephalopathy (Armstrong et al., 1995). An interesting feature of this study was that memory retrieval deficits were particularly prominent, and thus were thought to represent a potentially sensitive clinical marker of white matter neuropathology (Armstrong et al., 1995). Memory retrieval deficits are proposed to be a central feature of white matter dementia (Filley, 1998).

The tendency for many milder forms of radiation leukoencephalopathy to resolve spontaneously testifies to the resiliency of white matter if the damage is not extensive. Recovery can be excellent if axons are not damaged. Corticosteroids are used by many clinicians for cases of acute and early delayed reaction, although their efficacy is difficult to determine because most patients recover with supportive care alone. Treatment for the more serious late delayed reaction has been disappointing. Clinical reports of radiation necrosis responding to heparin and warfarin have been presented (Glantz et al., 1994), but this evidence must be regarded as preliminary. Strategies at present focus on minimizing potential toxicity by limiting the dose of irradiation as much as possible. In those with inattention, apathy, and related cognitive deficits related to irradiation, methylphenidate has reportedly been of symptomatic benefit (Weizner et al., 1995).

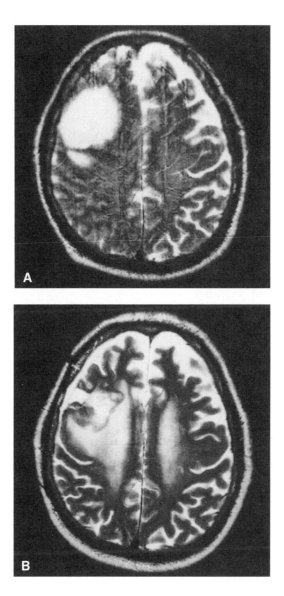

Figure 9-1. T2-weighted MRI scans of patient with a right frontal glioblastoma multiforme *A,* before, and *B,* after radiation and BCNU chemotherapy. Although the tumor size has de-creased, leukoencephalopathy has developed.

Therapeutic Drugs

The introduction of new drugs into clinical practice inevitably entails the advent of new toxicities. Many new agents have recently been used for the treatment of cancer, and with the improved care for cancer patients that permits higher doses of antineoplastic drugs and longer survival periods, toxic effects are often accentuated (Gilbert, 1998). Cancer chemotherapeutic drugs constitute the major category of medications capable of inducing drug-related leukoencephalopathy, but certain immunosuppressive drugs and antimicrobials have also been implicated. As is the case with other white matter disorders, advances in neuroimaging techniques, especially MRI, have rapidly propelled this field forward.

Chemotherapeutic Agents

Many drugs for the treatment of cancer may produce a leukoencephalopathy that is clinically, neuropathologically, and neuroradiologically similar to that produced by radiation. The clinical effects of these drugs closely resemble those of radiation leukoencephalopathy: lassitude, drowsiness, confusion, memory loss, and dementia (Lee et al., 1986). In practice, radiation and chemotherapy are often administered together, so the toxic effects on the brain are compounded. Similarly, the neuroimaging appearance of cancer drug neurotoxicity can closely mimic that of radiation. Combined treatment produces more severe leukoencephalopathy, particularly if the chemotherapy is given by the intrathecal or intraventricular routes (Lee et al., 1986).

The first antineoplastic drug recognized to produce leukoencephalopathy was methotrexate, which may be associated with the syndrome when given intravenously or intrathecally (Gilbert, 1998) or even orally in rare cases (Worthley and McNeil, 1995). High-dose intravenous methotrexate causes leukoencephalopathy, which is manifested clinically by personality change, progressive dementia, and stupor (Allen et al., 1980). Leukovorin (folinic acid) may be helpful in the prevention and treatment of this syndrome (Cohen et al., 1990).

1,3-bis(2-chloroethyl)-1-nitrosourea (BCNU) is frequently used in the treatment of brain tumors because its lipid solubility promotes entry into the brain. It represents another cause of leukoencephalopathy, whether given intravenously (Burger et al., 1981) or intraarterially (Kleinschmidt-DeMasters and Geier, 1989). Dementia and a fatal outcome may ensue (Kleinschmidt-DeMasters and Geier, 1989).

A variety of other antineoplastic drugs may produce this syndome. Cytosine arabinoside, 5–fluorouracil, levamisole, fludarabine, cisplatin, thiotepa, interleukin-2, and interferon-alpha have all been implicated (Filley, 1999). In general, these drugs share similar clinical features of leukoencephalopathy and they are typically well visualized on MRI scans. The neuropathology, when available, documents variable degrees of cerebral demyelination and necrosis. Many cases are reversible, but more intense exposure seems to be associated with more severe leukoencephalopathy (Filley, 1999).

Immunosuppressive Agents

With the increasing popularity of organ transplantation, immunosuppressive drugs are used more frequently in the postoperative period. Cyclosporine is the most widely employed immunosuppresant for the prevention of graft rejection in transplant patients, and a reversible leukoencephalopathy has been observed with its use (Truwit et al., 1991). Another immunosuppressive drug, tacrolimus or FK-506, has been reported to cause a similar syndrome (Tomura et al., 1998). While generally reversible with discontinuation or reduction of dose, leukoencephalopathy from these agents is an important consideration as organ transplantation becomes increasingly feasible.

Antimicrobials

Amphotericin B has long been employed as a mainstay in the treatment of various fungal infections. This drug has recently been recognized to produce a frontally predominant leukoencephalopathy that features personality change, confusion, dementia, and akinetic mutism that may culminate in a fatal outcome (Devinsky et al., 1987; Walker and Rosenblum, 1992). Hexachlorophene is an antiseptic detergent shown to be a cerebral white matter toxin in infants and children who had therapeutic (Shuman et al., 1975) or accidental (Martinez et al., 1974) exposure. Most recently, parenteral therapy with herbal extracts, often used to prevent or treat viral infections, caused a reaction resembling acute disseminated encephalomyelitis in two patients (Schwarz et al., 2000). While it is impossible to know the specific agent responsible for the clinical picture in such cases because herbal remedies typically contain many substances, this report highlights the potential of "natural" and seemingly harmless medications to have substantial untoward effects.

Drugs of Abuse

Injury to the nervous system from drugs of abuse has been difficult to characterize because drug abusers are often exposed to more than one agent, and neuropathologic studies of individuals with single exposures are rare. However, with the use of MRI, and in some cases neuropathologic examination, a group of abused drugs with selective effects on white matter has been identified.

Toluene

This organic hydrocarbon, also known as methlybenzene, is the major solvent in spray paints, and is also found in many other readily obtainable household products. Exposure to toluene, in addition to many other organic solvents, thus occurs in workers in many occupations and in the general public (Kornfeld, 1996). Although concern exists about low-level exposure to organic solvents including toluene in the workplace, toxic effects have been difficult to document in this setting. In contrast, high-level exposure to toluene has provided persuasive data about the neurotoxic effects of this drug (Hormes et al., 1986). Abuse of toluene is practiced by the intentional inhalation of solvent vapors derived mainly from spray paint, which induces euphoria without a dramatic withdrawal state. If exposure is heavy and prolonged, a striking neurologic syndrome appears in which dementia is the most prominent feature of a picture that also includes ataxia, corticospinal dysfunction, and cranial nerve abnormalities (Hormes et al., 1986). These effects may be persistent in many abusers even after abstinence is achieved. The pattern of dementia in these individuals fits that described in subcortical dementia (Hormes et al., 1986), and, more specifically, the profile of white matter dementia (Filley, 1998).

The first MRI studies of toluene dementia proved invaluable in documenting diffuse leukoencephalopathy in the cerebrum and cerebellum (Fig. 9-2). A range of findings can be seen, including increased periventricular white matter, signal intensity on T2-weighted images, loss of differentiation between the gray and white matter, and diffuse cerebral atrophy (Rosenberg et al., 1988a). These findings have been amply confirmed by other observers (Caldemeyer et al., 1993; Xiong et al., 1993; Yamanouchi et al., 1997). Some cases have shown additional T2 hypointensities in the thalamus and basal ganglia; initially attributed to iron deposition, these changes may actually reflect the partitioning of toluene in lipids within these areas (Unger et al., 1994). The white matter changes in toluene abuse appear to account for cognitive loss, as the severity of cerebral white matter involvement on MRI was found to be strongly correlated with the degree of neuropsychological impairment in affected individuals (Filley et al., 1990).

Neuropathologic studies of toluene leukoencephalopathy were soon able to confirm the selectivity of white matter involvement. Postmortem studies consistently disclosed widespread white matter changes in the brain sparing cortical and subcortical gray matter as well as axons (Rosenberg et al., 1988b; Kornfeld et al., 1994). True demyelination was not observed; rather, an increase in very long chain fatty acids in the cerebral white matter suggested a neuropathologic commonality with adrenoleukodystrophy (Kornfeld et al., 1994).

Whereas the neurobehavioral sequelae of extended toluene abuse are clear, the impact of low-level occupational exposure to toluene and other solvents remains uncertain. Workers exposed in industrial settings often have many neurobehavioral complaints that could be a result of solvent exposure (Hartman, 1988). However, these symptoms, typically including fatigue, poor concentration, memory loss, depression, and sleep disturbance, are nonspecific and frequently are not accompanied by neurologic findings or evidence of neuropsychological dysfunction. Moreover, determining a cause-and-effect relationship is very difficult because many individuals are exposed to multiple solvents, experience depression or anxiety, have concurrent alcohol or other drug issues, or are involved in litigation to obtain compensation for alleged toxic injury. The issue has been controversial since the 1970s, when the first description of the so-called "chronic painters' syndrome" appeared from Scandinavia (Arlien-Soborg et al., 1979). Since then, much

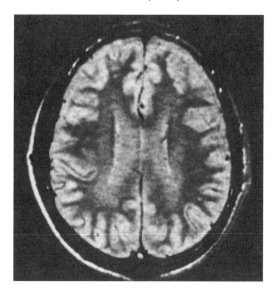

Figure 9-2. T2-weighted MRI scan of a patient with dementia secondary to chronic toluene inhalation. Diffuse leukoencephalopathy is present in the cerebral white matter.

has been written about this condition, also called chronic toxic encephalopathy and the psychoorganic syndrome, and opinions on its existence range from supportive (White and Feldman, 1987; Baker, 1994) to skeptical (Rosenberg, 1995; Albers et al., 2000).

Among individuals with this problem, consistent patterns of neuropsychological impairment in attention, memory, and visuospatial dysfunction have been noted in many studies (Baker, 1994), but methodological problems with this research have also been stressed. These include uncertainty about the degree of exposure, dose–response relationships, and confounding problems such as alcoholism (see below), psychiatric disorders, and compensation issues (Rosenberg, 1995). Neuroimaging scans have not usually been helpful in detecting low-level solvent neurotoxicity, as CT studies of solvent-exposed workers typically fail to show cerebral atrophy (Treibig and Lang, 1993). Magnetic resonance imaging may assist in this area, however, as one study showed diffuse white matter hyperintensity in individuals exposed to industrial solvents when compared to age-matched control subjects (Thuomas et al., 1996). The use of event-related potentials (ERPs) may also be of some use in this context, as delayed P300 latency has been documented in individuals exposed to mixtures of solvents including toluene (Morrow et al., 1992). Neuropsychological testing offers a sensitive means of detecting deficits, but interpretation of the results may be problematic. Accurate diagnosis of individuals in this setting is far from straightforward, and many cases of alleged cognitive impairment after occupational solvent exposure are unconvincing after careful neurobehavioral evaluation. Thus, although the leukoenceph-alopathy of toluene abuse remains the best example of solvent-induced neurobe-havioral dysfunction, and one of the most instructive varieties of white matter de-mentia (Filley, 1998), similar effects from low-level exposure to toluene or other solvents remain to be substantiated. Prospective, controlled studies will be needed to establish if neurotoxicity occurs in this setting, and the threshold of exposure above which this can be expected.

Ethanol

Inclusion of ethanol on a list of white matter toxins may at first glance appear puz-zling. Many of the effects of alcohol on the nervous system are widely taught to be nutritional in origin, and a toxic effect on the white matter—indeed the nervous system as a whole—is still conjectural (Charness et al., 1989). Even if there is a neurotoxic effect, the damage may occur in gray matter areas in addition to white matter (Charness et al., 1989). However, considerable evidence supports the no-tion that ethanol is a white matter toxin that can produce significant neurobehav-ioral effects.

Abusers of alcohol are vulnerable to many neurologic and systemic complica-tions that can disturb cognition. Many individuals, for example, manifest cogni-tive impairment or dementia as a result of hepatic encephalopathy, infection, sub-dural hematoma, or traumatic brain injury. However, in sober alcoholics who do not have these problems, neuropsychological deficits can still be detected in 50%–70% of cases (Charness et al., 1989). A traditional view maintains that the cogni-tive dysfunction in these individuals can be satisfactorily explained by nutritional or metabolic disorders, the best known of which is Korsakoff's psychosis, the amnestic syndrome caused by dietary thiamine (vitamin B1) deficiency (Victor, 1993). Alternatively, it has been noted that many alcoholics have cognitive deficits in addition to amnesia, as well as cerebral atrophy on neuroimaging studies, and as a result the category of alcoholic dementia has been invoked to explain these findings (Lishman, 1981, 1990). The controversy has not been resolved, primarily because of the lack of a distinctive brain histopathology in alcoholism that can be used to support the concept of alcoholic dementia (Victor, 1993). Specifically, a direct toxic effect of ethanol on cerebral neurons has been difficult to demonstrate (Victor, 1993).

The assumption that neurons are the target of ethanol neurotoxicity, however, may be incorrect. Rather, substantial reason exists to support the belief that alco-hol may have toxic effects on myelin that can result in cognitive impairment or de-mentia. Early CT studies found that cerebral atrophy in alcoholics could be par-tially reversed with abstinence, in parallel with improvement in cognitive function (Carlen et al., 1978); because structural improvement was observed, the tissue damage could have taken place in the white matter, which has a more robust ca-pacity to restore its integrity because of remyelination. This possibility was sup-ported by an MRI study that found a significant and selective increase in cerebral white matter volume among alcoholics who achieved abstinence for 3 months compared to similar patients who did not; an alternative explanation of brain re-hydration in abstainers was deemed unlikely because the study was initiated ap-proximately 1 month after the patients' last drink, and thus well past the acute withdrawal period (Shear et al., 1994). Other investigators found MRI white matter changes in 40% of sober alcoholics who had no other complications of al-coholism (Gallucci et al., 1989). With more advanced MRI using diffusion tensor imaging (DTI), another group showed microstructural changes in the white matter of alcoholics (Pfefferbaum et al., 2000). Neuropathologic studies have been con-sistent with this hypothesis, demonstrating a disproportionate loss of white matter in chronic alcoholics (Harper et al., 1981; de la Monte, 1988). Moreover, animal experiments showed a selective vulnerability of the white matter in dogs exposed to alcohol (Hansen et al., 1991). A recent review concluded that alcohol damages white matter more than gray matter through a change in myelination, and that this process is reversible in some cases (Harper, 1998). A toxic effect on oligodendro-cytes has been suggested by some investigators (Lancaster, 1994).

Clinical evidence for white matter damage in alcoholism can also be found. Neuropsychological studies of alcoholics who do not have Korsakoff's psychosis demonstrate prominent attentional (Ratti et al., 1999) and executive dysfunction (Ihara et al., 2000), consistent with neuropathologic studies identifying the pre-frontal white matter as most significantly reduced (Kril et al., 1997). More direct support comes from studies of subtle white matter damage as demonstrated by DTI that correlates with decrements in attention and working memory in alco-holics (Pfefferbaum et al., 2000).

Evidence from other neurologic problems related to ethanol can also be in-voked. In Marchiafava-Bignami disease, an uncommon dementia syndrome most often seen in chronic alcoholics, the primary neuropathology is widespread necro-sis of the corpus callosum and subcortical white matter (Merritt and Weissman, 1945; Ferracci et al., 1999; Ruiz-Martinez et al., 1999; Kohler et al., 2000). Even in alcoholics who have neither Marchiafava-Bignami disease nor Korsakoff's psy-chosis, atrophy of the corpus callosum can be seen on MRI, which implicates a leukotoxic effect of ethanol (Hommer et al., 1996; Oishi et al., 1999). Moreover, with abstinence, patients with Marchiafava-Bignami disease may show reversal of callosal changes on neuroimaging studies in parallel with clinical improvement (Gass et al., 1998). The fetal alcohol syndrome is another ethanol-related problem, and delayed myelination and agenesis of the corpus callosum have been observed in addition to a number of other developmental defects (Lancaster, 1994). These observations suggest that future studies to examine correlations between cognitive impairment and white matter damage in alcoholism and its complications would be revealing.

Heroin

Abuse of heroin, when injected intravenously, has been known for some time as a cause of hypoxic-ischemic leukoencephalopathy (Ginsburg et al., 1976). More re-cently, leukoencephalopathy has been observed in abusers who inhale heroin vapor to avoid the infectious risks of parenteral drug administration, a process known as "chasing the dragon." The procedure involves heating the heroin on aluminum foil so that inhalable heroin pyrolysate is produced. The first reports of this form of leukoencephalopathy originated from the Netherlands two decades ago (Wolters et al., 1982), and the syndrome has since been found in Italy, Switzerland, and the United States (Kreigstein et al., 1999). Inattention, memory impairment, dementia, gait disorder, ataxia, and akinetic mutism have been observed, and the outcome is typically poor (Wolters et al., 1982). Symmetric white matter involvement is seen on MRI, which correlates with a spongiform leukoencephalopathy at autopsy (Wolters et al., 1982). The toxic agent is unknown, but recent findings of elevated brain lactate and swollen mitochondria have suggested a mitochodrial insult within oligodendrocytes (Kriegstein et al., 1999). If so, then antioxidants may be of use in the treatment of this syndrome (Kriegstein et al., 1999).

Cocaine

This drug is known for causing many neurologic and psychiatric sequelae including seizures, infarction, hemorrhage, vasculitis, anxiety, paranoia, and psychosis. Recent reports have documented a significant increase in white matter hyperintensities on MRI among cocaine-dependent individuals who do not have these complications (Bartzokis et al., 1999). The mechanism of this leukoencephalopathy is thought to relate to vasospasm producing ischemia in the white matter (Bartzokis et al., 1999). Cocaine may also have other white matter effects, as magnetic resonance spectroscopy studies in asymptomatic cocaine abusers showed elevated white matter creatine and myoinositol, possibly indicating involvement of glial cells (Chang et al., 1997).

3,4-Methylenedioxymethamphetamine

This drug, 3,4-methylenedioxymethamphetamine (MDMA), is also known as "ecstacy," and has become a recent and popular addition to the recreational drug list. It is an amphetamine with psychoactive properties that has been most strongly linked to damage of central serotonin neurons (Bolla et al., 1998). However, a case of severe toxic leukoencephalopathy after exposure to MDMA has been reported (Bertram et al., 1999). Myelin damage may occur because of oxidative stress related to serotonergic axonal injury (Sprague et al., 1998).

Psilocybin

A case has been reported of multifocal cerebral demyelination after ingestion of mushrooms presumed to contain psilocybin (Spengos et al., 2000). Although the possibility of immune demyelination could not be ruled out, oligoclonal bands were absent in the cerebrospinal fluid, and the syndrome occurred after each of two exposure incidents in the same patient (Spengos et al., 2000).

Environmental Toxins

Environmental chemicals may produce selective white matter injury. Carbon monoxide heads this list because of its well documented toxic potential and the frequency with which significant exposure comes to clinical attention.

Carbon Monoxide

Carbon monoxide (CO) in the atmosphere mainly results from vehicular fuel combustion, but is also a by-product of home and industrial energy consumption. Accidental or suicidal exposure to CO is common, and the usual injury to the brain is one of hypoxic damage to the neocortex, hippocampus, basal ganglia, and cerebellum leading to immediate and lasting disability in survivors. Other exposed individuals, however, manifest a different clinical course featuring an initial period of recovery and then delayed neurological deterioration with parkinsonism, dementia, and abulia caused by widespread cerebral demyelination, a syndrome first described many decades ago (Grinker, 1926). This syndrome was further clarified by Plum and colleagues, who reported five cases of hypoxia, two with CO poisoning, who developed a similar syndrome approximately 2 weeks after apparent recovery and in whom cerebral demyelination was the consistent finding at autopsy (Plum et al., 1962).

Modern neuroimaging studies have shown expected changes in affected patients: low attenuation in the white matter on CT scans and increased white matter signal on MRI (Chang et al., 1992; Fig. 9-3). In another study of CO poisoning, fluid attentuated inversion recovery imaging was used to document slight demyelination that was clinically asymptomatic (Murata et al., 1995), suggesting that mild forms of this syndrome may occur, and that a threshold of white matter injury is necessary for clinical manifestations to appear. At the other end of the clinical spectrum, demyelination is severe enough to produce white matter damage within the basal ganglia, which leads to Parkinsonism (Sohn et al., 2000). An interesting idea about the pathogenesis of this syndrome is that individuals with reduced activity of the enzyme arylsulfatase A ("pseudodeficiency")—which is completely or nearly absent in patients with metachromatic leukodystrophy—may be predisposed to posthypoxic demyelination (Gottfried et al., 1997). This genetic trait may render the white matter more vulnerable to posthypoxic demyelination even though individuals with pseudodeficiency of arylsulfatase A are considered clinically normal.

Arsenic

Arsenic neurotoxicity was common in the preantibiotic era when treatment of neurosyphilis with arsphenamine produced a hemorrhagic encephalitis that presented as acute encephalopathy (Beckett et al., 1986). Today, arsenic poisoning is rare, although it can occur with exposure to insecticides and rodenticides, and in certain occupations (Freeman and Couch, 1978); suicide has also been attempted with arsenic (Fincher and Koerker, 1987). The most familiar neurotoxicity of this metal

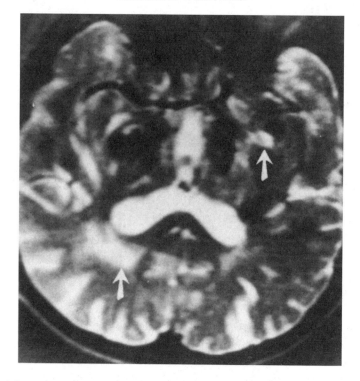

Figure 9-3. T2-weighted MRI scan of a patient with areas of demyelination (*arrows*) that appeared as a delayed effect of carbon monoxide poisoning. (Reprinted with permission from Pomeranz SJ. Craniospinal magnetic resonance imaging. Philadelphia: W.B. Saunders, 1989.)

is peripheral neuropathy (Freeman and Couch, 1978), but acute (Beckett et al., 1986) and prolonged (Freeman and Couch, 1978) cases of encephalopathy have been noted. The neuropathology involves multiple regions of necrosis and hemorrhage in the cerebral white matter (Cole et al., 1966). Treatment with chelating agents may be effective (Beckett et al. 1986; Fincher and Koerker, 1987; Freeman and Couch, 1978).

Carbon Tetrachloride

This is a hydrocarbon extensively used as a fire-extinguishing agent, fumigant, solvent, degreaser, gasoline additive, refrigerant, and paint thinner. The kidneys and liver are the main targets of toxicity, but neurotoxicity can occur as well. Diffuse perivenous hemorrhagic white matter lesions in the cerebrum, cerebellum, and brainstem have been documented in a case of a man who developed confusion, stupor, and coma before expiring from exposure to carbon tetrachloride (Luse and Wood, 1967).

References

Albers JW, Wald JJ, Garabrant DH, et al. Neurologic evaluation of workers previously diagnosed with solvent-induced toxic encephalopathy. J Occup Env Med 2000; 42: 410–423.

Allen JC, Rosen G, Mehta BM, Horten B. Leukoencephalopathy following high-dose Iv methotrexate chemotherapy with leukovorin rescue. Cancer Treat Rep 1980; 64: 1261–1273.

Arlien-Soborg P, Bruhn P, Glydensted C, Melgaard B. Chronic painters' syndrome. Chronic toxic encephalopathy in house painters. Acta Neurol Scand 1979; 60: 149–156.

Armstrong C, Ruffer J, Corn B, et al. Biphasic patterns of memory deficits following moderate-dose partial brain irradiation: neuropsychologic outcome and proposed mechanisms. J Clin Oncol 1995; 13: 2263–2271.

Baker EL. A review of recent research on health effects of human occupational exposure to organic solvents. J Occup Med 1994; 36: 1079–1092.

Bartzokis G, Goldstein IB, Hance DB, et al. The incidence of T2-weighted MR imaging signal abnormalities in the brain of cocaine-dependent patients is age-related and region-specific. AJNR 1999; 20: 1628–1635.

Beckett WS, Moore JL, Keough JP, Bleecker ML. Acute encephalopathy due to occupational exposure to arsenic. Br J Ind Med 1986; 43: 66–67.

Bertram M, Egelhoff T, Schwarz S, Schwab S. Toxic leukoencephalopathy following "ecstacy" ingestion. J Neurol 1999; 246: 627–618.

Bolla KI, McCann UD, Ricaurte GA. Memory impairment in abstinent MDMA ("Ecstacy") users. Neurology 1998; 51: 1532–1537.

Burger PC, Kamenar E, Schold SC, et al. Encephalomyelopathy following high-dose BCNU therapy. Cancer 1981; 48: 1318–1327.

Caldemeyer KS, Pascuzzi RM, Moran CC, Smith RS. Toluene abuse causing reduced MR signal intensity in the brain. AJR 1993; 161: 1259–1261.

Carlen PL, Wortzman G, Holgate RC, et al. Reversible cerebral atrophy in recently abstinent chronic alcoholics measured by computed tomography scans. Science 1978; 200: 1076–1078.

Chang KH, Han MN, Kim HS, et al. Delayed encephalopathy after carbon monoxide intoxication: MR imaging features and distribution of cerebral white matter lesion. Radiology 1992; 184: 117–122.

Chang L, Mehringer CM, Ernst T, et al. Neurochemical alterations in asymptomatic abstinent cocaine users: a proton magnetic resonance spectroscopy study. Biol Psychiatry 1997; 42: 1105–1114.

Charness ME, Simon RP, Greenberg DA. Ethanol and the nervous system. N Engl J Med 1989; 321: 442–454.

Cheung M, Chan AS, Law SC, et al. Cognitive function of patients with nasopharyngeal carcinoma with and without temporal lobe radionecrosis. Arch Neurol 2000; 57: 1347–1352.

Cohen IJ, Stark B, Kaplinsky C, et al. Methotrexate leukoencephalopathy is treatable with high-dose folinic acid: a case report and analysis of the literature. Ped Hem Oncol 1990; 7: 79–87.

Cole M, Scheulein M, Kerwin D. Arsenical encephalopathy due to use of Milibis. Arch Int Med 1966; 17: 706–711.

Constine LS, Knoski A, Ekholm S, et al. Adverse effects of brain irradiation correlated with MR and CT imaging. Int J Radiat Oncol Biol Phys 1988; 15: 319–330.

Corn BW, Yousem DM, Scott DB, et al. White matter changes are correlated significantly with radiation dose. Cancer 1994; 10: 2828–2835.

Crossen JR, Garwood D, Glatstein E, Neuwelt EA. Neurobehavioral sequelae of cranial irradiation in adults: a review of radiation-induced encephalopathy. J Clin Oncol 1994; 12: 627–642.

DeAngelis LM, Delattre J-Y, Posner JB. Radiation-induced dementia in patients cured of brain metastases. Neurology 1989; 39: 789–796.

de la Monte SM. Disproportionate atrophy of cerebral white matter in chronic alcoholics. Arch Neurol 1988; 45: 990–992.

Devinsky O, Lemann W, Evans AC, et al. Akinetic mutism in a bone marrow transplant recipient following total body irradiation and amphotericin B chemoprophylaxis. Arch Neurol 1987; 44: 414–417.

Ferracci F, Conte F, Gentile M, et al. Marchiafava-Bignami disease: computed tomographic scan, 99mTc HMPAO-SPECT, and FLAIR MRI findings in a patient with subcortical aphasia, alexia, bilateral agraphia, and left-handed deficit of constructional ability. Arch Neurol 1999; 56: 107–110.

Filley CM. The behavioral neurology of cerebral white matter. Neurology 1998; 50: 1535–1540.

Filley CM, Rosenberg NL, Heaton RK. White matter dementia in chronic toluene abuse. Neurology 1990; 40: 532–534.

Filley CM. Toxic leukoencephalopathy. Clin Neuropharmacol 1999; 22: 249–260.

Fincher RE, Koerker RM. Long-term survival in acute arsenic encephalopathy. Am J Med 1987; 82: 549–552.

Fletcher JM, Copeland DR. Neurobehavioral effects of central nervous system prophylactic treatment of cancer in children. J Clin Exp Neuropsychol 1988; 10: 495–538.

Freeman JW, Couch JR. Prolonged encephalopathy with arsenic poisoning. Neurology 1978; 28: 853–855.

Gallucci M, Amicarelli I, Rossi A, et al. MR imaging of white matter lesions in uncomplicated chronic alcoholism. J Comput Assist Tomogr 1989; 13: 395–398.

Gass A, Birtsch C, Oster M, et al. Marchiafava-Bignami Disease: reversibility of neuroimaging abnormality. J Comp Assist Tomogr 1998; 22: 503–504.

Gilbert MR. The neurotoxicity of cancer chemotherapy. Neurologist 1998; 4: 43–53.

Ginsberg MD, Hedley-Whyte TE, Richardson EP. Hypoxic-ischemic leukoencephalopathy in man. Arch Neurol 1976; 33: 5–14.

Glantz MJ, Burger PC, Friedman AH, et al. Treatment of radiation-induced nervous system injury with heparin and warfarin. Neurology 1994; 44: 2020–2027.

Gottfried JA, Meyer SA, Shungu DC, et al. Delayed posthypoxic demyelination. Association with arylsulfatase A deficiency and lactic acidosis on proton MR spectroscopy. Neurology 1997; 49: 1400–1404.

Grinker RR. Parkinsonism following carbon monoxid poisoning. J Nerv Ment Dis 1926; 64: 18–28.

Hansen LA, Natelson BH, Lemere C, et al. Alcohol-induced brain changes in dogs. Arch Neurol 1991; 48: 939–942.

Harper C. The neuropathology of alcohol-specific brain damage, or does alcohol damage the brain? J Neuropathol Exp Neurol 1998; 57: 101–110.

Harper CG, Kril JJ, Holloway RL. Brain shrinkage in chronic alcoholics: a pathological study. Br Med J 1981; 290: 501–504.

Hartman DE. Neuropsychological toxicology. New York: Pergamon Press, 1988.

Hommer D, Momenan R, Rawlings R, et al. Decreased corpus callosum size among alcoholic women. Arch Neurol 1996; 53: 359–363.

Hormes JT, Filley CM, Rosenberg NL. Neurologic sequelae of chronic solvent vapor abuse. Neurology 1986; 36: 698–702.

Ihara H, Berrios GE, London M. Group and case study of the dysexecutive syndrome in alcoholism without amnesia. J Neurol Neurosurg Psychiatry 2000; 68: 731–737.

Kleinschmidt-DeMasters BK, Geier JM. Pathology of high-dose intraarterial BCNU. Surg Neurol 1989; 31: 435–443.

Kohler CG, Ances BM, Coleman AR, et al. Marchiafava-Bignami Disease: literature review and case report. Neuropsychiatry Neuropsychol Behav Neurol 2000; 13: 67–76.

Kornfeld M. Leukoencephalopathies due to exogenous factors with features of leukodystrophy: central nervous system damage caused by exposure to solvent vapors (toluene). In: Moser HW, ed. Handbook of Clinical Neurology. Vol.22 (66). Neurodystrophies and neurolipidoses. Amsterdam: Elsevier, 1996: 721–733.

Kornfeld M, Moser AB, Moser HW, et al. Solvent vapor abuse leukoencephalopathy. Comparison to adrenoleukodystrophy. J Neuropathol Exp Neurol 1994; 53: 389–398.

Kreigstein AR, Shungu DC, Millar WS, et al. Leukoencephalopathy and raised brain lactate from heroin vapor inhalation ("chasing the dragon"). Neurology 1999; 53: 1765–1773.

Kril JJ, Halliday GM, Svoboda MD, Cartwright H. The cerebral cortex is damaged in chronic alcoholics. Neuroscience 1997; 79: 983–998.

Lancaster FE. Alcohol and white matter development—a review. Alcohol Clin Exp Res 1994; 18: 644–647.

Lee Y-Y, Nauert C, Glass JP. Treatment-related white matter changes in cancer patients. Cancer 1986; 57: 1473–1482.

Lishman WA. Cerebral disorder in alcoholism. Syndromes of impairment. Brain 1981; 104: 1–20.

Lishman WA. Alcohol and the brain. Br J Psychiatry 1990; 156: 635–644.

Luse SA, Wood WG. The brain in fatal carbon tetrachloride poisoning. Arch Neurol 1967; 17: 304–312.

Martinez AJ, Boehm R, Hadfield MG. Acute hexachlorophene encephalopathy: clinico-neuropathological correlation. Acta Neuropathol 1974; 28: 93–103.

Merritt HH, Weissman AD. Primary degeneration of the corpus callosum (Marchifava-Bignami's disease). J Neuropathol Exp Neurol 1945; 4: 155–163.

Meyers CA, Geara F, Wong PF, Morrison WH. Neurocognitive effects of therapeutic irradiation for base of skull tumors. Int J Radiat Oncol Biol Phys 2000; 46: 51–55.

Moore BD, Copeland DR, Ried H, Levy B. Neurophysiological basis of cognitive deficits in long-term survivors of childhood cancer. Arch Neurol 1992; 49: 809–817.

Morrow LA, Steinhauer SR, Hodgson MJ. Delay in P300 latency in patients with organic solvent exposure. Arch Neurol 1992; 49: 315–320.

Mulhern RK, Reddick WE, Palmer SL, et al. Neurocognitive deficits in medulloblastoma survivors and white matter loss. Ann Neurol 1999; 46: 834–841.

Murata T, Itoh S, Koshino Y, et al. Serial cerebral MRI with FLAIR sequences in acute carbon monoxide poisoning. J Comput Assist Tomogr 1995; 19: 631–634.

Oishi M, Mochizuki Y, Shikata E. Corpus callosum atrophy and cerebral blood flow in chronic alcoholics. J Neurol Sci 1999; 162: 51–55.

Pfefferbaum A, Sullivan EV, Hedehus M, et al. In vivo detection and functional correlates of white matter microstructural disruption in chronic alcoholism. Alcohol Clin Exp Res 2000; 24: 1214–1221.

Plum F, Posner JB, Hain RF. Delayed neurologic deterioration after hypoxia. Arch Int Med 1962; 110: 18–25.

Ratti MT, Soragna D, Sibilla L, et al. Cognitive impairment and cerebral atrophy in "heavy drinkers." Prog Neuropsychopharmacol Biol Psychiatry 1999; 23: 243–258.

Rosenberg NK, Kleinschmidt-DeMasters BK, Davis KA, et al. Toluene abuse causes diffuse central nervous system white matter changes. Ann Neurol 1988b; 23: 611–614.

Rosenberg NL. Neurotoxicity of organic solvents. In: Rosenberg NL, ed. Occupational and environmental neurology. Stoneham, MA: Butterworth-Heinemann, 1995: 71–113.

Rosenberg NL, Spitz MC, Filley CM, et al. Central nervous system effects of chronic toluene abuse—clinical, brainstem evoked response and magnetic resonance imaging studies. Neurotoxicol Teratol 1988a; 10: 489–495.

Ruiz-Martinez J, Perez-Balsa AM, Ruibal M, et al. Marchiafava-Bignami disease with widespread extracallosal lesions and favourable course. Neuroradiology 1999; 41: 40–43.

Schultheiss TE, Kun LE, Ang KK, Stephens LC. Radiation response of the central nervous system. Int J Radiat Oncol Biol Phys 1995; 31: 1093–1112.

Schwartz S, Knauth M, Schwab S, et al. Acute disseminated encephalomyelitis after parenteral therapy with herbal extracts: a report of two cases. J Neurol Neurosurg Psychiatry 2000; 69: 516–518.

Shear PK, Jernigan TL, Butters N. Volumetric magnetic resonance imaging quantification of longitudinal brain changes in abstinent alcoholics. Alcohol Clin Exp Res 1994: 18: 172–176.

Sheline GE, Wara WM, Smith V. Therapeutic irradiation and brain injury. Int J Radiat Oncol Biol Phys 1980; 6: 1215–1228.

Shuman RM, Leech RW, Alford EC. Neurotoxicity of hexachlorophene in humans: a clinicopathological study of 46 premature infants. Arch Neurol 1975; 32: 320–325.

Sohn YH, Jeong Y, Kim HS, et al. The brain lesion responsible for parkinsonism after carbon monoxide poisoning. Arch Neurol 2000; 57: 1214–1218.

Spengos K, Schwartz A, Hennerici M. Multifocal cerebral demyelination after magic mushroom abuse. J Neurol 2000; 247: 224–225.

Sprague JE, Everman SL, Nichols DE. An integrated hypothesis for the serotonergic axonal loss induced by 3,4-methylene-dioxymethamphetamine. Neurotoxicology 1998; 19: 427–441.

Taphoorn MJ, Schiphost AK, Snoek FJ, et al. Cognitive functions and quality of life in patients with low-grade gliomas: the impact of radiotherapy. Ann Neurol 1994; 36: 48–54.

Thuomas K-Ä, Möller C, Ödkvist LM, et al. MR imaging in solvent-induced chronic toxic encephalopathy. Acta Radiol 1996; 37: 177–179.

Tomura N, Kurosawa R, Kato K, et al. Transient neurotoxicity associated with FK-506: MR findings. J Comput Assist Tomogr 1998; 22: 505–507.

Triebig G, Lang C. Brain imaging techniques applied to chronically solvent-exposed workers: current results and clinical evaluation. Environ Res 1993; 61: 239–250.

Truwit CL, Denaro CP, Lake JR, DeMarco T. MR imaging of reversible cyclosporin A-induced neurotoxicity. AJNR 1991; 12: 651–659.

Unger E, Alexander A, Fritz T, et al. Toluene abuse: physical basis for hypointensity of the basal ganglia on T2-weighted images. Radiology 1994; 193: 473–476.

Valk PE, Dillon WP. Radiation injury of the brain. AJNR 1991; 12: 45–62.

Victor M. Persistent altered mentation due to ethanol. Neurol Clin 1993; 11: 639–661.

Walker RW, Rosenblum MK. Amphotericin B-associated leukoencephalopathy. Neurology 1992; 42: 2005–2010.

Weitzner MA, Meyers CA, Valentine AD. Methylphenidate in the treatment of neurobe-havioral slowing associated with cancer and cancer treatment. J Neuropsychiatry Clin Neurosci 1995; 7: 347–350.

Wenz F, Steinvorth S, Lohr F, et al. Acute central nervous system (CNS) toxicity of total body irradiation (TBI) measured using neuropsychological testing of attention functions. Int J Radiat Oncol Biol Phys 1999; 44: 891–894.

White RF, Feldman RG. Neuropsychological assessment of toxic encephalopathy. Am J Ind Med 1987; 11: 395–398.

Wolters EC, van Wijngaarden GK, Stam FC, et al. Leucoencephalopathy after inhaling "heroin" pyrolysate. Lancet 1982; 2: 1233–1237.

Worthley SG, McNeil JD. Leukoencephalopathy in a patient taking low dose oral methotrexate therapy for rheumatoid arthritis. J Rheumatol 1995; 22: 335–337.

Xiong L, Matthes JD, Li J, Jinkins JR. MR imaging of "spray heads": toluene abuse via aerosol paint inhalation. AJNR 1993; 14: 1195–1199.

Yamanouchi N, Okada S, Kodama K, et al. Effects of MRI abnormalities in WAIS-R performance in solvent abusers. Acta Neurol Scand 1997; 34–39.

10

Metabolic Disorders

A number of disorders in the general category of metabolic dysfunction can result in white matter disease of the brain. Although there is considerable overlap between metabolic and toxic disturbances (Chapter 9), the disorders considered in this chapter can be seen as stemming from a metabolic derangement in which clinical, neuroimaging, or neuropathologic evidence of leukoencephalopathy has been observed. The pathophysiology of these diverse disorders is unclear in most cases, but a disturbance of brain metabolism, based on nutritional or other factors, is present in each. Highlighting a theme that recurs in the white matter disorders, many of these conditions are reversible if the metabolic derangement is corrected before irreversible damage develops. Neurobehavioral aspects of these disorders have been gradually characterized and consistent findings have emerged, although precise correlations between white matter lesions and neurobehavioral features are largely unavailable as yet.

Cobalamin Deficiency

One of the most commonly sought causes of reversible dementia is deficiency of cobalamin (vitamin B_{12}). Cobalamin deficiency has been noted in up to 40% of older individuals, and in those who are deficient, as many as 50% have been reported to manifest cerebral symptoms (Goebels and Soyka, 2000). Although classically associated with pernicious anemia, it is now clear that neurologically significant cobalamin deficiency can occur in patients who have no anemia or macro-cytosis (Lindenbaum et al., 1988). Thus routine screening of serum vitamin B_{12} levels in older persons has been recommended (Pennypacker et al., 1992). Controversy exists, however, about the level of cobalamin that indicates significant tissue depletion. It is generally agreed that levels below 100 pg/ml regularly produce neurologic manifestations, and that those above 300 pg/ml are normal. B_{12} levels that fall between these numbers are difficult to interpret, and many recommend the measurement of serum homocysteine and methylmalonic acid in these patients; if one or both of these metabolites are elevated above the normal range, clinically significant cobalamin deficiency can be assumed (Pennypacker et al., 1992).

In cobalamin-deficient patients, peripheral neuropathy is the most common neurologic syndrome, affecting 70% of those with symptoms referable to the nervous system (Healton et al., 1991). In the central nervous system, the familiar syndrome of subacute combined degeneration is also well known as a myelopathy caused by deficient intake of vitamin B_{12}. Relatively little, however, is known about the cerebral manifestations of this disorder.

The neurobehavioral manifestations of cobalamin deficiency are protean. Neuropsychiatric dysfunction has been frequently described (Shorvon et al., 1980), and psychosis appears to be particularly common (Hutto, 1997). A recent study of community-dwelling older women found that metabolically significant cobalamin deficiency conferred a twofold increase in the risk of severe depression (Penninx et al., 2000). Cognitive loss and dementia have also been documented (Meadows et al., 1994; Larner et al. 1999), and the pattern of deficits in these syndromes, which often includes cognitive slowing and confusion along with depression, has been regarded as consistent with subcortical dementia (Tenuisse et al., 1996; Larner et al., 1997).

Although neuropathologic observations of the brain in cobalamin deficiency have long been available (Woltman, 1918; Adams and Kubik, 1944), it is not well recognized that white matter lesions can occur in the brain that are identical to those in the spinal cord. The cerebral lesions usually develop later in the course than cord lesions do, and are characterized by perivascular degeneration of myelinated fibers with sparing of cortical and subcortical gray matter (Adams and Kubik, 1944). Monkeys deprived of cobalamin show white matter changes in the cerebrum that are indistinguishable from those seen in B_{12}-deficient humans (Agamanolis et al., 1976). The underlying pathophysiology of cobalamin deficiency is unknown, but a disturbance of fatty acid synthesis leading to abnormal myelin has been postulated (Shevell and Rosenblatt, 1992).

The cerebral white matter lesions seen neuropathologically have been nominated as responsible for the mental changes in individuals with cobalamin deficiency (Adams and Kubik, 1944). Recent case studies with magnetic resonance imaging (MRI) scans have supported this claim, noting that clinical and neuroradiologic improvement of leukoencephalopathy may occur in parallel with cobalamin replacement (Chatterjee et al., 1996; Stojsavljević et al., 1997). Figure 10-1 shows the MRI appearance of metabolic leukoencephalopathy from cobalamin deficiency before and after treatment. Additional, although indirect, evidence of struc-

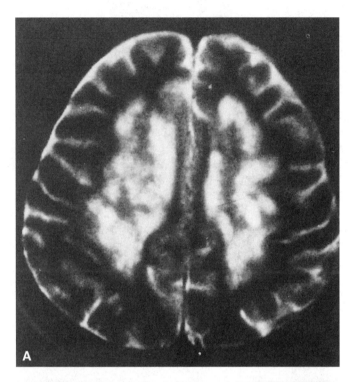

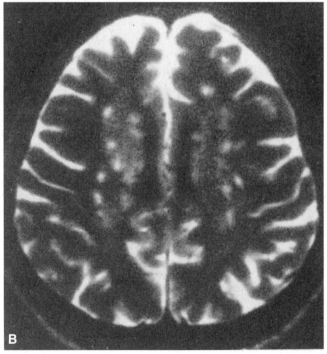

tural white matter involvement in this disease comes from a report of improvement in P300 latency following treatment with cobalamin (Oishi and Moshizuki, 1998).

However, it must be recognized that a variety of biochemical disturbances occur in the brain and may contribute to the neurobehavioral picture of this disorder (Penninx et al., 2000). The biochemistry of cobalamin metabolism is complex, and many factors may contribute to dementia. One area deserving further attention is the effect of hyperhomocysteinemia, which is strongly associated with clinically significant cobalamin deficiency (Lindenbaum et al., 1988). Elevated homocysteine has recently been recognized as an independent risk factor for cerebrovascular disease (Fassbender et al., 1999), and vascular white matter lesions related to elevated homocysteine may also occur in cobalamin deficiency.

Treatment with cobalamin has been observed to benefit neurobehavioral syndromes in some individuals with vitamin B_{12} deficiency. Whether there is true reversibility has been debated, as some investigators describe very few responders (Clarfield, 1988) whereas others report a substantial number (Lindenbaum et al., 1988). It is also unclear how much recovery actually takes place in many patients who are said to be improved. Nevertheless, well-documented examples of significant cognitive and neuroimaging recovery with cobalamin treatment (Meadows et al., 1994; Chatterjee et al., 1996; Stojsavljević et al., 1997) suggest that reversible dementia results from white matter involvement in some individuals with cobalamin deficiency. Further prospective studies with MRI correlations of patients with cobalamin deficiency will be necessary to expand on these findings.

Folate Deficiency

Folate (folic acid) deficiency is another nutritional problem that is pursued frequently in clinical practice, and the measurement of folate continues to be one of the common entries on the list of tests for the routine dementia work-up. Despite this practice, cases of neurologically affected individuals who have folate deficiency are rarely discovered. Nevertheless, some evidence suggests that folate deficiency can cause white matter injury and associated neurobehavioral dysfunction. The syndrome is encountered mostly in alcoholics, and occasionally in individuals taking anticonvulsant drugs and in those with inborn errors of folate metabolism. An interference with the normal synthesis of myelin is suspected (Guettat et al., 1997).

Figure 10-1. T2-weighted MRI scans of a patient with cobalamin deficiency. Diffuse leukoencephalopathy is severe before B_{12} replacement (*A*), whereas after 44 months of treatment with vitamin B_{12} (*B*), the white matter changes are much improved. (Reprinted with permission from Stojsavljević et al. A 44-month clinical-brain MRI follow-up in a patient with B_{12} deficiency. Neurology 1997; 49: 878–881.)

Similar to cobalamin deficiency, the clinical features of folate deficiency may be diverse. Neuropsychiatrically, a tendency for mood disorder has been noted (Hutto, 1997). Dementia has been observed in several cases (Strachan and Henderson, 1967), although the evidence for direct causation by folate deficiency is equivocal (Hutto, 1997). Neuropathologic and neuroimaging studies have been few. An autopsy case of a 2-year-old girl who died from an inborn error of folate metabolism showed striking demyelination throughout the brain and spinal cord (Clayton et al., 1986). An adult with chronic alcoholism studied with brain MRI indicated that leukoencephalopathy can be encountered with folate deficiency (Guettat et al., 1997). Treatment with folate is not always effective but may prove beneficial in some cases; one patient with subacute combined degeneration of the cord and dementia from folate deficiency had an impressive recovery from both syndromes with folate replacement (Pincus et al., 1972).

Central Pontine Myelinolysis

Central pontine myelinolysis (CPM) is a demyelinative disorder of the pons caused by the overly rapid correction of hyponatremia (Karp and Laureno, 2000). Additional areas of demyelination, called extrapontine myelinolysis (Wright et al., 1979), may be seen in the cerebral white matter, thalamus, basal ganglia, and cerebellum, and affect about 10% of CPM patients (Charness et al., 1989). Patients with alcoholism are particularly vulnerable to CPM (Karp and Laureno, 2000). Clinical manifestations include lethargy, confusion, behavioral changes, dysarthria, dysphagia, pseudobulbar palsy, extraocular muscle weakness, and seizures within a few days of overly zealous sodium correction, and the patient may soon progress to stupor and coma. Behavioral changes suggesting a psychiatric disorder may be prominent (Price and Mesulam, 1987; Chalela and Kattah, 1999). The disease can be prevented or minimized by limiting correction of hyponatremia to 10 mEq/L on the first day of treatment (Karp and Laureno, 2000). Initially considered uniformly fatal, CPM is now known to be a disease from which most patients experience substantial recovery (Karp and Laureno, 2000). One case report suggested a beneficial effect of intravenous immunoglobulins (IVIG) in CPM, but spontaneous recovery could not be ruled out (Finsterer et al., 2000).

Neuropathologically, there is myelin loss in affected regions without inflammation, and sparing of axon cylinders and neuronal cell bodies (Wright et al., 1979). Some similarities between this disorder and delayed posthypoxic demyelination (Chapter 9) have been noted, but myelinolysis in CPM is not thought to result from hypoxia (Karp and Laureno, 2000). Rather, CPM is a syndrome of osmotic demyelination caused by a rapid rise in serum sodium (Kleinschmidt-DeMasters and Norenberg, 1981), and thus qualifies as a metabolic disease of white matter. Computed tomography (CT) or MRI scans often disclose a striking focal abnormality in the central pons (Miller et al., 1988; Fig. 10-2), and there can be patchy white matter disease in extrapontine areas (Rippe et al., 1987). The various neurobehavioral deficits in CPM may be related to white matter lesions interfering with the integrity of ascending neurotransmitter systems (Price and Mesulam, 1987).

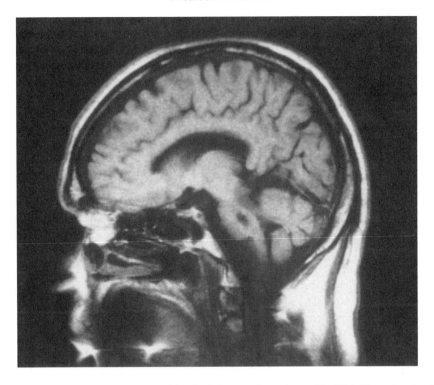

Figure 10-2. Midsagittal T1-weighted MRI scan of a patient with CPM. There is a focal area of white matter loss in the pons.

Hypoxia

Hypoxic injury to the brain is common with a wide range of systemic diseases that share the capacity to reduce oxygen delivery. In Chapter 9, the toxicity of carbon monoxide is discussed as one example of hypoxic brain injury, and the syndrome of delayed cerebral demyelination was reviewed. In this section, other causes of hypoxia that produce an identical clinical picture are considered. Later, in Chapter 11, similar clinical syndromes related to cerebral ischemia are discussed. Whereas the final results of hypoxia and ischemia are virtually indistinguishable in many respects, these separate considerations will be maintained to point out the variety of clinical settings in which white matter can sustain hypoxic-ischemic damage.

In addition to hypoxia from carbon monoxide poisoning, cerebral hypoxia related to surgery and anesthesia, drug overdose, anaphylaxis, strangulation, and seizure disorder can also produce a syndrome of delayed cerebral demyelination (Ginsburg, 1979). It should be recognized that delayed posthypoxic demyelination is a relatively rare phenomenon, occurring in a minority of individuals affected with hypoxia (Ginsburg, 1979). The more common sites for hypoxic injury are in the gray matter of the neocortex, hippocampus, basal ganglia, and cerebellum (Cervos-

Navarro and Diemer, 1991). However, despite its rarity, posthypoxic demyelination may cause a devastating clinical picture including confusion, memory loss, dementia, stupor, and coma; patients may not survive this disorder, and long-term outcome in those who do is frequently poor. Neuroimaging studies have supported the initial clinical–pathologic observations in this syndrome, with white matter degeneration observed on MRI beginning 21 days after hypoxic injury and progressing thereafter (Takahashi et al., 1993). Treatment for this syndrome has been supportive only, but some cases have shown substantial recovery (Plum et al., 1962).

Hypertensive Encephalopathy

A sudden sharp rise in blood pressure can bring about a syndrome of headache, nausea, vomiting, papilledema, and confusion known as hypertensive encephalopathy. In severe cases, stupor and coma can supervene. Both CT (Fisher et al., 1985) and MRI scans (Hauser et al., 1988) in affected patients show white matter lesions that can resolve with treatment of the hypertension, as do the mental status changes (Hauser et al., 1988). The pathophysiology of this syndrome is unclear, but it is thought that vasogenic edema in the white matter accounts for the neuroimaging changes. The changes in mental status also seem to be related to the edema, although clinical–neuropathologic correlations are unavailable because of the prompt recovery of most individuals with antihypertensive treatment.

Recently, cases of reversible posterior leukoencephalopathy have been reported that appear to be similar to hypertensive encephalopathy (Hinchey et al., 1996). In these patients, reversible confusion and visual deficits evolve in parallel with mainly occipital white matter changes; headache, nausea, vomiting, and seizures may also be present. As in hypertensive encephalopathy, vasogenic edema is postulated. The etiology is thought to relate to a brain capillary leak that stems from hypertension and medication effects. Similar to other disorders involving vasogenic edema, recovery is typical, because, as opposed to cases of cytotoxic edema, no neuronal injury has occurred. In view of leukoencephalopathy that may be seen with cylosporine and tacrolimus (Chapter 9), it is noteworthy that immunosuppressive drugs of this group are frequently implicated in reversible posterior leukoencephalopathy (Hinchey et al., 1996).

Eclampsia

Eclampsia is a disorder of pregnancy that has much in common with hypertensive encephalopathy. Hypertension is a core feature of eclampsia, along with variable mental status changes, peripheral edema, proteinuria, and occasionally seizures. An MRI picture identical to that of hypertensive encephalopathy can occur in eclampsia, with a predilection for the posterior hemispheric white matter (Sanders et al., 1991). Neurobehavioral and visual disturbances are thought to derive from lesions in these locations (Sanders et al., 1991). The mechanism of brain involvement may again relate to vasogenic edema secondary to a breakdown of the blood–brain barrier; infarction is unlikely in view of the typical reversibility of the syndrome (Hinchey et al., 1996).

High Altitude Cerebral Edema

A final entry in the category of metabolic white matter disorders is high altitude cerebral edema (HACE)—a rapidly evolving and potentially fatal neurologic syndrome of confusion and ataxia seen in individuals who are at high altitudes (Hackett et al., 1998). The disorder is considered the most severe type of the more common acute mountain sickness, which features headache, fatigue, malaise, nausea, dizziness, anorexia, and sleep disturbance but no neurologic abnormalities (Klocke et al., 1998). Hypoxia is the initiating stimulus of HACE, and the disorder is associated with MRI white matter hyperintensities that are thought to reflect vasogenic edema (Hackett et al., 1998). Clinical and MRI recovery from HACE is ordinarily complete after removal from high altitude and provision of supportive care, further supporting the likelihood that vasogenic edema is the cause of the white matter changes.

Less severe altitudinal hypoxia may also prove harmful. Climbers who ascend to high altitude without the use of supplemental oxygen may develop MRI white matter hyperintensities (Garrido et al., 1993), and subtle neuropsychological deficits can occur in these individuals (Kramer et al., 1993). Thus, hypoxia at high altitude may account for cognitive and white matter abnormalities even in healthy persons who sustain relatively mild degrees of oxygen deprivation. Further study of this phenomenon is warranted.

References

Adams RD, Kubik CS. Subacute degeneration of the brain in pernicious anemia. N Engl J Med 1944; 231: 1–9.

Agamanolis DP, Chester EM, Victor M, et al. Neuropathology of experimental vitamin B_{12} deficiency in monkeys. Neurology 1976; 26: 905–914.

Cervos-Navarro J, Diemer NH. Selective vulnerability in brain hypoxia. Crit Rev Neurobiol 1991; 6: 149–182.

Chalela J, Kattah J. Catatonia due to central pontine and extrapontine myelinolysis: case report. J Neurol Neurosurg Psychiatry 1999; 67: 692–693.

Clarfield AM. The reversible dementias: do they reverse? Ann Int Med 1988; 109: 476–486.

Charness ME, Simon RP, Greenberg DA. Ethanol and the nervous system. N Engl J Med 1989: 321: 442–454.

Chatterjee A, Yapundich R, Palmer CA, et al. Leukoencephalopathy associated with cobalamin deficiency. Neurology 1996; 46: 832–834.

Clayton PT, Smith I, Harding B, et al. Subacute combined degeneration of the cord, dementia, and Parkinsonism due to an inborn error of folate metabolism. J Neurol Neurosurg Psychiatry 1986; 49: 920–927.

Fassbender K, Mielke O, Bertsch T, et al. Homocysteine in cerebral macroangiopathy and microangiopathy. Lancet 1999; 353: 1586–1587.

Finsterer J, Engelmayer E, Trnka E, Stiskal M. Immunoglobulins are effective in pontine myelinolysis. Clin Neuropharmacol 2000; 23: 110–113.

Fisher M, Maister B, Jacobs R. Hypertensive encephalopathy: diffuse reversible white matter CT abnormalities. Ann Neurol 1985: 18: 268–270.

Garrido E, Castello A, Ventura JL, et al. Cortical atrophy and other brain magnetic resonance imaging (MRI) changes after extremely high altitude climbs without oxygen. Int J Sports Med 1993: 14: 232–234.

Ginsburg MD. Delayed neurological deterioration following hypoxia. Adv Neurol 1979; 26: 21–47.

Goebels N, Soyka M. Dementia associated with vitamin B_{12} deficiency: presentation of two cases and review of the literature. J Neuropsychiatry Clin Neurosci 2000; 12: 389–394.

Guettat L, Gille M, Delbecq CQ, Depre A. Folic acid deficiency with leukoencephalopathy and chronic axonal neuropathy of sensory predominance. Rev Neurol 1997; 153: 351–353.

Hackett PH, Yarnell PR, Hill R, et al. High-altitude cerebral edema evaluated with magnetic resonance imaging. Clinical correlation and pathophysiology. JAMA 1998; 280: 1920–1925.

Hauser RA, Lacey DM, Knight MR. Hypertensive encephalopathy. Magnetic resonance imaging of reversible cortical and white matter lesions. Arch Neurol 1988; 45: 1078–1083.

Healton EB, Savage DG, Brust JC, et al. Neurologic aspects of cobalamin deficiency. Medicine 1991; 70: 229–245.

Hinchey J, Chaves C, Appignani B, et al. A reversible posterior leukoencephalopathy syndrome. N Engl J Med 1996; 334: 494–500.

Hutto BR. Folate and cobalamin in psychiatric illness. Comp Psychiatry 1997; 38: 305–314.

Karp BI, Laureno R. Central pontine and extrapontine myelinolysis after correction of hyponatremia. Neurologist 2000; 6: 255–266.

Kleinschmidt-DeMasters BK, Norenberg MD. Rapid correction of hyponatremia causes demyelination: relation to central pontine myelinolysis. Science 1981; 211: 1068–1070.

Klocke DL, Decker WW, Stepanek J. Altitude-related illnesses. Mayo Clin Proc 1998; 73: 988–993.

Kramer AF, Coyne JT, Strayer DL. Cognitive function at high altitude. Hum Factors 1993; 35: 329–344.

Larner AJ, Janssen JC, Cipolotti L, Rossor MN. Cognitive profile in dementia associated with B_{12} deficiency due to pernicious anaemia. J Neurol 1999; 246: 317–319.

Lindenbaum J, Healton EB, Savage DG, et al. Neuropsychiatric disorders caused by cobalamin deficiency in the absence of anemia or macrocytosis. N Engl J Med 1988; 318: 1720–1728.

Meadows M-E, Kaplan RF, Bromfield EB. Cognitive recovery with vitamin B_{12} therapy: a longitudinal neuropsychological assessment. Neurology 1994; 44: 1764–1765.

Miller GM, Baker HL, Okazaki H, et al. Central pontine myelinolysis and its imitators: MR findings. Radiology 1988; 168: 795–802.

Oishi M, Mochizuki Y. Improvement of P300 latency by treatment of B_{12} deficiency. J Clin Neurophysiol 1998; 15: 173–174.

Penninx BWJH, Guralnik JM, Ferrucci L, et al. Vitamin B_{12} deficiency and depression in physically disabled older women: epidemiologic evidence from the Women's Health and Aging Study. Am J Psychiatry 2000; 157: 715–721.

Pennypacker LC, Allen RH, Kelly JP, et al. High prevalence of cobalamin deficiency in elderly outpatients. J Am Geriatr Soc 1992; 40: 1197–1204.

Pincus JH, Reynolds EH, Glaser GH. Subacute combined system degeneration with folate deficiency. JAMA 1972; 221: 496–497.

Plum F, Posner JB, Hain RF. Delayed neurologic deterioration after hypoxia. Arch Int Med 1962; 110: 18–25.

Price BH, Mesulam M-M. Behavioral manifestations of central pontine myelinolysis. Arch Neurol 1987; 44: 671–673.

Rippe DJ, Edwards MK, D-Amour PG, et al. MR imaging of central pontine myelinolysis. J Comput Assist Tomogr 1987; 11: 724–726.

Sanders TG, Clayman DA, Sanchez-Ramos J, et al. Brain in eclampsia: MR imaging with clinical correlation. Radiology 1991; 180: 475–478.

Shevell MI, Rosenblatt DS. The neurology of cobalamin. Can J Neurol Sci 1992; 19: 472–486.

Shorvon SD, Carney MWP, Chanarin I, Reynolds EH. The neuropsychiatry of megaloblastic anaemia. Br Med J 1980; 281: 1036–1038.

Stojsavljević N, Lević Z, Drulović J, Dragutinović G. A 44–month clinical-brain MRI follow-up in a patient with B_{12} deficiency. Neurology 1997; 49: 878–881.

Strachan RW, Henderson JG. Dementia and folate deficiency. Quart J Med 1967; 36: 189–204.

Takahashi S, Higano S, Ishii K, et al. Hypoxic brain damage: cortical laminar necrosis and delayed changes in white matter at sequential MR imaging. Radiology 1993; 189: 449–456.

Tenuisse S, Bollen AE, van Gool WA, Walstra GJM. Dementia and subnormal levels of vitamin B_{12}: effects of replacement therapy on dementia. J Neurol 1996; 243: 522–529.

Woltman HW. Brain changes associated with pernicious anemia. Arch Intern Med 1918; 21: 791–843.

Wright DJ, Laureno R, Victor M. Pontine and extrapontine myelinolysis. Brain 1979; 102: 361–385.

11

Vascular Diseases

Vascular disease is one of the major concerns of clinical neuroscience and medicine. Stroke continues to be the third leading cause of death in the United States, and represents an enormous source of disability from neurologic and neurobehavioral dysfunction. Many controversies persist in the area of vascular disease, but one that has captured much recent attention concerns the importance of the white matter. A lively debate in neurology has centered on the origin and significance of white matter changes that are frequently seen on the neuroimaging scans of older individuals. These findings have prompted a renewed examination of the concept of vascular dementia, which continues to undergo revision. In this chapter, a number of clinical entities in which white matter vascular disease occurs are reviewed, with particular attention to the neurobehavioral implications of these lesions.

Binswanger's Disease

In 1894, the German neuropathologist Otto Binswanger introduced an idea on white matter disease and dementia that has sparked more than a century of controversy. In a three-part article discussing the differential diagnosis of general paresis of the insane, he presented a series of eight patients, of whom one had marked white matter atrophy sparing the cortex and basal ganglia on gross neuropathologic examination, and introduced the term encephalitis subcorticalis chronica progressiva as a disorder of white matter related to insufficient blood supply

(Blass et al., 1991). In so doing, Binswanger made the seminal proposal that ischemic damage to white matter alone could result in mental impairment.

Eight years later, Alzheimer presented additional cases with histologic observations supporting Binswanger's idea that arteriosclerotic white matter disease could produce dementia (Alzheimer, 1902). Alzheimer also introduced the term Binswanger's disease (BD) for this disorder (Roman, 1987), and as time passed, this designation appeared more regularly in the medical literature, although not without controversy. In a major review in 1962, for example, Olszewski translated the articles of Binswanger and Alzheimer and presented two new cases; he emphasized the importance of lacunar infarction in this disease, and offered the alternative name of subcortical arteriosclerotic encephalopathy (Olszewski, 1962). The existence of BD has been vigorously challenged because of the limited neuropathologic data provided in the initial report (Hachinski, 1991). Much energy has been expended on whether the disease exists and if so, whether it should be attributed to Binswanger (Caplan, 1995). However, recent reviews have generally endorsed the terminology using the eponym (Babikian and Ropper, 1987; Fisher, 1989; Caplan, 1995; Hurley et al., 2000), and the name BD continues to receive steady, if somewhat grudging acceptance. Formal diagnostic clinical criteria have been proposed (Bennett et al., 1990), and reference to the term BD is sufficiently common to support its use on a regular basis.

Binswanger's disease can thus be regarded as a form of vascular dementia characterized by prominent involvement of the cerebral white matter. The incidence and prevalence of the disease are not known because no definitive premortem diagnostic test is available; although white matter changes on neuroimaging scans are necessary for the diagnosis, they are not sufficient because they can be seen in other diseases and in normal aging. Despite this diagnostic uncertainty, the disorder nevertheless may be common. Autopsy studies have suggested that as much as 4% of the general population and 35% of dementia patients have the lesions of BD at postmortem examination (Santamaria Ortiz and Knight, 1994). A population-based, prospective study of older individuals with neuropathologic documentation will be required to assess its true prevalence, but BD is a dementing disease that may be more common than is currently appreciated.

Clinically, the disease is associated with hypertension or other vascular risk factors, and presents in mid- to late life with progressive neurologic and neurobehavioral features, often, but not always, with a stepwise course (Babikian and Ropper, 1987; Fisher, 1989; Caplan, 1995). Elemental neurologic features include the subacute onset of focal pyramidal or extrapyramidal signs, acute lacunar syndromes, gait disorder, pseudobulbar signs, and sometimes seizures. Neurobehavioral manifestations include apathy, inertia, abulia, memory impairment, visuospatial dysfunction, and poor judgement and insight. The diagnosis may be difficult in early stages of BD, when all of these features may be subtle. In particular, mental status alterations can be misleading. Frequently, apathy and inertia may be mistaken for the cognitive slowing that is a common feature of normal aging (Chapter 3). In addition, depression is common in BD (Bennett et al., 1994), but may not be appreciated as a feature of the disease in the absence of prominent neurologic dysfunction. Convincing neurologic signs become more apparent as the disease progresses, but early detection is important because of the possibility of treating affected patients before more disabling features develop.

Neuropathologic observations form the foundation for understanding the origin of dementia in BD. The long penetrating arterioles of the deep cerebral white matter are invariably affected by hyalinization of the vessel walls that narrows but usually does not occlude the lumen (Babikian and Ropper, 1987). Ischemia thus develops in the deep white matter, and this same process may also involve the brainstem (Pullicino et al., 1995). In addition, modern formulations have acknowledged that lacunar infarction is present in cerebral areas as well; the finding of lacunar infarction has even led some to equate BD with the lacunar state (Román, 1987). In any case, the cortex is spared from this process, and the subcortical gray matter is less affected than the white matter (Caplan, 1995). Microscopically, findings in early cases may be limited to myelin pallor, but in advanced cases, loss of myelin, axons, and oligodendrocytes is common along with astrocytic gliosis and frank cavitation of the white matter; the subcortical U fibers are typically spared (Babikian and Ropper, 1987).

The neuroradiology of BD is controversial because of lingering doubt about the nosologic status and diagnosis of the disease. With the advent of magnetic resonance imaging (MRI), the initial identification of white matter changes led many to assume that these changes established the presence of BD (Kinkel et al., 1985), but it soon became apparent that white matter changes did not always produce dementia. At present, BD is definitively diagnosed only when appropriate clinical and neuropathologic criteria are met; MRI is supportive if it reveals variable combinations of white matter ischemia and infarcts on T2–weighted scans (Fig. 11-1). In addition to conventional MRI, the application of diffusion-weighted MRI (DWMRI; Choi et al., 2000) and magnetization transfer imaging (MTI; Tanabe et al., 1999) promises to improve the detection and quantitation of white matter changes in BD and the lacunar state, and thus permit more detailed brain–behavior correlations in these disorders.

The precise characterization of cognitive dysfunction in BD is still under study. Babikian and Ropper (1987) emphasized memory loss, confusion, apathy, and changes in mood and behavior that were usually unaccompanied by aphasia, apraxia, and movement disorder. Roman (1987) referred to BD as a subcortical dementia on the basis of the frequency of personality change, forgetfulness and confusion, and the relative rarity of aphasia, apraxia, and agnosia. Stuss and Cummings (1990) endorsed this proposal, adding that the clinical profile of BD reflects dysfunction of the frontal-subcortical axis. Thus, the disease forms a contrast to the cortical syndrome that is often seen with multi-infarct dementia, another form of vascular dementia. Several clinical series have supported this claim, using either mental status or neuropsychological examinations in patients with BD to demonstrate deficits in attention, memory, visuospatial ability, and abstract thinking with relative sparing of language, praxis, and gnosis (Kinkel et al., 1985; Sacquena et al., 1989; Lee et al., 1989). In contrast, when cortical deficits are encountered in patients with BD, concomitant Alzheimer's disease (AD) should be considered (Derix et al.,

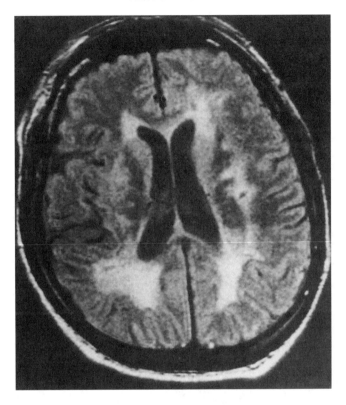

Figure 11-1. Mildly T2-weighted MRI scan of a patient with Binswanger's disease. There is diffuse ischemic white matter disease around the lateral ventricles. (Reprinted with permission from Caplan LR. Caplan's stroke. A clinical approach. 3rd ed. Boston: Butterworth-Heinemann, 2000.)

1987). The available neuropsychological evidence thus suggests that cognitive and emotional dysfunction in BD can best be attributed to subcortical pathology.

The contribution of the white matter disease burden to dementia in BD is a more difficult issue, and the pathogenesis of cognitive dysfunction is not completely settled. As an initial observation germane to this question, recent studies in stroke patients have suggested that part of the clinical picture can be explained by the effects of single lacunar infarctions, after which neurobehavioral deficits may be functionally limiting (van Zandvoort et al., 1998). Thus, even an isolated white matter lacune may produce substantial cognitive loss. Less obvious but probably equally important is the impact of slowly accumulating white matter ischemia. Animal studies have demonstrated a high vulnerability of cerebral white matter to experimental ischemia (Pantoni et al., 1996). Correlations of white matter changes with infarction and ischemia have been made in BD (Révész et al., 1989), and lowered intelligence quotient (IQ) scores have also been correlated with white matter lesions (Loizou et al., 1981). In a quantitative study of vascular dementia patients using MRI, Liu and colleagues (1992) found a strong correlation between white matter lesion area and dementia. Other investigators have suggested that dementia develops when 25% or more of the cerebral white matter is affected (Román et al., 1993). Most recently, studies of MTI in patients with BD have found a significant correlation between cognitive function and decreased magnetization transfer ratio in periventricular white matter (Hanyu et al., 1999).

Additional indirect evidence for white matter involvement in BD affecting cognition is helpful. Caplan and Schoene (1978) and Babikian and Ropper (1987) pointed out a resemblance between the clincal features of BD and normal pressure hydrocephalus, another disease primarily affecting cerebral white matter (Chapter 14). Exploring this possible connection further, Gallassi and colleagues (1991) found similar neuropsychological features in these two diseases. A neuropsychological study of BD found poor concentration, apathy, and cognitive slowing that were interpreted as reflecting prominent frontal lobe disturbance (Bogucki et al., 1991), consistent with white matter dysfunction. Cases have also appeared documenting the onset of psychiatric dysfunction before the advent of cognitive deterioration and neurologic signs (Lawrence and Hillam, 1995), a sequence that has been noted in other white matter disorders (Chapter 17). Although further study of neurobehavioral features is clearly needed, the pattern of deficits and preserved areas is consistent with the profile suggested by the term white matter dementia (Filley, 1998). However, detailed quantitative comparisons of white matter involvement with cortical and particularly subcortical gray matter disease are still required to determine the relative contributions of these tissues in causing dementia.

Treatment of BD is limited by the ambiguity of its pathogenesis. Most authorities advocate control of blood pressure and other vascular risk factors for both prevention and treatment of the disease, but few data are available to guide clinical practice. The role of antiplatelet agents and anticoagulation remains undefined. An encouraging recent trial of the vasodilator nimodipine in subcortical vascular dementia, a new term that encompasses both BD and the lacunar state (Pantoni et al., 2000) merits futher investigation of this agent. Caplan (1995) has raised the interesting possibility that hemorrheologic factors and hyperfibrinogenemia may contribute to microcirculatory impairment of blood flow and offer possibilities for treatment. Symptomatic treatment of apathy and associated cognitive deficits may be possible with stimulant drugs such as methylphenidate (Watanabe et al., 1995).

The many controversies surrounding BD serve to highlight uncertainties about the neurobehavioral implications of white matter disease in general. This issue is well illustrated by cerebrovascular disease. Whereas neurologists have long understood the potential for cortical infarcts to impact cognitive function, this principle has not been as readily applicable to vascular lesions of the white matter. Clinicians rightly point out that single white matter lacunes and ischemic white matter hyperintensities on MRI often have no obvious cognitive correlates. However, the clinical–pathologic entity of BD is gaining increasing credibility as a disease of the cerebral white matter that can have marked effects on behavior, and therefore merits attention as a prototype white matter dementia (Filley, 1998).

Cerebral Autosomal Dominant Arteriopathy with Subcortical Infarcts and Leukoencephalopathy

The concept of white matter ischemic damage as a source of neurobehavioral impairment has been illuminated in the last decade by the discovery of a new disease called cerebral autosomal dominant arteriopathy with subcortical infarcts and leukoencephalopathy (CADASIL; Tournier-Lasserve et al., 1993). This disease is a genetic form of vascular dementia that bears a close resemblance to BD clinically but is caused by genetic mutation rather than cerebral arteriosclerosis. Credit for the first clinical recognition of this disease goes to van Bogaert (1955), who first described a disease similar to BD in two sisters. Several large pedigrees around the world have now been used to confirm that CADASIL maps to chromosome 19q12 (Tournier-Lasserve et al., 1993). A number of different mutations at this locus appear to be responsible. Although this disease qualifies as a genetic disorder (Chapter 5), CADASIL is discussed in this chapter because it is most readily understood in the context of BD.

Clinically, patients with CADASIL are reminiscent of those with BD in many respects. Stroke, dementia, mood disorders, and migraine with aura have been cited as the most frequent clinical features, and the age of onset is mid- to late adulthood (Chabriat et al., 1995). White matter disease on MRI is regularly encountered, even in presymptomatic persons, and takes the form of scattered subcortical lesions that progress with time into confluent leukoencephalopathy (Harris and Filley, 2001; Fig. 11-2). Neurobehavioral dysfunction in the absence of significant elemental neurologic deficits may dominate the clinical course, and early neuropsychiatric dysfunction has been observed to precede the gradual appearance of cognitive decline and dementia (Filley et al., 1999). The profile of cognitive dysfunction may feature abulia, sustained attention deficit, impaired memory retrieval, sparing of language, and perseveration, a pattern consistent with white matter dementia (Filley et al., 1999; Harris and Filley, 2001).

The diagnosis of CADASIL is often problematic. The disease should be considered in normotensive adults who have leukoencephalopathy and clinical features of the disease, and a family history consistent with autosomal dominant inheritance is also helpful. Definitive diagnosis requires blood testing for confirmation of a genetic mutation in the Notch 3 region of chromosome 19 (Tournier-Lasserve et al., 1993). In some cases, ultrastructural changes consisting of granular osmiophilic inclusions in vascular smooth muscle can be seen using electron microscopy of skin obtained by biopsy, but these changes are not always present.

The pathogenesis of neurobehavioral dysfunction in CADASIL is being clarified. Although many cases have a mixture of subcortical white and gray matter disease, careful perusal of published reports shows that dementia can be seen in those with exclusive white matter involvement (Hedera and Friedland, 1997). Studies using conventional MRI have demonstrated that cognitive decline can be correlated with white matter lesion burden in CADASIL (Dichgans et al., 1999). As in BD, both infarction and ischemia appear to contribute to cognitive dysfunction. Recent studies with DWMRI have disclosed that ultrastructural changes in

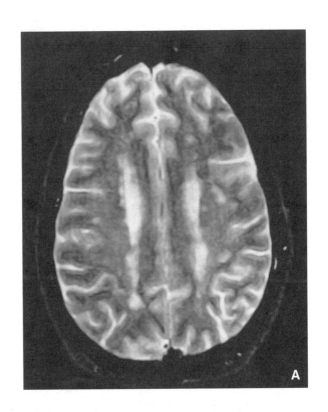

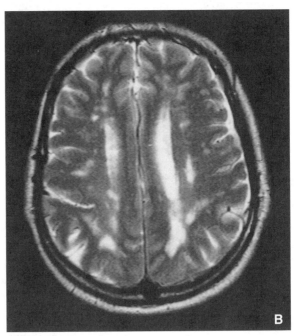

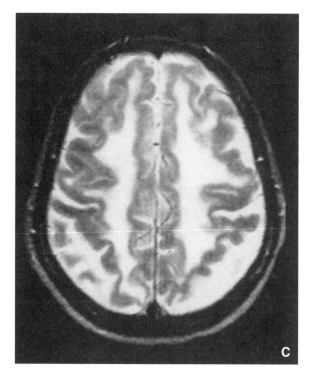

Figure 11-2. T2-weighted MRI scans of three members of a
family with CADASIL: *A,* proband; *B,* his father; and *C,* his
paternal grandmother. Leukoencephalopathy is present on all
scans but is most severe in the oldest patient.

white matter outside of infarcts, both in areas of hyperintensity on T2–weighted
scans and in the normal appearing white matter, also contribute to cognitive loss
(Chabriat et al., 1999). Thus, both infarction and ischemia alone (incomplete infarction) seem to have deleterious effects on cognitive function in this disease.

With regard to the impact of specific regions of white matter disease, the frontal
and temporal lobes have been found to be the regions most affected in CADASIL,
and damage in these areas correlates with attentional, memory, visuospatial, and
conceptual dysfunction (Yousry et al., 1999). This predilection for frontal and
temporal lobe involvement may also help explain the early neuropsychiatric dysfunction that may occur in CADASIL (Filley et al., 1999; Harris and Filley, 2001);
the tendency for cognitive loss to develop later in the disease course has been encountered in other cerebral white matter disorders as well (Filley and Gross,
1992). Longitudinal follow-up of affected individuals with CADASIL will be required to establish this sequence more securely.

Treatment of CADASIL is presently limited to supportive care and prevention
of other risk factors that can worsen the white matter burden already associated

with the disease. The presence of CADASIL does not preclude the possibility of cerebrovascular disease occurring for other reasons. In addition, counseling of family members at risk is advisable because the gene may be passed on to off-spring by presymptomatic individuals who will later develop clinical features of CADASIL. In this respect, the disease is very similar to Huntington's disease, an-other autosomal dominant disease that typically manifests in adulthood.

Leukoaraiosis

As is true of all the disorders considered in this book, the advent of modern neu-roimaging in the last 3 decades has had an enormous impact on vascular white matter disease (Román, 1996). Hence, it has become commonplace for clinicians to encounter unexpected white matter changes on neuroimaging scans of older persons, which are routinely but somewhat tentatively ascribed to ischemia. These changes are so common in older persons with apparently intact cognitive and emo-tional functions that they are often explained solely as a feature of normal aging. Even when the neuroimaging findings are extensive, there is some reluctance to diagnose a specific disorder because of their near ubiquitous presence in seem-ingly normal older individuals. However, this finding has been interpreted by some as a problem of epidemic proportions in the elderly that mandates a vigorous ef-fort by the medical community (van Gijn, 1998).

In 1987, Hachinski and colleagues introduced the term leukoaraiosis to describe white matter changes frequently seen on CT and especially on MRI scans of older persons with or without symptoms and signs of cerebral impairment (Hachinski et al., 1987). These changes take the form of low density white matter areas on CT and white matter hyperintensities on MRI; the descriptor "unidentified bright ob-jects" is often invoked to refer to the MRI changes (Román, 1996; Fig. 11-3). The intent of using leukoaraiosis was to provide a purely descriptive word for these changes, which at that time and still today are not completely understood with re-gard to their pathogenesis and clinical correlates (Hachinski et al., 1987). The cau-tion embodied by the term was appropriate, as some investigators immediately made the premature assumption that these changes represented BD (Kinkel et al., 1985). However, with further work, both the origin and significance of leukoarai-osis became more clear, and in light of more complete information, it is now plau-sible to consider their relationship to more established clinical entities such as BD and CADASIL.

The likely origin of leukoaraiosis does in fact appear to be cerebral ischemia (Pantoni and Garcia, 1997). Clinical studies have found strong associations between leukoaraiosis and cerebrovascular risk factors such as hypertension, diabetes melli-tus, cardiac disease, and prior history of stroke (Gerard and Weisberg, 1986; Inzitari et al., 1987). Cerebral blood flow studies have generally shown reduced white mat-ter perfusion while gray matter is normal (Markus et al., 2000). Consistent with these observations, several neuropathologic studies have found arteriosclerotic changes within areas of leukoaraiosis (Awad et al., 1986; Leifer et al., 1990; Fazekas et al.,

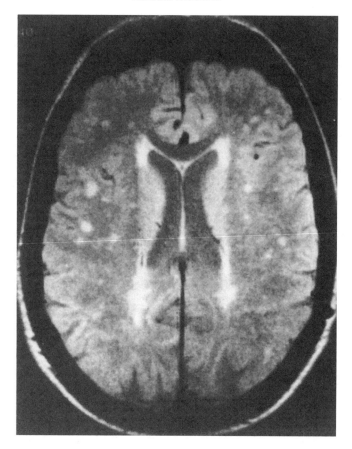

Figure 11-3. Mildly T2-weighted MRI scan of an aymptomatic older individual with leukoaraiosis. Scattered white matter hyperintensities are seen thoughout the cerebrum. (Reprinted with permission from Brant-Zawadski M, Norman D, eds. Magnetic resonance imaging of the central nervous system. New York: Raven Press, 1987.)

1993). The small penetrating arterioles supplying the white matter show narrowing of the lumen secondary to the accumulation of hyaline material (Pantoni and Garcia, 1997), findings very similar to those seen in BD (Caplan, 1995). Other similarities include a range of white matter lesions from localized ischemia to cavitation, the presence of lacunar infarction in some cases, and the sparing of the subcortical U fibers (Pantoni and Garcia, 1997). Many believe that recurrent transient hypotension producing incomplete infarction in the white matter is at the basis of leukoaraiosis (Pantoni and Garcia, 1997). Despite the vaidity of these considerations, however, leukoaraiosis remains a neuroradiologic finding that in a given patient may represent nonvascular conditions such as dilation of perivascular Virchow-Robin spaces (état criblé) or periventricular rims, caps, and halos—all of which are benign—or the demyelinative plaques of multiple sclerosis (MS) (Merino and Hachinski, 2000).

The neurobehavioral significance of leukoaraiosis has been vigorously disputed, but in light of more data a coherent view is emerging. Early studies using conventional MRI and neuropsychological testing frequently found no correlation of white matter changes with cognitive dysfunction (Filley et al., 1989; Rao et al., 1989). Subsequent research found that such correlations could be made, and the main cognitive domains affected appeared to be attention and cognitive speed (Junqué et al, 1990; van Swieten et al., 1991; Schmidt et al., 1993; Ylikoski et al., 1993). The resolution of these inconsistent results may be provided by considering the degree of white matter change. Boone and colleagues (1992) found that a threshold of 10 cm^2 of affected white matter was required before cognitive dysfunction could be detected. In this respect, leukoaraiosis recalls a similar observation in MS that a certain threshold of demyelination must be reached before cognitive impairment occurs (Chapter 6). Recent large-scale studies of older individuals have continued to find strong correlations between the severity of leukoaraiosis and cognitive dysfunction (Longstreth et al., 1996; de Groot et al., 2000). The application of diffusion tensor MRI has recently disclosed diminished anisotropy in patients with leukoaraiosis, suggesting that details of pathogenesis and progression can be further elucidated with this technique (Jones et al., 1999).

Moreover, additional neurologic morbidity and even mortality may be associated with leukoaraiosis. Longstreth and colleagues (1996) found a significant association of leukoaraiosis with gait disorder, and Briley and colleagues (2000) found that leukoaraiosis increases morbidity and mortality in part because of a higher risk of falls. Because of the wide distribution of white matter and the probability of multifocal white matter involvement interfering with the operations of many distributed neural networks, it is not surprising that leukoaraoisis of sufficient magnitude can disrupt elemental as well as higher neurologic functions.

Thus, it would seem that leukoaraiosis in an otherwise intact older person may be asymptomatic, or if more advanced, associated with neurologic deficits including cognitive impairments and gait disorder. These conclusions, combined with neuroradiologic and neuropathologic commonalities, lend support to the notion that leukoaroisis may lie on the same clinical–pathologic spectrum as BD (Filley et al., 1988; van Swieten et al., 1991; Román, 1996). If so, one important implication is that vigorous treatment of leukoaraiosis, perhaps by modifcation of vascular risk factors, may significantly deter the onset of age-related cognitive decline. Whereas it may be unjustified to proclaim a "silent epidemic" of leukoaraiosis as an imminent harbinger of widespread dementia in the elderly population (van Gijn, 1998), there are sufficient reasons to move forward with studies addressing the hypothesis that leukoaraiosis is a precursor of BD.

Cerebral Amyloid Angiopathy

Cerebral amyloid angiopathy (CAA) is an idiopathic disorder, distinct from the systemic amyloidoses, characterized by the deposition of amyloid in the cerebral and leptomeningeal vasculature. Best known for its propensity to cause intracerebral and subarachnoid hemorrhage, CAA is also associated with dementia. The disorder can be seen in patients with AD (Mandybur, 1975), and may cause multiple strokes that worsen the dementia severity (Caplan, 2000). Thus, CAA may contribute to the higher frequency of white matter changes in patients with AD (Filley et al., 1989; Brun and Englund, 1986), and account for the more severe clinical course that this additional burden implies (Janota, et al., 1989). In some individuals, CAA may produce a prominent leukoencephalopathy as its only manifestation (Janota et al., 1989; Loes et al., 1990; Imaoka et al., 1999), and these white matter changes may in fact represent BD (Yoshimura et al., 1992; Caplan, 2000). As in those with BD, the leukoencephalopathy likely accounts for dementia in these patients. Although CAA is usually associated with dementia because of intracerebral hemorrhage, multiple strokes, or AD, the disorder may also lead to dementia because of leukoencephalopathy.

White Matter Disease of Prematurity

The increasing survival of premature infants due to improved perinatal care in the last several decades has brought to light two important disorders of the white matter that occur very early in development: periventricular leukomalacia and periventricular hemorrhage (Perlman, 1998). These problems, which often lead to cerebral palsy and mental retardation, are major determinants of poor long-term neurologic and neurobehavioral outcome in these infants (Perlman, 1998; Stewart et al., 1999). Although details of pathogenesis in these disorders remain controversial, enough similarities with adult vascular white matter disease exist to justify their discussion in this chapter. Evidence continues to mount that primary damage to white matter in the developmental period has enormous implications for neurobehavioral function throughout later life.

Periventricular leukomalacia occurs in 4%–15% of premature infants and features both focal and diffuse cerebral white matter injury (Perlman, 1998). Cognitive impairment and spastic diplegia are recognized sequelae. Neuropathologically, the focal lesions represent areas of necrosis, and the diffuse involvement reflects loss of myelin and glial cells; all lesions are essentially confined to white matter, as the cortex and subcortical gray matter are virtually unaffected (Banker and Larroche, 1962; DeReuck et al., 1972; Young et al., 1982). Cyst formation follows in many cases within a few weeks, particularly in focal areas of necrosis. Cranial ultrasound has been instrumental in detecting the areas of focal necrosis and cyst formation, and MRI has also been used to assess diffuse injury (Van de Bor et al., 1992). Conventional MRI studies demonstrate increased signal in the cerebral white matter on T2–weighted scans (Fig. 11-4), and recent studies have also suggested that DWMRI can detect diffuse white matter involvement even when conventional MRI is normal (Inder et al., 1999). Cognitive impairment is correlated with increased lateral ventricular volume, which is a marker of white matter injury (Melhem et al., 2000). Neuropsychological studies of the pattern of cognitive impairment have generally shown a greater effect on nonverbal than on verbal

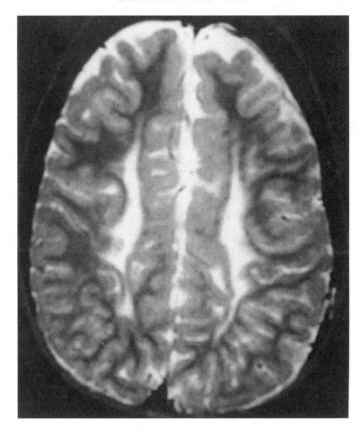

Figure 11-4. T2-weighted MRI scan of a patient with periventricular leukomalacia. The cerebral white matter lesions are bilateral and symmetric. (Reprinted with permission from Atlas SW, ed. Magnetic resonance imaging of the brain and spine. 2nd ed. Philadelphia: Lippincott-Raven, 1996.)

skills (Fedrizzi et al., 1996), possibly caused by the greater proportion of affected white matter in the right hemisphere than in the left (Chapter 2). Many investigators have attributed the white matter injury to reduced blood flow from hypotension (Banker and Larroche, 1962; DeReuck et al., 1972; Young et al., 1982), but the exact mechanism of periventricular leukomalacia remains uncertain because inflammatory and infectious factors have been implicated in addition to ischemic insult (Kuban, 1998). Delayed myelination leading to ventriculomegaly has also been suggested to occur in these infants (Leviton and Gilles, 1996). The possibility has been raised that cerebral white matter ischemia may interfere with normal myelination by diverting stem cells into reactive astrocytes and reducing the population of oligodendrocytes available to synthesize myelin (Squier and Keeling,

1991). Treatment has been supportive, but a recent report describing a protective effect of betamethasone is encouraging (Baud et al., 1999).

Periventricular hemorrhage affects 10%–15% of infants weighing less than 1000 grams at birth (Perlman, 1998). Hemorrhage of this kind remains a major source of long-term neurobehavioral sequelae in affected individuals. This is typically a unilateral periventricular white matter hemorrhage that arises from the ependymal germinal matrix and frequently ruptures into the adjacent lateral ventricle (Kuban, 1999). The germinal matrix is a transitional region absent at term, but in prematurity it is vulnerable to hypertension in both arterial and venous vessels that is presumed to underlie the pathogenesis of this injury (Perlman, 1998). The diagnosis is usually made by ultrasound, but white matter damage may also be detected by MRI in later life (Stewart et al., 1999). Cognitive and motor deficits are frequent in survivors (Guzzetta et al., 1986; Stewart et al., 1987), and with extensive hemorrhage, there is little chance for normal cognitive or motor function later in life (Guzzetta et al., 1986). Antenatal corticosteroids can significantly reduce the incidence of periventricular hemorrhage in premature infants (Crowley, 1995), and indomethacin appears promising for prevention of this complication in the postnatal period (Perlman, 1998).

Migraine

A final vascular disorder of the white matter deserving comment is migraine. Although not usually considered a structural disease of the brain, migraine can rarely be associated with cerebral infarction (Tietjen, 2000). Magnetic resonance imaging white matter changes, however, are seen with some regularity in migraineurs; in one series of 129 consecutive migraine patients, 19% had deep white matter abnormalities on T2–weighted scans (Pavese et al., 1994). Preliminary evidence suggests that these changes are more frequent in individuals with classic migraine (Soges et al., 1998), and some investigators have suggested that these represent areas of microinfarction (Ferbert et al., 1991). In addition, migraine associated with prolonged aura and white matter lesions may represent an unusual phenotype of CADASIL (Ceroni et al., 2000; see above).

The clinical significance of white matter lesions in migraine is unclear, and major cognitive deficits have not been demonstrated. However, clinically normal young men with a small degree of white matter hyperintensity on MRI have been found to have reduced attentional capacity (Lewine et al., 1993). Thus, in those migraine patients who have white matter changes, the usual lesion burden is probably below the threshold for neurobehavioral features to be clinically manifest, but subtle decrements may be detectable on careful neuropsychological testing. These considerations once again raise the possibility that white matter lesions may be associated with a wide variety of neurobehavioral changes, which may include attentional compromise at the mild end of the spectrum.

References

Alzheimer A (1902). Mental disturbances of arteriosclerotic origin (Förstl H, Howard R, Levy R, tr.). Neuropsychiatry Neuropsychol Behav Neurol 1992; 5: 1–6.

Awad I, Johnson PC, Spetzler RF, Hodak JA. Incidental subcortical lesions identified on magnetic resonance imaging in the elderly. II. Postmortem pathological correlations. Stroke 1986: 17: 1090–1097.

Babikian V, Ropper AH. Binswanger's disease: a review. Stroke 1987; 18: 2–12.

Banker BQ, Larroche JC. Periventricular leukomalacia in infancy. Arch Neurol 1962; 7: 386–410.

Baud O, Foix-L'Helias L, Kaminski M, et al. Antenatal glucocorticoid treatment and cystic periventricular leukomalacia in very premature infants. N Engl J Med 1999; 341: 1190–1196.

Bennett DA, Gilley DW, Lee S, Cochran EJ. White matter changes: neurobehavioral manifestations of Binswanger's disease and clinical correlates in Alzheimer's Disease. Dementia 1994; 5: 148–152.

Bennett DA, Wilson RS, Gilley DW, Fox JH. Clinical diagnosis of Binswanger's Disease. J Neurol Neurosurg Psychiatry 1990; 53: 961–965.

Blass JP, Hoyer S, Nitsch R. A translation of Otto Binswanger's article, "The delineation of the generalized progressive paralyses." Arch Neurol 1991; 48: 961–972.

Bogucki A, Janczewska E, Koszewska I, et al. Evaluation of dementia in subcortical arteriosclerotic encephalopathy (Binswanger's Disease). Eur Arch Psychiatry Clin Neurosci 1991; 241: 91–97.

Boone KB, Miller BL, Lesser IM, et al. Neuropsychological correlates of white-matter lesions in healthy elderly subjects. A threshold effect. Arch Neurol 1992; 49: 549–554.

Briley DP, Haroon S, Sergent SM, Thomas S. Does leukoaraiosis predict morbidity and mortality? Neurology 2000; 54: 90–94.

Brun A, Englund E. A white matter disorder in dementia of the Alzheimer's disease: a pathoanatomical study. Ann Neurol 1986; 19: 253–262.

Caplan LR. Binswanger's disease—revisited. Neurology 1995; 45: 626–633.

Caplan LR. Caplan's stroke. A clinical approach. 3rd ed. Boston: Butterworth-Heinemann, 2000.

Caplan LR, Schoene WC. Clinical features of subcortical arteriosclerotic encephalopathy (Binswanger disease). Neurology 1978; 28: 1206–1215.

Ceroni M, Poloni TE, Tonietti S, et al. Migraine with aura and white matter abnormalities: Notch3 mutation. Neurology 2000; 54: 1869–1871.

Chabriat H, Pappata S, Poupon C, et al. Clinical severity in CADASIL related to ultrastructural damage in white matter. In vivo study with diffusion tensor MRI. Neurology 1999; 30: 2637–2643.

Chabriat H, Vahedi K, Iba-Zizen MT, et al. Clinical spectrum of CADASIL: a study of 7 families. Lancet 1995; 346: 934–939.

Choi SH, Na DL, Chung CS, et al. Diffusion-weighted MRI in vascular dementia. Neurology 2000; 54: 83–89.

Crowley P. Antenatal corticosteroid therapy: a meta-analysis of the randomized trials. Am J Obstet Gynecol 1995; 173: 322–335.

De Groot JC, de Leeuw F-E, Oudkerk M, et al. Cerebral white matter lesions and cognitive function: the Rotterdam Scan study. Ann Neurol 2000; 47: 145–151.

DeReuck J, Chatta AS, Richardson EP. Pathogenesis and evolution of periventricular leukomalacia in infancy. Arch Neurol 1972; 27: 229–236.

Derix MMA, Hijdra A, Verbeeten BE. Mental changes in subcortical arteriosclerotic encephalopathy. Clin Neurol Neurosurg 1987; 89: 71–78.

Dichgans M, Filippi M, Brüning R, et al. Quantitative MRI in CADASIL. Correlation with disability and cognitive performance. Neurology 1999; 52: 1361–1367.

Fazekas F, Kleinert R, Offenbacher H, et al. Pathologic correlates of incidental MRI white matter signal hyperintensities. Neurology 1993; 43: 1683–1689.

Fedrizzi E, Inverno M, Bruzzone MG, et al. MRI features of cerebral lesions and cognitive functions in preterm spastic diplegia children. Pediatr Neurol 1996; 15: 207–212.

Ferbert A, Busse D, Thron A. Microinfarction in classic migraine? A study with magnetic imaging findings. Stroke 1991, 22: 1010–1014.

Filley CM, Davis KA, Schmitz SP, et al. Neuropsychological performance and magnetic resonance imaging in Alzheimer's disease and normal aging. Neuropsychiatry Neuropsychol Behav Neurol 1989; 2: 81–91.

Filley CM, Franklin GM, Heaton RK, Rosenberg NL. White matter dementia: clinical disorders and implications. Neuropsychiatry Neuropsychol Behav Neurol 1988; 1: 239–254.

Filley CM, Gross KF. Psychosis with cerebral white matter disease. Neuropsychiatry Neuropsychol Behav Neurol 1992; 5: 119–125.

Filley CM. The behavioral neurology of cerebral white matter. Neurology 1998; 50: 1535–1540.

Filley CM, Thompson LL, Sze C-I, et al. White matter dementia in CADASIL. J Neurol Sci 1999; 163; 163–167.

Fisher CM. Binswanger's encephalopathy. J Neurol 1989; 236: 65–79.

Gallassi R, Morreale A, Montagna P, et al. Binswanger's disease and normal-pressure hydrocephalus. Clinical and neuropsychological comparison. Arch Neurol 1991; 48: 1156–1159.

Gerard G, Weisberg LA. MRI periventricular lesions in adults. Neurology 1986; 36: 998–1001.

Guzzetta F, Shackleford GD, Volpe S, et al. Periventricular intraparenchymal echodensities in the premature newborn: critical determinant of neurologic outcome. Pediatrics 1986; 78: 995–1006.

Hachinski VC. Binswanger's disease: neither Binswanger's nor a disease. J Neurol Sci 1991; 103: 1.

Hachinski VC, Potter P, Merskey H. Leuko-araiosis. Arch Neurol 1987; 44: 21–23.

Harris JG, Filley CM. CADASIL: Neuropsychological findings in three generations of an affected family. J Int Neuropsychol Soc, 2001; 7: 768–774.

Hanyu H, Asano T, Sakurai H, et al. Magnetization transfer ratio in cerebral white matter lesions of Binswanger's Disease. J Neurol Sci 1999; 166: 85–90.

Hedera P, Friedland RP. Cerebral autosomal dominant arteriopathy with subcortical infarcts and leukoencepahlopathy: study of two American families with predominant dementia. J Neurol Sci 1997; 146: 27–33.

Hurley RA, Tomimoto H, Akiguchi I, et al. Binswanger's Disease: an ongoing controversy. J Neuropsychiatry Clin Neurosci 2000; 12: 301–304.

Imaoka K, Kobayashi S, Fujihara S, et al. Leukoencephalopathy with cerebral amyloid angiopathy: a semiquantitative and morphometric study. J Neurol 1999; 246: 661–666.

Inder T, Huppi PS, Zientara GP, et al. Early detection of periventricular leukomalacia by diffusion-weighted magnetic resonance imaging techniques. J Pediatr 1999; 134: 631–634.

Inzitari D, Diaz F, Fox A, et al. Vascular risk factors and leuko-araiosis. Arch Neurol 1987; 44: 42–47.

Janota I, Mirsen TR, Hachinski VC, et al. Neuropathologic correlates of leuko-araiosis. Arch Neurol 1989; 46: 1124–1128.

Jones DK, Lythgoe D, Horsfield MA, et al. Characterization of white matter damage in ischemic leukoaraiosis with diffusion tensor MRI. Stroke 1999; 30: 393–397.

Junqué C, Pujol J, Vendrell P, et al. Leuko-araiosis on magnetic resonance imaging and speed of mental processing. Arch Neurol 1990; 47: 151–156.

Kinkel WR, Jacobs L, Polachini I, et al. Subcortical arteriosclerotic encephalopathy (Binswanger's Disease). Arch Neurol 1985; 42: 951–959.

Kuban K, Sanocka U, Leviton A, et al. White matter disorders of prematurity: association with intraventricular hemorrhage and ventriculomegaly. J Pediatr 1999; 134: 539–546.

Kuban KCK. White-matter disease of prematurity, periventricular leukomalacia, and ischemic lesions. Dev Med Child Neurol 1998; 40: 571–573.

Lawrence RM, Hillam JC. Psychiatric symptomatology in early-onset Binswanger's disease: two case reports. Behav Neurol 1995; 8: 43–46.

Lee A, Yu YL, Tsoi M, et al. Subcortical arteriosclerotic encephalopathy—a controlled psychometric study. Clin Neurol Neurosurg 1989; 91: 235–241.

Leifer D, Buonanno FS, Richardson EP. Clinicopathologic correlates of cranial magnetic resonance imaging of periventricular white matter. Neurology 1990; 40: 911–918.

Leviton A, Gilles F. Ventriculomegaly, delayed myelination, white matter hypoplasia, and "periventricular" leukomalacia: how are they related? Pediatr Neurol 1996; 15: 127–136.

Lewine R, Hudgins P, Risch SC, Walker EF. Lowered attention capacity in young, medically healthy men with magnetic resonance brain hyperintensity signals. Neuropsychiatry Neuropsychol Behav Neurol 1993; 6: 38–42.

Liu CK, Miller BL, Cummings JL, et al. A quantitative MRI study of vascular dementia. Neurology 1992; 42: 138–143.

Loes DJ, Biller J, Yuh WTC, et al. Leukoencephalopathy in cerebral amyloid angiopathy: MR imaging in four cases. AJNR 1990; 11: 485–488.

Loizou LA, Kendall BE, Marshall J. Subcortical arteriosclerotic encephalopathy: a clinical and radiological investigation. J Neurol Neurosurg Psychiatry 1981; 44: 294–304.

Longstreth WT, Manolio TA, Arnold A, et al. Clinical correlates of white matter findings on cranial magnetic resonance imaging of 3301 elderly people. The Cardiovascular Health Study. Stroke 1996; 27: 1274–1282.

Mandybur TI. The incidence of cerebral amyloid angiopathy in Alzheimer's disease. Neurology 1975; 25: 120–126.

Markus HS, Lythgoe DJ, Ostegaard L, et al. Reduced cerebral blood flow in white matter in ischaemic leukoaraiosis demonstrated using quantitative exogenous contrast based perfusion MRI. J Neurol Neurosurg Psychiatry 2000; 69: 48–53.

Melhem ER, Hoon AH, Ferrucci JT, et al. Periventricular leukomalacia: relationship between lateral ventricular volume on brain MR images and severity of cognitive and motor impairment. Radiology 2000; 214: 199–204.

Merino JG, Hachinski V. Leukoaraiosis. Reifying rarefaction. Arch Neurol 2000; 57: 925–926.

Olszewski J. Subcortical arteriosclerotic encephalopathy: review of the literature on the so-called Binswanger's disease and presentation of two cases. World Neurol 1962; 3: 359–374.

Pantoni L, Garcia JH. Pathogenesis of leukoaraiosis. A review. Stroke 1997; 28: 652–659.

Pantoni L, Garcia JH, Gutierrez JA. Cerebral white matter is highly vulnerable to ischemia. Stroke 1996; 27: 1641–1647.

Pantoni L, Rossi R, Inzitari D, et al. Efficacy and safety of nimodipine in subcortical vascular dementia: a subgroup analysis of the Scandinavian Multi-Infarct Dementia Trial. J Neurol Sci 2000; 175: 124–134.

Pavese N, Canapicchi R, Nuti A, et al. White matter MRI hyperintensities in a hundred and twenty-nine consecutive migraine patients. Cephalalgia 1994; 14: 342–345.

Perlman JM. White matter injury in the preterm infant: an important determination of abnormal neurodevelopment outcome. Early Hum Dev 1998; 53: 99–120.

Pullicino P, Ostrow P, Miller L, et al. Pontine ischemic rarefaction. Ann Neurol 1995; 37: 460–466.

Rao SM, Mittenberg W, Bernardin L, et al. Neuropsychological test findings in subjects with leukoaraiosis. Arch Neurol 1989; 46: 40–44.

Révész T, Hawkins CP, du Boulay EPGH, et al. Pathological findings correlated with magnetic resonance imaging in subcortical arteriosclerotic encephalopathy (Binswanger's disease). J Neurol Neurosurg Psychiatry 1989; 52: 1337–1344.

Román GC. Senile dementia of the Binswanger type. A vascular form of dementia in the elderly. JAMA 1987; 258: 1782–1788.

Román GC. From UBOs to Binswanger's disease. Impact of magnetic resonance imaging on vascular dementia research. Stroke 1996; 27: 1269–1273.

Román GC, Tatemichi TK, Erkinjuntti T, et al. Vascular dementia: diagnostic criteria for research studies. Report of the NINDS-AIREN International Workshop. Neurology 1993; 43: 250–260.

Sacquena T, Guttmann S, Giuliani S, et al. Binswanger's disease: a review of the literature and a personal contribution. Eur Neurol 1989; 29 (suppl 2): 20–22.

Santamaria Ortiz J, Knight PV. Binswanger's disease, leukoaraiosis and dementia. Age Ageing 1994; 23: 75–81.

Schmidt R, Fazekas F, Offenbacher H, et al. Neuropsychologic correlates of MRI white matter hyperintensities: a study of 150 normal volunteers. Neurology 1993; 43: 2490–2494.

Soges LJ, Cacayorin ED, Petro GR, Ramachandran TS. Migraine: Evaluation by MR. AJNR 1988; 9: 425–429.

Squier M, Keeling JW. The incidence of prenatal brain injury. Neuropathol Appl Neurobiol 1991; 17: 29–38.

Stewart AL, Reynolds EO, Hope PL, et al. Probability of neurodevelopmental disorders estimated from ultrasound appearance of brains of very preterm infants. Dev Med Child Neurol 1987; 29: 3–11.

Stewart AL, Rifkin L, Amess PN, et al. Brain structure and neurocognitive and behavioural function in adolescents who were born very preterm. Lancet 1999; 353: 1653–1657.

Stuss DT, Cummings JL. Subcortical vascular dementias. In: Cummings JL, ed. Subcortical dementia. New York: Oxford University Press, 1990: 145–163.

Tanabe JL, Ezekiel F, Jagust WJ, et al. Magnetization transfer ratio of white matter hyperintensities in subcortical vascular dementia. AJNR 1999; 20: 839–844.

Tietjen GE. The relationship of migraine and stroke. Neuroepidemiology 2000; 19: 13–19.

Tournier-Lasserve E, Joutel A, Melki J, et al. Cerebral autosomal dominant arteriopathy with subcortical infarcts and leukoencephalopathy maps to chromosome 19q12. Nature Gen 1993; 3: 256–259.

van Bogaert L. Encéphalopathie sous corticale progressive (Binswanger) à évolution rapide chez des soeurs. Méd Hellen 1955; 24: 961–972.

van de Bor M, den Ouden L, Guit GL. Value of cranial ultrasound and magnetic resonance imaging in predicting neurodevelopmental outcome in preterm infants. Pediatrics 1992; 90: 196–199.

van Gijn J. Leukoaraiosis and vascular dementia. Neurology 1998; 51(suppl 3): S3–S8.

van Sweiten JC, Geyskes GG, Derix MMA, et al. Hypertension in the elderly is associated with white matter lesions and cognitive decline. Ann Neurol 1991; 30: 825–830.

van Zandvoort MJE, Kapelle LJ, Algra A, De Haan EHF. Decreased capacity for mental effort after single supratentorial lacunar infarct may affect performance in everyday life. J Neurol Neurosurg Psychiatry 1998; 65: 697–702.

Ylikoski R, Ylikoski A, Erkinjuntti T, et al. white matter changes in healthy elderly persons correlate with attention and speed of mental processing. Arch Neurol 1993; 50: 818–824.

Yoshimura M, Yamanouchi H, Kuzuhara S, et al. Dementia in cerebral amyloid angiopathy: a clinicopathological study. J Neurol 1992; 239: 441–450.

Young RSK, Hernandez MJ, Yagel SK. Selective reduction of blood flow to white matter during hypotension in newborn dogs: a possible mechanism of periventricular leukomalacia. Ann Neurol 1982: 12: 445–448.

Yousry TA, Seelos K, Mayer M, et al. Characteristic MR lesion pattern and correlation of T1 and T2 lesion volume with neurologic and neuropsychological findings in cerebral autosomal dominant arteriopathy with subcortical infarcts and leukoencephalopathy (CADASIL). AJNR 1999; 20: 91–100.

Watanabe MD, Martin EM, DeLeon OA, et al. Successful methylphenidate treatment of apathy after subcortical infarcts. J Neuropsychiatry Clin Neurosci 1995; 7: 502–504.

12

Traumatic Disorders

Trauma to the brain can occur because of accidents, assaults, sporting contests, or intentional therapeutic maneuvers. This problem is one of the most urgent in neurology and medicine, as traumatic brain injury (TBI) from motor vehicle accidents and other events constitutes one of the most prevalent and tragic neurologic disorders. The neuropathologic changes in the brain caused by trauma are complex, and understanding their clinical consequences is a formidable task. Nevertheless, the white matter of the brain is significantly damaged in TBI, and considering this category of injury from a neurobehavioral perspective is instructive.

Traumatic Brain Injury

Traumatic brain injury has recently been the recipient of considerable and much deserved interest in neurology. This welcome development follows a long period when, despite its high prevalence and substantial impact on society, TBI could legitimately be termed a silent epidemic (Goldstein, 1990) because of the relatively little attention devoted to it by the neuroscientific community. Traumatic brain injury may of course be an immediately fatal event, as in many motor vehicle accidents, and death from TBI may occur acutely, even in the setting of competitive sports (Kelly et al., 1991). Many individuals survive TBI, and it is sobering to consider the statistic that TBI ranks as the most common etiology of major neurologic disability in the United States (Alexander, 1987). The problems faced by many patients and their families and caregivers are particularly burdensome given the high incidence of TBI in young adults, who may be required to cope with major neurobehavioral sequelae for decades. These deficits in cognition and especially emotional status are typically the most problematic, far outpacing physical disability. The substantial initial recovery of physical functions often misleads clinicians and other observers to predict a good neurobehavioral outcome that may not in fact occur (Filley, 1995).

The clinical presentation of TBI necessarily includes an impairment of mental status. The diagnosis is often obvious from the history or signs of trauma to the head or other areas, but with more mild or remote injuries, physical signs may be absent and the evaluation of the mental state becomes paramount. In all cases, TBI involves some loss of neurobehavioral function, ranging from confusion and amnesia from concussion (Kelly et al., 1991) to the vegetative state following severe injury (Adams et al., 2000). Those individuals with mild injuries usually recover, whereas more severe injury leads to lifelong deficits in attention, memory, and comportment (Filley, 1995). Evidence developed over the last half century has established that the most important factor underlying the neurobehavioral sequelae of TBI is injury to the cerebral white matter.

A consideration of TBI as a white matter disorder requires a review of fundamental neuropathology and pathophysiology. Although the range of neuropathology found in TBI is broad, including focal cortical contusions, hypoxic-ischemic lesions, and extra-axial hemorrhages, clinical and experimental studies have implicated injury to white matter as most prominent (Strich, 1956; Adams et al., 1982; Gennarelli et al., 1982; Alexander, 1995). This lesion was first described as "diffuse degeneration of the cerebral white matter" in patients with severe posttraumatic dementia (Strich, 1956), and later by the similar descriptor "shearing injury" (Strich, 1961), but the currently favored term is diffuse axonal injury (DAI), by which is implied widespread injury to axons within the white matter of the injured brain (Adams et al., 1982). Thus, although the term DAI points to the axon as the primary site of injury, it serves for our purposes to highlight the damage to white matter that is clinically demonstrable and produces major neurobehavioral sequelae.

Variable degrees of DAI have been shown to be present in both severe (Adams et al., 1982) and mild TBI (Oppenheimer, 1968). In the series of Nevin (1967), white matter neuropathology was present in all individuals who survived more than 1 week after severe TBI, and an identical pattern of DAI has been demonstrated in experimental animals (Gennarelli et al., 1982). Diffuse axonal injury is characterized by its microscopic features, which include axonal retraction balls, microglial clusters, and Wallerian degeneration in white matter fiber tracts (Gennarelli et al., 1982). The pathophysiology of DAI involves shearing forces produced in the brain by sudden acceleration and deceleration (Alexander, 1995). Rotational forces appear to be most deleterious. These shearing forces act mainly upon long fiber systems in the brain that are most vulnerable to mechanical disruption. Injury to blood vessels producing multiple hemorrhagic foci is common as well. The extent of DAI correlates with clinical measures of severity, including the Glasgow Coma Scale, the length of unconsciousness, and the duration of post-traumatic amnesia (Alexander, 1995). In very severe cases, damage to the subcortical white matter plays a major role in the pathogenesis of the vegetative state (Adams et al., 2000). Thus, the essential difference between mild and severe forms of TBI is the degree of DAI (Alexander, 1995). Areas most prominently affected by TBI are the dorsal midbrain, the corpus callosum, and the hemispheric white matter (Fig. 12-1; Filley, 1995).

Neuroimaging studies have generally supported neuropathologic findings emphasizing the importance of white matter damage in TBI (Fig. 12-2). Early reports using computed tomography (CT) demonstrated small focal hemorrhages in the white matter of TBI patients (Zimmerman et al., 1978). The increased sensitivity of magnetic resonance imaging (MRI) was later shown by observations that a substantial number of brain-injured individuals with normal CT scans have white matter lesions on MRI (Mittl et al., 1994). In a prospective study, DAI was found to be the most common primary lesion in TBI identified neuroradiologically, followed by cortical contusions (Gentry et al., 1988). On MRI, DAI lesions are seen in the hemispheric white matter, corpus callosum, and dorsal midbrain, the same sites identified from neuropathologic studies (Gentry et al., 1988). Correlations between white matter changes on MRI and neuropsychological function, however, have often been modest (Levin et al., 1992), prompting the suggestion that the microscopic lesions of DAI may be undetectable with conventional MRI (Mittl et al.,

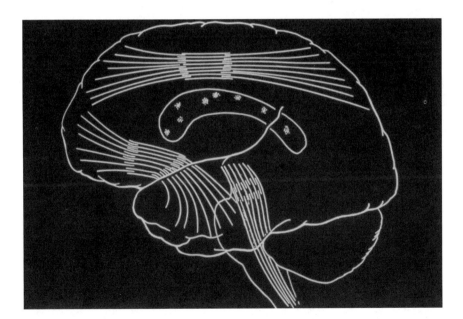

Figure 12-1. Schematic drawing of white matter regions in the brain that are most susceptible to diffuse axonal injury in TBI: the brainstem, cerebral hemispheres, and corpus callosum.

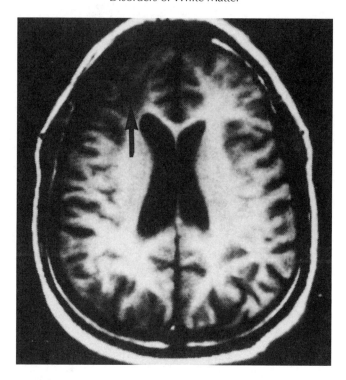

Figure 12-2. Heavily T1-weighted MRI scan of a patient with prior TBI showing right frontal DAI (*arrow*) and associated enlargement of the adjacent right lateral ventricle. (Reprinted with permission from Pomeranz SJ. Craniospinal magnetic resonance imaging. Philadelphia: W.B. Saunders, 1989.)

1994). Newer, more sensitive MRI techniques were then predicted to prove helpful in improving white matter–behavior correlations (Smith et al., 1995). Consistent with this prediction, the normal appearing white matter in TBI patients was studied with magnetic resonance spectroscopy (MRS), which revealed reduced *N*-acetyl aspartate that correlated with the severity of TBI (Garnett et al., 2000), and magnetization transfer imaging (MTI), which detected abnormalities that correlated with cognitive impairment (Bagley et al., 2000; McGowan et al., 2000). These data provide further support for the importance of DAI in the pathogenesis of neurobehavioral dysfunction in TBI.

The specific clinical impact of DAI can be difficult to determine in many cases because there are other neurologic and systemic injuries in TBI that also contribute to overall outcome. For example, patients with diffuse injury and superimposed cortical lesions fare worse than those with diffuse injury alone (Filley et al., 1987). However, some data are useful in developing a profile of neurobehavioral deficits that can be tentatively ascribed to DAI. As a general rule, attention, memory, and executive function are most affected in TBI (Wilson and Wyper, 1992). These disturbances also tend to dominate in patients with mild TBI who go on to develop the postconcussion syndrome (Alexander, 1995). Deficits in these domains are consistent with the preponderance of white matter lesions on MRI found in the frontal and temporal lobes (Levin et al., 1987). Sustained attention or concentration may be particularly affected, in contrast to simple attention as assessed by the digit span (Kaufmann et al., 1993). Memory loss has been associated with ventricular dilation that is most likely a result of white matter volume loss (Anderson and Bigler, 1995). Disconnection effects related to corpus callosum atrophy have been found with the use of dichotic listening tests (Levin et al., 1989; Benavidez et al., 1999). An interesting observation is that TBI patients may display relative preservation of procedural memory in comparison to declarative memory (Ewert et al., 1989). Additional examination of memory also reveals that this sparing of procedural memory may be accompanied by specific difficulty with memory retrieval (Timmerman and Brouwer, 1999), a pattern consistent with the proposed category of white matter dementia (Filley, 1998). Executive dysfunction has been documented in TBI, and may reflect damage to white matter connections of the dorsolateral prefrontal cortices to posterior structures (Filley, 1995). In contrast to these areas of deficit, language is relatively preserved after TBI. Studies using Wechsler Adult Intelligence Scale (WAIS) verbal and performance intelligence quotient (IQ) scores after TBI have shown that language abilities are less affected and recover more quickly than nonverbal skills (Mandleberg and Brooks, 1975). Personality and emotional changes, however, are frequent. Disinhibition may be disabling in itself because of the social disruption that limits or precludes reintegration into society (Filley et al., 1987), and depression occurs in nearly half of TBI patients (van Reekum et al., 2000). Thus a complex amalgam of neurobehavioral deficits is typical of TBI, and because of the common denominator of DAI and a clinical profile that matches that of other white matter disorders (Filley, 1998), there is good reason to regard the white matter neuropathology as responsible for a major component of the neurobehavioral disability experienced by all TBI patients.

The treatment of patients with TBI involves a complex series of interventions ranging from acute intensive care and neurosurgical procedures to outpatient rehabilitation and counseling. The optimization of recovery from TBI requires attention to many issues that follow from the entire range of neurologic and systemic injuries that individuals may sustain. In terms of white matter, however, it is worth pointing out that specific pharmacologic treatment based on white matter neuropathology may be warranted. Diffuse axonal injury in the cerebral white matter may have a selective effect on the cholinergic system, as shown in animal models (Schmidt and Grady, 1995), and the use of cholinergic drugs such as donepezil may be beneficial (Arciniegas et al., 1999). This kind of therapy would be most promising in the long-term treatment of TBI, when the acute management has been completed and community reintegration and optimal postinjury adjustment are the goals. Drugs of this sort can be expected to help in TBI only if some axons are intact and capable of enabling neurotransmission, an assumption that seems reasonable in most cases. As in other white matter disorders, the possibility of sparing irreplaceable neuronal elements in TBI may portend a better prognosis and improved treatment potential than in primary diseases of the neurons themselves. Caution is warranted, however, as there are few data supporting the pharmacotherapy of chronic TBI at this time. A controlled study of the stimulant methylphenidate in patients with closed head injury, for example, did not support the use of this drug for individuals with TBI (Speech et al., 1993).

Shaken Baby Syndrome

The shaken baby syndrome is a tragic reminder of the potential for the physical abuse of young children. This syndrome, first described in the 1960s as the battered-child syndrome (Kempe et al., 1961) and later as the whiplash shaken infant syndrome (Caffey, 1974), is now known to result from major rotational forces applied to the infant brain (Duhaime et al., 1998). In addition to injury from shaking, most abused infants have evidence of blunt impact to the head as well (Duhaime et al., 1998). Nonaccidental trauma causing the shaken baby syndrome occurs mostly in the first 3 years of life, and is the most common cause of traumatic death in infancy (Duhaime et al., 1998). Common clinical features include lethargy, irritability, seizures, retinal hemorrhages, cutaneous bruising, and coma (Duhaime et al., 1998). Nearly all patients have subdural or subarachnoid hemorrhage, and death may occur from intracranial hypertension (Duhaime et al., 1998). Severe mental retardation may follow as a lifelong condition in those who survive (Caffey, 1974). Typical neuropathologic findings include subdural and subarachnoid blood, cortical contusions most common in the frontal lobes, and DAI in the corpus callosum and hemispheric white matter (Duhaime, et al., 1998). This syndrome thus closely resembles TBI in general, and the pattern of white matter damage is similar to that seen in brain-injured adults. In addition to mechanical trauma, autopsy studies have suggested that hypoxia-ischemia may also contribute to white matter injury (Shannon et al., 1998). The contribution of this white matter damage to neurobehavioral disturbance appears to be important, although, as in TBI generally, there is other neuropathologic injury that should be considered.

Corpus Callosotomy

A final entry in the list of traumatic disorders of white matter is corpus callosotomy, in which intentional severing of the largest white matter tract in the brain is the goal. Corpus callosotomy is a surgical lesion that serves as a useful contrast to congenital callosal agenesis (Chapter 5). A discussion of this procedure and its effects is included at this point because, of all the acquired callosal lesions, corpus callosotomy offers the most useful data on the role of corpus callosum in behavior. Acquired callosal lesions may also occur with demyelinative, infectious, toxic, vascular, and neoplastic disorders, which are discussed elsewhere in this volume.

Sectioning of the corpus callosum is a neurosurgical procedure undertaken for the relief of selected cases of severe epilepsy. Patients who qualify for this procedure typically have frequent generalized seizures that are medically intractable, and bilateral epileptogenic foci that preclude the possibility of resective surgery such as temporal lobectomy (Sauerwein and Lassonde, 1997). In some cases, section of the anterior callosum is sufficient for seizure control, but in others, complete callosotomy is necessary (Sauerwein and Lassonde, 1997). From these patients, who are commonly referred to as having a "split brain," much has been learned about the functional specializations of the cerebral hemispheres. There is no doubt that the two sides of the cerebrum have different roles, the most obvious being the lateralization of language to the left and visuospatial function to the right in most people. In health, the corpus callosum serves to unite the two hemispheres anatomically and functionally, and when callosal damage occurs, a variety of deficits can be observed (Bogen, 1993; Gazzaniga, 2000).

As corpus callosotomy is a therapeutic intervention, it is gratifying that observations have often been made on how mild its effects may be, and how split brain patients may exhibit remarkably normal daily lives (Bogen, 1993). In fact, enhanced social adjustment and neuropsychological improvement are frequently seen, largely because of improved seizure control (Nordgren et al., 1991; Rougier et al., 1997; Lassonde and Sauerwein, 1997). Improvement may be most notable in those less than 13 years of age, in keeping with the presumably greater plasticity of the brain in younger individuals (Lassonde and Sauerwein, 1997).

However, disconnection signs can be demonstrated, especially immediately following surgery and in older patients. As a general rule, disconnection effects in callosotomy patients are more apparent than in those individuals with callosal agenesis (Chiarello, 1980; Gazzaniga, 2000). Broadly stated, cerebral disconnection is characterized by the absence of interhemispheric transfer of information derived from a stimulus presented unilaterally, and a wealth of experimental data has been gathered in support of this formulation (Gazzaniga et al., 1962; Seymour et al., 1994). Neurologists have long been aware of neurobehavioral deficits stemming from disorders of the corpus callosum, and these have provided some of the best examples of disconnection syndromes (Geschwind, 1965). History taking may reveal evidence of intermanual conflict and the alien hand syndrome (Bogen, 1993). On examination, patients with callosal damage from callosotomy or other neuropathology can display left-hand tactile anomia, agraphia, and apraxia, and left hemialexia, all of which suggest that left hemisphere language and praxis systems are disconnected from the right hemisphere (Bogen, 1993).

It has also been observed that callosotomy patients are frequently able to compensate for disconnection effects. One research question in this area has therefore been the mechanism of interhemispheric transfer of information in the absence of a complete corpus callosum. Data on the possibility of transfer by other commissures have been controversial, and some critics have claimed instead that residual information transfer takes place via preserved callosal fibers that were not severed in the process of surgery (Funnell et al., 2000). In any case, the importance of the corpus callosum in the integration of bihemispheric brain activities is fully supported by these studies.

A major impact of research on the clinical effects of corpus callosum lesions has been to introduce a range of questions on the nature of consciousness and the mind in general. The relative paucity of signs observable by standard neurologic methods should not obscure the fact that deficits can be detected with careful neurobehavioral and neuropsychological examination. Whereas few serious adverse sequelae follow this seemingly radical brain operation, the disconnection effects of commissurotomy testify to the role of the commissural white matter in higher function. Indeed, consciousness itself may depend critically on the corpus callosum in that it permits the subjective experience of integrated awareness known to all normal humans (Gazzaniga, 2000).

References

Adams JH, Graham DI, Jennett B. The neuropathology of the vegetative state after an acute brain insult. Brain 2000; 123: 1327–1338.

Adams JH, Graham DI, Murray, LS, Scott G. Diffuse axonal injury due to nonmissile head injury: an analysis of 45 cases. Ann Neurol 1982; 12: 557–563.

Alexander MP. The role of neurobehavioral syndromes in the rehabilitation and outcome of closed head injury. In: Levin HS, Grafman J, Eisenberg HM, eds. Neurobehavioral recovery from head injury. New York: Oxford University Press, 1987: 191–205.

Alexander MP. Mild traumatic brain injury: pathophysiology, natural history, and clinical management. Neurology 1995; 45: 1252–1260.

Anderson CV, Bigler ED. Ventricular dilation, cortical atrophy, and neuropsychological outcome following traumatic brain injury. J Neuropsychiatry Clin Neurosci 1995; 7: 42–48.

Arciniegas DB, Adler LE, Topkoff J, et al. Attention and memory dysfunction after traumatic brain injury: cholinergic mechanisms, sensory gating, and a hypothesis for further investigation. Brain Injury 1999; 13: 1–13.

Bagley LJ, McGowan JC, Grossman RI, et al. Magnetization transfer imaging of traumatic brain injury. J Magn Res Imaging 2000; 11: 1–8.

Benavidez DA, Fletcher JM, Hannay HJ, et al. Corpus callosum damage and interhemispheric transfer of information following closed head injury in children. Cortex 1999; 35: 315–336.

Bogen JE. The callosal syndromes. In: Heilman KM, Valenstein E, eds. Clinical neuropsychology. 3rd ed. New York: Oxford University Press, 1993: 337–407.

Caffey J. The whiplash shaken infant syndrome: manual shaking by the extremities with whiplash-induced intracranial and intraocular bleedings, linked with residual permanent brain damage and mental retardation. Pediatrics 1974: 54: 396–403.

Chiarello C. A house divided? Cognitive functioning with callosal agenesis. Brain Lang 1980; 11: 128–158.

Duhaime A-C, Christian CW, Rorke LB, Zimmerman RA. Nonaccidental head injury in infants—the "shaken baby syndrome." N Engl J Med 1998; 338: 1822–1829.

Ewert L, Levin HS, Watson MG, Kalisky Z. Procedural memory during posttraumatic amnesia in survivors of severe closed head injury. Implications for rehabilitation. Arch Neurol 1989; 46: 911–916.

Filley CM. Neurobehavioral anatomy. Niwot, CO: University Press of Colorado, 1995.

Filley CM. The behavioral neurology of cerebral white matter. Neurology 1998; 50: 1535–1540.

Filley CM, Cranberg LD, Alexander MP, Hart EJ. Neurobehavioral outcome after closed head injury in childhood and adolescence. Arch Neurol 1987; 44: 194–198.

Funnell MG, Corballis PM, Gazzaniga MS. Cortical and subcortical interhemispheric interactions following partial and complete callosotomy. Arch Neurol 2000; 57: 185–189.

Garnett MR, Blamire AM, Rajagopalan B, et al. Evidence for cellular damage in normal-appearing white matter correlates with injury severity in patients following traumatic brain injury. A magnetic resonance spectroscopy study. Brain 2000; 123: 1403–1409.

Gazzaniga MS. Cerebral specialization and interhemispheric communication. Does the corpus callosum enable the human condition? Brain 2000; 123: 1293–1326.

Gazzaniga MS, Bogen JE, Sperry RW. Some functional effects of sectioning the cerebral commissures in man. Proc Natl Acad Sci USA 1962: 48: 1765–1769.

Gennarelli TA, Thibault LE, Adams JH, et al. Diffuse axonal injury and traumatic coma in the primate. Ann Neurol 1982; 12: 564–574.

Gentry LR, Godersky JC, Thompson B. MR imaging of head trauma: review of the distribution and radiopathologic features of traumatic lesions. AJNR 1988; 150: 663–672.

Geschwind N. Disconnexion syndromes in animals and man. Brain 1965; 88: 237–294, 585–644.

Goldstein M. Traumatic brain injury: a silent epidemic. Ann Neurol 1990; 27: 327.

Kaufmann PM, Fletcher JM, Levin HS, et al. Attentional disturbance after pediatric closed head injury. J Child Neurol 1993; 8: 348–353.

Kelly JP, Nichols JS, Filley CM, et al. Concussion in sports. Guidelines for the prevention of catastrophic outcome. JAMA 1991; 266: 2867–2869.

Kempe CH, Silverman FN, Steele BF, et al. The battered-child syndrome. JAMA 1961; 181: 17–24.

Lassonde M, Sauerwein C. Neuropsychological outcome of corpus callosotomy in children and adolescents. J Neurosurg Sci 1997; 41: 67–73.

Levin HS, Amparo E, Eisenberg HM, et al. Magnetic resonance imaging and computerized tomography in relation to the neurobehavioral sequelae of mild and moderate head injuries. J Neurosurg 1987; 66: 706–713.

Levin HS, High WM, Williams DL, et al. Dichotic listening and manual performance in relation to magnetic resonance imaging after closed head injury. J Neurol Neurosurg Psychiatry 1989; 52: 1162–1169.

Levin HS, Williams DH, Eisenberg HM, et al. Serial MRI and neurobehavioral findings after mild to moderate closed head injury. J Neurol Neurosurg Psychiatry 1992; 55: 255–262.

Mandleberg IA, Brooks DN. Cognitive recovery after severe head injury. 1: Serial testing on the Wechsler Adult Intelligence Scale. J Neurol Neurosurg Psychiatry 1975; 38: 1121–1126.

McGowan JC, Yang JH, Plotkin RC, et al. Magnetization transfer imaging in the detection of injury associated with mild head trauma. AJNR 2000; 21: 875–880.

Mittl RL, Grossman RI, Hiehle JF, et al. Prevalence of MR evidence of diffuse axonal injury in patients with mild head injury and normal head CT findings. AJNR 1994; 15: 1583–1589.

Nevin NC. Neuropathological changes in the white matter following head injury. J Neuropathol Exp Neurol 1967; 26: 77–84.

Nordgren RE, Reeves AG, Viguera AC, Roberts DW. Corpus callosotomy for intractable seizures in the pediatric age group. Arch Neurol 1991; 48: 364–372.

Oppenheimer DR. Microscopic lesions in the brain following head injury. J Neurol Neurosurg Psychiatry 1968; 31: 299–306.

Rougier A, Claverie B, Pedespan JM, et al. Callosotomy for intractable epilepsy: overall outcome. J Neurosurg Sci 1997; 41: 51–57.

Sauerwein HC, Lassonde M. Neuropsychological alterations after split-brain surgery. J Neurosurg Sci 1997; 41: 59–66.

Schmidt RH, Grady MS. Loss of forebrain cholinergic neurons following fluid-percussion injury: implications for cognitive impairment in closed head injury. J Neurosurg 1995; 83: 496–502.

Seymour SE, Reuter-Lorenz PA, Gazzaniga MS. The disconnection syndrome. Basic findings reaffirmed. Brain 1994; 117: 105–115.

Shannon P, Smith CR, Deck J, et al. Axonal injury and the neuropathology of the shaken baby syndrome. Acta Neuropathol 1998; 95: 625–631.

Smith DH, Meaney DF, Lenkinski RE, et al. New magnetic resonance imaging techniques for the evaluation of traumatic brain injury. J Neurotrauma 1995; 12: 573–577.

Speech TJ, Rao SM, Osmon DC, Sperry LT. A double-blind controlled study of methylphenidate treatment in closed head injury. Brain Inj 1993; 7: 333–338.

Strich SJ. Diffuse degeneration of the cerebral white matter in severe dementia following head injury. J Neurol Neurosurg Psychiatry 1956; 19: 163–185.

Strich SJ. Shearing injury of nerve fibres as a cause of brain damage due to head injury. Lancet 1961; 2: 443–448.

Timmerman ME, Brouwer WH. Slow information processing after very severe closed head injury: impaired access to declarative knowledge and intact application and acquisition of procedural knowledge. Neuropsychologia 1999; 37: 467–478.

van Reekum R, Cohen T, Wong J. Can traumatic brain injury cause psychiatric disorders? J Neuropsychiatry Clin Neurosci 2000; 12: 316–327.

Wilson JTL, Wyper D. Neuroimaging and neuropsychological functioning following closed head injury: CT, MRI, and SPECT. J Head Trauma Rehab 1992; 7: 29–39.

Zimmerman RA, Bilaniuk LT, Gennarelli T. Computed tomography of shearing injuries of the white matter. Radiology 1978; 127: 393–396.

13

Neoplasms

A discussion of brain tumors that selectively damage white matter may appear to be very limited. Brain tumors do not as a rule affect one discrete region, and instead show a tendency to involve widespread areas of both gray and white matter. This characteristic, combined with the associated edema and mass effect that frequently occur, often render correlations of tumor location with neurobehavioral status tentative at best. Even early in the clinical course, when the more limited extent of the tumor might predict a more focal location, correlations of lesion site with clinical status can be problematic. However, many neoplasms actually arise from white matter structures, and exert major effects on white matter throughout their clinical course. These tumors, both diffuse and focal, are discussed in this chapter to illustrate that neoplastic white matter involvement can be a source of neurobehavioral dysfunction.

Gliomatosis Cerebri

Gliomatosis cerebri is a diffusely infiltrative glial cell neoplasm of the brain. Although this rare disease has been reported in only about 150 cases (Ponce et al., 1998), it serves the purposes of this book because it is the best example of a neoplastic disorder confined to the cerebral white matter throughout most of its course. Moreover, because the diagnosis has mainly been possible only at autopsy, the incidence of the disease may be underestimated, and advancing neuroimaging techniques may increase its recognition during life (Keene et al., 1999).

Gliomatosis cerebri usually appears in adulthood, although it may arise at any age. The insidious onset of mental status changes is the most frequent presentation, and headache, motor dysfunction, and seizures may also occur (Couch and Weiss, 1974; Artigas et al., 1985). Diagnosis in life is difficult because the clinical presentation is consistent with a wide range of diseases featuring diffuse white matter involvement, and even with cerebral biopsy there may be confusion about the classification of this lesion. The clinical course is quite variable, with survival durations reported from weeks to many years (Couch and Weiss, 1974; Artigas et al., 1985), but a fatal outcome has been typical. Surgery, chemotherapy, and radiotherapy may be partially effective, but no curative treatment has been found; one recent case showed a dramatically positive response to radiotherapy (Shintani et al., 2000).

In contrast to gliomas that tend to be single or multicentric, gliomatosis cerebri involves infiltration of contiguous areas of the cerebrum. Although gray matter structures may be affected, the major neuropathologic burden falls on the white matter, where there is destruction of the myelin sheath with suprisingly little damage to neurons and axons (Artigas et al., 1985). Thus, there is widespread white matter infiltration with relatively preserved cerebral architecture. Periventricular white matter often undergoes additional damage because of the hydrocephalus and increased intracranial pressure that can develop from aqueductal stenosis or tumor overgrowth (Couch and Weiss, 1974). The origin of the abnormal cells in gliomatosis cerebri has been disputed, and the small number of cases has hindered thorough study. Nevin, who first described the disease, believed it to be a blastomatous malformation of glial cells (Nevin, 1938). Many authorities, however, believe that gliomatosis cerebri represents a true neoplasm. Microscopic examination and immunohistochemical studies have suggested that the lesion is a glial cell tumor usually composed of neoplastic astrocytes (Duffy et al., 1980), but occasionally made up of oligodendrocytes (Balko et al., 1992) or transitional cells between the two (Artigas et al., 1985). The progressive nature of the disorder and its partial response to chemotherapy and radiation are clinical points favoring this view.

Modern neuroimaging has improved the detection of gliomatosis cerebri, although there are no pathognomonic neuroradiologic features. Computed tomography (CT) can reveal low-density white matter changes reminiscent of demyelination or dysmyelination (Geremia et al., 1988) and there may be enhancement late in the course (Hayek and Valvanis, 1982). Magnetic resonance imaging (MRI) has generally proven more sensitive in detecting the white matter changes of this disease (del Carpio-O'Donovan et al., 1996; Fig. 13-1). Poor gray–white matter demarcation has been reported as one sign of neoplastic invasion (Koslow et al., 1992), and more recent MRI studies have documented widespread high signal in the white matter on T2-weighted images, prominently involving the frontal lobes and the corpus callosum (Keene et al., 1999). Magnetic resonance spectroscopy of gliomatosis cerebri has shown features similar to those of gliomas, but no specific MR spectra have been identified (Pyhtinen, 2000). Functional neuroimaging studies using positron emission tomography have shown hypometabolism in the cerebral cortex consistent with disconnection of the cortex from subcortical structures (Plowman et al., 1998).

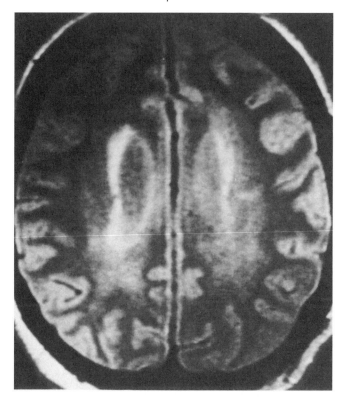

Figure 13-1. Proton density MRI scan of a patient with gliomatosis cerebri. Diffuse tumor infiltration in the centrum semiovale is apparent. (Reprinted with permission from Atlas SW, ed. Magnetic resonance imaging of the brain and spine. 2nd ed. Philadelphia: Lippincott-Raven, 1996.)

The neurobehavioral changes associated with gliomatosis cerebri have been only partially characterized, and there is no study of neuropsychological function in affected patients. This paucity of information is largely due to the rarity of the disease; a review in 1985 could locate only 58 cases in the literature from which to draw conclusions about the clinical features of gliomatosis cerebri (Artigas et al., 1985). Moreover, few reports contain substantial detail on neurobehavioral aspects of this disease. However, despite these shortcomings, personality and mental status changes are repeatedly stated to be the most striking findings in patients with gliomatosis cerebri, whether in the initial or later stages of the disease (Artigas et al., 1985; Couch and Weiss, 1974; Sarhaddi et al., 1973). The mental changes are typically described as confusion, disorientation, and memory loss, and focal cortical signs including aphasia are rarely noted. Neuropsychiatric dysfunction, typically described as personality change, is also frequently cited as an initial or early manifestation. One case report described a man with autopsy-proven gliomatosis cerebri who developed depression and then schizophrenia-like psychosis for nearly 2 years before progressive dementia ensued (Vassallo and Allen, 1995). Although the presence of gray matter involvement in many cases must be considered, these clinical features are consistent with that which would be expected with diffuse white matter involvement. Moreover, the frequent presence of neuropsychiatric dysfunction can plausibly be attributed in large part to involvement of the frontal lobe white matter (Filley and Gross, 1992).

Diffusely Infiltrative Gliomas

Gliomas are malignant neoplasms that arise from glial cells. The three major gliomas that affect the brain are the astrocytoma, the oligodendroglioma, and the ependymoma. Although it is well known that these tumors exert widespread effects as they expand and produce vasogenic edema, in fact they arise principally from the cerebral white matter because of the relative abundance of astrocytes, oligodendrocytes, and ependymal cells in myelinated regions of the brain (Adams and Graham, 1989). Thus, despite the more florid manifestations such as headache, seizures, and focal neurologic deficits that indicate cortical and diffuse brain involvement, the initial features of gliomas are less obvious. It is likely, in fact, that the often cited but subtle symptoms of inertia, forgetfulness, inattention, confusion, and personality change in patients with gliomas (Galasko et al., 1988; Victor and Ropper, 2000) reflect early white matter involvement. Not only is the white matter directly damaged by the neoplasm, but diffusion MRI studies have disclosed additional involvement because of deviation of fibers in the normal appearing white matter adjacent to tumors (Wieshmann at al., 2000). Although the recognition of nonspecific, initial mental features of glioma is a major challenge to clinicians, this phase of the natural history of gliomas deserves more attention because of the potential opportunity for early detection and improved treatment of these devastating tumors.

Another clinical feature of gliomas that directly implicates the white matter is that the dissemination appears to follow association pathway trajectories in a rapid and preferential manner (Giese and Westphal, 1996; Geer and Grossman, 1997). This finding may help explain the poor survival of patients with brain malignancies in whom locally applied therapy has only limited efficacy (Geer and Grossman, 1997). In addition, the knowledge that gliomas tend to spread along white matter tracts may assist in the analysis of the clinical effects of malignancies, especially as they disrupt distributed neural networks connected by association pathways. Understanding of the means of tumor spread along white matter tracts may thus have an important impact on the clinical manifestations of malignant brain tumors and the approach to their treatment.

The most commom glioma in the brain is the astrocytoma, followed by the oligodendroglioma and the ependymoma (Adams and Graham, 1989). Astrocytomas occur anywhere in cerebrum (Adams and Graham, 1989), whereas oligodendrogliomas often favor the frontal lobes (Mørk et al., 1985; Ludwig et al., 1986) and ependymomas cluster around the lateral ventricles (Adams and Graham, 1989). Among their many clinical effects, cognitive dysfunction from the effects of gliomas has long been recognized by clinicians.

Astrocytomas vary considerably in their degree of malignancy, and the most severe form, glioblastoma multiforme, is typically fatal within months. One patient with a bitemporal glioblastoma multiforme presented with florid mania within months of her death (Filley and Kleinschmidt-DeMasters, 1995). In more benign astrocytomas, cognitive function may be primarily affected, with impairments in attention and memory overshadowing language and intelligence deficits (Ater et al., 1996). Figure 13-2 shows the MRI scan of a patient with an astrocytoma that displayed a striking predilection for the white matter.

The tendency of oligodendrogliomas to affect the frontal lobe white matter may be easily seen on MRI (Fig. 13-3). In light of this common localization, it is noteworthy that in a large series of proven oligodendrogliomas, dementia was

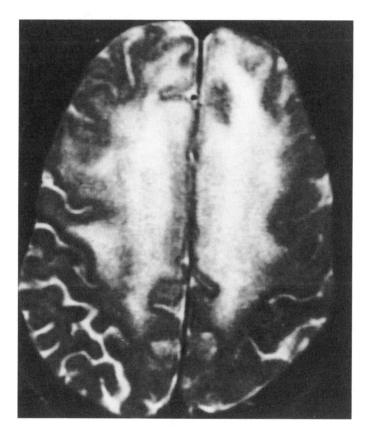

Figure 13-2. T2-weighted MRI scan of a patient with an astrocytoma. The cerebral white matter is diffusely involved. (Reprinted with permission from Osborn AG. Diagnostic neuroradiology. St. Louis: Mosby Year Book, 1994.)

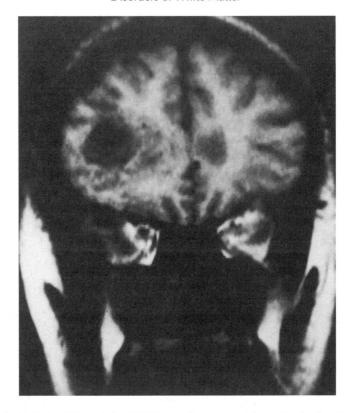

Figure 13-3. Coronal T1-weighted MRI scan of a patient with an oligodendroglioma. The tumor is demonstrated in the white matter of both frontal lobes. (Reprinted with permission from Ramsey RR, ed. Neuroradiology. 3ʳᵈ ed. Philadelphia: W.B. Saunders, 1996.)

present in 46% of patients and psychosis in 19% (Ludwig et al., 1986). The relative prominence of dementia and psychosis in patients with this tumor is consistent with a general trend in the brain tumor literature: frontal and temporal lobe tumors tend to present with neurobehavioral manifestations far more often than do parietal, occipital, and posterior fossa tumors (Filley and Kleinschmidt-DeMasters, 1995).

Ependymomas are rare, and cognitive function in affected patients has been little studied. It is possible, however, to speculate that the periventricular origin of ependymomas might produce cognitive deficits similar to those of multiple sclerosis. An interesting case demonstrating a dramatic decline in performance intelligence quotient (IQ) with the growth of a right parietal ependymoma in a young man illustrates the potential of this tumor to affect cognition by producing damage to cerebral white matter (Sands et al., 2000).

Neuropsychological data on the cognitive effects of glioma patients taken as a group are relatively sparse (Weitzner and Meyers, 1997), particularly in those who are untreated. In general, glioma patients manifest deficits in attention and concentration (Taphoorn et al., 1992), memory (Salander et al., 1995), and frontal lobe function (Taphoorn et al., 1992). Lateralized verbal and nonverbal test reductions associated with left and right hemisphere gliomas, respectively, have also been noted (Scheibel et al., 1996). Improvement in cognitive function among glioma patients given methylphenidate indirectly suggests that primary damage may be in the white matter, where ascending dopaminergic fibers may be disrupted by the neoplasm (Meyers et al, 1998).

These studies, however, are all compromised by the difficulty in correlating neuropsychological deficits with white matter neuropathology in glioma patients because of coexisting gray matter damage in most, and the variable effects of radiation and chemotherapy on white matter (Chapter 9). A thoughtful study addressing both these issues is that of Anderson and colleagues (1990), in which untreated glioma patients who all had white matter involvement were analyzed with neuroimaging and neuropsychological testing. The results indicated that glioma patients manifested cognitive deficits expected on the basis of tumor location, although the deficits were generally milder than those of stroke patients with lesions in comparable brain regions (Anderson et al., 1990). This study provides some support for the role of white matter neuropathology in the neurobehavioral manifestations of gliomas, although more precise behavior–white matter correlations are still desirable.

Primary Cerebral Lymphoma

Primary cerebral lymphoma is a rare form of non-Hodgkin's lymphoma that arises in the brain. The term primary central nervous system lymphoma is used to refer to this tumor in the brain or spinal cord, but to emphasize its neurobehavioral effects, primary cerebral lymphoma will be used henceforth. These tumors account for approximately 1% to 2% of all primary brain tumors (O'Neill and Illig, 1989), but are much more common among patients with acquired immunodeficiency syndrome (AIDS) (Beral et al., 1991). Primary cerebral lymphoma has in fact become one of the routine considerations in AIDS patients who present with neurobehavioral dysfunction (Snider et al., 1983), and it is the fourth leading cause of death in these individuals (O'Neill and Illig, 1989).

This tumor, formerly referred to as reticulum cell sarcoma, microglioma, or immunoblastic sarcoma, is now known as primarily a B-cell lymphoma that typically arises in the central white matter of the brain, with lesser involvement of deep gray matter (O'Neill and Illig, 1989). Less than 10% of primary cerebral lymphomas are of T-cell origin (Abrey, 2000; Kleinschmidt-DeMasters et al., 1992). Cognitive loss and personality changes are the most common initial features (Abrey, 2000), and the clinical presentation often involves lethargy, confusion, and memory loss (Remick et al., 1990). Neuropsychiatric dysfunction has also been described (Kleinschmidt-DeMasters et al., 1992). Rapidly progressive dementia in the setting of diffuse cerebral white matter infiltration may occur (Carlson, 1996). Treatment of primary cerebral lymphoma can provide substantial palliative relief but is not curative. Corticosteroids are initially helpful in reducing the edema around the tumor, and this response can be helpful diagnostically. Definitive treatment with radiation and chemotherapy is capable of significantly increasing survival, whereas surgery is reserved for diagnostic purposes because aggressive tumor resection does not improve on the outcome with medical therapy (Abrey, 2000).

Neuropathologically, there is diffuse angiocentric growth of malignant lymphocytes (Abrey, 2000), and focal vascular occlusion with infarction can contribute to neurobehavioral decline (Kleinschmidt-DeMasters et al., 1992). The tumor has a predilection, however, for the frontal lobe white matter, corpus callosum, and periventricular white matter (Abrey, 2000). The tumor may also present with diffuse infiltration reminiscent of gliomatosis cerebri, prompting the term lymphomatosis cerebri (Bakshi et al., 1999).

Neuroimaging has become instrumental in the the diagnosis of primary cerebral lymphoma. Computed tomography typically shows a central hyperdense mass that enhances with contrast, and ring-enhancing lesions are not unusual (Whiteman et al., 1993). On MRI, the lesion has the unusual feature of being isointense or hypointense on all sequences, unless necrosis has developed and the T2-weighted images show hyperintensity (Johnson et al., 1997). Both solid and ring-like lesions can be seen on MRI, and both enhance with gadolinium (Johnson et al., 1997). Figure 13-4 displays the CT scan of a patient with primary cerebral lymphoma.

This tumor has not been subjected to detailed study regarding relationships between white matter involvement and neurobehavioral status. Available information, however, is consistent with the likelihood that white matter disease burden contributes to the mental status deficits of affected patients (Abrey, 2000; Kleinschmidt-DeMasters et al., 1992).

Focal White Matter Tumors

Focal neoplastic invasion of the cerebral white matter occurs occasionally, and more specific neurobehavioral deficits can arise as a result. A number of case reports and clinical series of patients with isolated tumors involving discrete areas of white matter have appeared. Although caution is advised when employing patients with brain tumors to study precise brain–behavior relationships because of uncertainty about the location and extent of the lesion (Anderson et al., 1990), these cases can provide important neurobehavioral insights (Filley and Kleinschmidt-DeMasters, 1995; Filley et al., 1999).

One region of interest that has received considerable attention is the fornix, a tract of the limbic system linking the hippocampus and the diencephalon that is implicated in human memory formation. Although rare reports have been presented claiming that isolated tumors such as an astrocytoma (Tucker et al., 1988) and a spongioblastoma unipolare (Heilman and Sypert, 1977) can cause amnesia through damage to one or both fornices, controversy has persisted because it is difficult in such cases to exclude damage to adjacent regions in the temporal lobe or

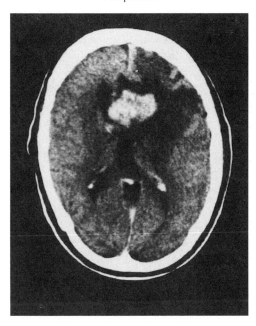

Figure 13-4. CT scan of a patient with primary cerebral lymphoma. The tumor involves the anterior corpus callosum and both frontal lobes. (Reprinted with permission from Filley CM, Kleinschmidt-DeMasters BK. Neurobehavioral presentations of brain neoplasms. West J Med 1995; 163: 19–25. 1995.)

thalamus. In a recent detailed study of 12 patients with surgical removal of third ventricle colloid cysts, Aggleton and colleagues (2000) used careful MRI analyses and found that only those patients with bilateral fornix interruption had significant memory impairment. To date, this study provides the largest number of well-studied cases with fornix lesions, and strongly suggests that damage to the fornices can interfere with recent memory. These results are consistent with functional imaging studies showing the existence of a medial temporal–diencephalic memory system (Fazio et al., 1992) in which the fornices play a crucial role.

The amyloidoma is a very rare tumor that exclusively affects the cerebral white matter. This neoplasm is characterized by the focal accumulation of large deposits of amyloid in the absence of systemic amyloidosis (Cohen et al., 1992; Vidal et al., 1992). Lesions are often solitary, but multiple amyloid deposits may also occur (Schröder et al., 1995). The tumor is relatively indolent, with one case reportedly surviving nearly 4 decades after onset (Linke et al., 1992). From the fewer than 20 reported cases of this disease, conclusions about brain–behavior relationships are necessarily limited, but personality change, psychosis, and dementia are all described in association with amyloidoma (Townsend et al., 1982; Cohen et al., 1992; Schroder et al., 1995; Lee et al., 1995), and some patients have mental signs as a component of a fluctuating course resembling multiple sclerosis (Linke et al., 1992). One woman with a solitary left parietal amyloidoma presented with "deteriorating mental function" for 1 year (Lee et al., 1995). A man with multiple amyloidomas, in whom the largest was in the left frontal lobe, had dementia with prominent frontal lobe features including inattentiveness, impulsivity, apathy, and witzelsucht (Cohen et al., 1992).

References

Abrey LE. Primary central nervous system lymphoma. Neurologist 2000; 6: 245–254.

Adams JH, Graham DI. An introduction to neuropathology. New York: Churchill Livingstone, 1989: 269–307.

Aggleton JP, McMackin D, Carpenter K, et al. Differential cognitive effects of colloid cysts of the third ventricle that spare or compromise the fornix. Brain 2000; 123: 800–815.

Anderson SW, Damasio H, Tranel D. Neuropsychological impairments associated with lesions caused by tumor or stroke. Arch Neurol 1990; 47: 397–405.

Artigas J, Cervos-Navarro J, Iglesias JR, Ebhardt G. Gliomatosis cerebri: clinical and histological findings. Clin Neuropathol 1985; 4: 135–148.

Ater JL, Moore BD, Francis DJ, et al. Correlation of medical and neurosurgical events with neuropsychological status in children at diagnosis of astrocytoma: utilization of a neurological severity score. J Child Neurol 1996; 11: 462–469.

Bakshi R, Mazziotta JC, Mischel PS, et al. Lymphomatosis cerebri presenting as a rapidly progressive dementia: clinical, neuroimaging, and pathologic findings. Dement Geriatr Aging Disord 1999; 10: 152–157.

Balko MG, Blisard KS, Samaha FJ. Oligodendroglial gliomatosis cerebri. Hum Pathol 1992; 23: 706–707.

Beral V, Peterman T, Berkelman R, Jaffe H. AIDS-associated non-Hodgkin lymphoma. Lancet 1991; 337: 805–809.

Carlson BA. Rapidly progressive dementia caused by nonenhancing primary lymphoma of the central nervous system. AJNR 1996; 17: 1695–1697.

Cohen M, Lanska D, Roessmann U, et al. Amyloidoma of the CNS. I. Clinical and pathologic study. Neurology 1992; 42: 2019–2023.

Couch JR, Weiss SA. Gliomatosis cerebri. Report of four cases and review of the literature. Neurology 1974; 24: 504–511.

del Carpio-O'Donovan R, Korah I, Salazar A, Melançon D. Gliomatosis cerebri. Radiology 1996; 198: 831–835.

Duffy PE, Huang YY, Rapport MM, Graf L. Glial fibrillary acidic protein in giant cell tumors of brain and other gliomas. Acta Neuropathol 1980; 52: 51–57.

Fazio F, Perani D, Gilardi MC, et al. Metabolic impairment in human amnesia: a PET study of memory networks. J Cereb Blood Flow Metab 1992; 12: 353–358.

Filley CM, Gross KF. Psychosis with cerebral white matter disease. Neuropsychiatry Neuropsychol Behav Neurol 1992; 5: 119–125.

Filley CM, Kleinschmidt-DeMasters BK. Neurobehavioral presentations of brain neoplasms. West J Med 1995; 163: 19–25.

Filley CM, Young DA, Reardon MS, Wilkening GN. Frontal lobe lesions and executive dysfunction in children. Neuropsychiatry Neuropsychol Behav Neurol 1999; 12: 156–160.

Galasko, Yuen K-O, Thal L. Intracranial mass lesions associated with late-onset psychosis and depression. Psychiatr Clin N Am 1988; 11: 151–166.

Geer CP, Grossman SA. Interstitial flow along white matter tracts: a potentially important mechanism for the dissemination of primary brain tumors. J Neurooncol 1997; 32: 193–201.

Geremia GK, Wollman R, Foust R. Computed tomography of gliomatosis cerebri. J Comput Assist Tomogr 1988; 12: 698–701.

Giese A, Westphal M. Glioma invasion in the central nervous system. Neurosurgery 1996; 39: 235–250.

Hayek J, Valvanis A. Computed tomography of gliomatosis cerebri. Comput Radiol 1982; 6: 93–98.

Heilman KM, Sypert GW. Korsakoff's syndrome resulting from bilateral fornix lesions. Neurology 1977; 27: 490–493.

Johnson BA, Fram EK, Johnson PC, Jacobowitz R. The variable MR appearance of primary cerebral lymphoma of the central nervous system: comparison with histopathologic features. AJNR 1997; 18: 563–572.

Keene DL, Jimenez C, Hsu E. MRI diagnosis of gliomatosis cerebri. Pediatr Neurol 1999; 20: 148–151.

Kleinschmidt-DeMasters BK, Filley CM, Bitter MA. Central nervous system angiocentric, angiodestructive T-cell lymphoma (lymphomatoid granulomatosis). Surg Neurol 1992; 37: 130–137.

Koslow SA, Claassen D, Hirsch WL, Jungreis CA. Gliomatosis cerebri: a case report with autopsy correlation. Neuroradiology 1992; 34: 331–333.

Lee J, Krol G, Rosenblum M. Primary amyloidoma of the brain: CT and MR presentation. AJNR 1995; 16: 712–714.

Linke RP, Gerhard L, Lottspeich F. Brain-restricted amyloidoma of immunoglobulin-light chain origin clinically resembling multiple sclerosis. Biol Chem Hoppe-Seyler 1992; 373: 1201–1209.

Ludwig CL, Smith MT, Godfrey AD, Armbrustmacher VW. A clinicopathological study of 323 patients with oligodendrogliomas. Ann Neurol 1986; 19: 15–21.

Meyers CA, Weitzner MA, Valentine AD, Levin VA. Methylphenidate therapy improves cognition, mood, and function of brain tumor patients. J Clin Oncol 1998; 16: 2522–2527.

Mørk SJ, Lindegaard K-F, Halvorsen TB, et al. Oligodendroglioma: incidence and biological behavior in a defined population. J Neurosurg 1985; 63: 881–889.

Nevin S. Gliomatosis cerebri. Brain 1938; 61: 170–191.

O'Neill BP, Illig JJ. Primary central nervous system lymphoma. Mayo Clin Proc 1989; 64: 1005–1020.

Plowman PN, Saunders CA, Maisey MN. Gliomatosis cerebri: disconnection of the cortical grey matter, demonstrated on PET scan. Br J Neurosurg 1998; 12: 240–244.

Ponce P, Alvarez-Santullano MV, Otermin E, et al. Gliomatosis cerebri: findings with computed tomography and magnetic resonance imaging. Eur J Radiol 1998; 28: 226–229.

Pyhtinen J. Proton MR spectroscopy in gliomatosis cerebri. Neuroradiology 2000; 42: 612–615.

Remick SC, Diamond C, Migliozzi JA, et al. Primary central nervous system lymphoma in patients with and without the acquired immune deficiency syndrome. A retrospective analysis and review of the literature. Medicine 1990; 69: 345–360.

Salander P, Karlsson T, Bergenheim T, Henriksson R. Long-term memory deficits in patients with malignant gliomas. J Neurooncol 1995; 25: 227–238.

Sands S, van Gorp WG, Finlay JL. A dramatic loss of non-verbal intelligence following a right parietal ependymoma: brief case report. Psychooncology 2000; 9: 259–266.

Sarhaddi S, Bravo E, Cyrus AE. Gliomatosis cerebri: a case report and review of the literature. South Med J 1973; 66: 883–888.

Scheibel RS, Meyers CA, Levin VA. Cognitive dysfunction following surgery for intracerebral glioma: influence of histopathology, lesion location, and treatment. J Neurooncol 1996; 30: 61–69.

Schröder R, Linke RP, Voges J, et al. Intracerebral A amyloidoma diagnosed by stereotactic biopsy. Clin Neuropathol 1995: 14: 347–350.

Shintani S, Tsuruoka S, Shiigai T. Serial positron emission tomography (PET) in gliomatosis cerebri treated with radiotherapy: a case report. J Neurol Sci 2000; 173: 25–31.

Snider WD, Simpson DM, Nielsen S, et al. Neurological complications of acquired immune deficiency syndrome: analysis of 50 patients. Ann Neurol 1983; 14: 403–418.

Taphoorn MJB, Heimans JJ, Snoek FJ, et al. Assessment of quality of life in patients treated for low-grade glioma: a preliminary report. J Neurol Neurosurg Psychiatry 1992; 55: 372–376.

Townsend JJ, Tomiyasu U, MacKay A, Wilson CB. Central nervous system amyloid presenting as a mass lesion. J Neurosurg 1982; 56: 439–442.

Tucker DM, Roeltgen DP, Tully R, et al. Memory dysfunction following unilateral transection of the fornix: a hippocampal disconnection syndrome. Cortex 1988; 24: 465–472.

Vassallo M, Allen S. An unusual cause of dementia. Postgrad Med J 1995; 71: 483–484.

Victor M, Ropper AH. Adams and Victor's principles of neurology. New York: McGraw-Hill, 2000.

Vidal RG, Ghiso J, Gallo G, et al. Amyloidoma of the CNS. II. Immunohistochemical and biochemical study. Neurology 1992; 42: 2024–2028.

Weishmann UC, Symms MR, Parker GJM, et al. Diffusion tensor imaging demonstrates deviation of fibres in normal appearing white matter adjacent to a brain tumor. J Neurol Neurosurg Psychiatry 2000; 68: 501–503.

Weitzner MA, Meyers CA. Cognitive functioning and quality of life in malignant glioma patients: a review of the literature. Psychooncology 1997; 6: 169–177.

Whiteman MLH, Post MJD, Bowen BC, Bell MD. AIDS-related white matter diseases. Neuroimaging Clin N Am 1993; 3: 331–359.

14

Hydrocephalus

The term hydrocephalus refers to the accumulation of excessive water in the head. Ordinarily the total volume of cerebrospinal fluid (CSF) within the neuraxis is approximately 140 cm^3, of which roughly 25 cm^3 are found in the four ventricles (Fishman, 1992). Higher ventricular volumes of CSF can develop either because additional CSF occupies space within a brain of normal size, or the parenchyma atrophies and CSF replaces the lost tissue (hydrocephalus ex vacuo). The cerebral white matter is implicated in both of these situations, either because an excessive volume of CSF may injure the periventricular regions or because changes in white matter contribute to the development of cerebral atrophy. These various situations, and their neurobehavioral sequelae, are considered in this chapter. Hydrocephalus occurring acutely in the context of mass lesions, trauma, infarction, and the like will not be reviewed because of methodological difficulties in studying the impact of specific white matter neuropathology in these settings.

Early Hydrocephalus

Early hydrocephalus is the development of hydrocephalus during gestation, infancy, or childhood. It thus encompasses cases of congenital and so-called occult tension hydrocephalus. In congenital hydrocephalus, an enlarged head reflects expanding CSF volume that increases the skull circumference because the sutures are unclosed in the first year of life, and in occult tension hydrocephalus, the head size remains stable because of closed sutures in spite of an intracranial process that causes hydrocephalus.

The common causes of early hydrocephalus include periventricular hemorrhage, the Arnold-Chiari malformation, aqueductal stenosis, and the Dandy-Walker syndrome. Infants affected in the first year of life present with an enlarging head and developmental delay. In occult tension hydrocephalus, insidious psychomotor retardation and difficulty with school performance may become apparent. Neuroimaging scans demonstrate ventriculomegaly, and magnetic resonance imaging (MRI) may show high signal in the periventricular white matter (Hoon and Melhem, 2000; Fig. 14-1). Although treatment with a shunt procedure may be beneficial, congenital hydrocephalus often produces severe mental retardation (Resch et al., 1996; Kirkinen et al., 1996). Alternatively, hydrocephalic children may remain asymptomatic until late adulthood, when they come to clinical attention with symptoms suggesting normal pressure hydrocephalus (see below); a beneficial response to shunt surgery may also be seen in these patients (Graff-Radford and Godersky, 1989).

The neuropathology of hydrocephalus falls most heavily upon the periventricular white matter and corpus callosum, where there is damage to axons and myelin from a combination of mechanical distortion and impaired cerebral blood flow (Del Bigio, 1993). The basal ganglia and thalamus may also be affected to a lesser

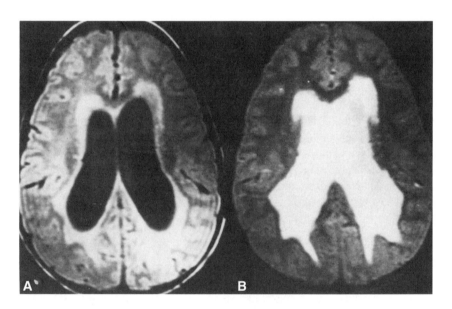

Figure 14-1. Proton density (*A*) and T2-weighted (*B*) MRI scans of a child with early hydrocephalus from aqueductal stenosis. Periventricular white matter changes are present on both images. (Reprinted with permission from Pomeranz SJ. Craniospinal magnetic resonance imaging. Philadelphia: W.B. Saunders, 1989.)

degree. Histologic changes are frequently absent in the cortex, although cortical damage can occur late in the course of prolonged hydrocephalus (Del Bigio, 1993). An animal model of neonatal hydrocephalus showed neuropathologic findings consistent with this pattern, as neonatal cats with kaolin-induced hydrocephalus had white matter changes including reactive gliosis, atrophy, and in some cases gross cavitation, with minimal cortical damage (Del Bigio et al., 1994).

The neurobehavioral impact of the white matter damage in early hydrocephalus has been investigated to a considerable degree. As a general rule, correlations of cognitive function are found with neuropathology in the cerebral white matter (van der Knaap et al., 1991; Fletcher et al., 1992). In some studies, these correlations are also seen with reductions in cortical gray matter, suggesting that the neuropathologic process may be severe enough in some patients to effect cortical dysfunction (Fletcher et al., 1996b). Mental retardation can be the presenting syndrome, but more often a less severe neurocognitive syndrome is encountered. In infants with congenital hydrocephalus, a significant correlation has been found between the degree of cerebral myelination as seen on MRI and intellectual development, implying that hydrocephalus retards myelination and thus cognitive development as well (van der Knaap et al., 1991).

More specifically, deficits in hydrocephalic children are typically seen in attention, memory, visuospatial ability, and frontal lobe function, with sparing of language (Mataró et al., 2000). A particularly common finding is a discrepancy between low performance intelligence quotient (PIQ) and relatively normal verbal IQ (VIQ), which has been attributed to white matter damage (Fletcher et al., 1992). In children with hydrocephalus, Fletcher and colleagues (1992) demonstrated significant ventriculomegaly and reduction in size of the corpus callosum and both internal capsules; lower VIQ was correlated with increased size of the left lateral ventricle while lower PIQ was correlated with increased right lateral ventricle size. These findings are consistent with a general trend for verbal intelligence and language to be better developed in early hydrocephalus than nonverbal intelligence (Dennis et al., 1981). Hydrocephalic children may in fact score as well as normals on many language measures, although close investigation may disclose subtle language deficits (Dennis et al., 1987). In contrast, visuospatial skills are regularly disrupted, and in one study this decrement was associated with reduced area of the corpus callosum (Fletcher et al., 1996a). Memory is also disturbed in early hydrocephalus, with evidence supporting deficits in both encoding and retrieval on both verbal and nonverbal tasks (Scott et al., 1998). In summary, currently available data on the pattern of neuropsychological deficits in children with early hydrocephalus are reasonably consistent with the profile of white matter dementia (Filley, 1998), in that there are deficits in attention, memory retrieval, visuospatial skills, and frontal lobe function with relative sparing of language. Discrepancies with the profile may indicate concurrent gray matter damage in some cases; for example, the presence of memory-encoding deficits may suggest that hippocampal regions are involved. Further neuroimaging studies, including the use of newer techniques, would be of interest in determining the relative contributions of white and gray matter to cognitive dysfunction.

Shunt procedures are routinely performed in the treatment of early hydro-cephalus. Cognitive recovery or improvement is often seen (Mataró et al., 2000), which may relate to the arrest of myelin destruction and the remyelination of some axons (Del Bigio, 1993). If axonal damage has occurred, recovery may be less complete, but early hydrocephalus is another example of the significant potential for white matter disorders to respond to medical or surgical therapy. As is gener-ally the case with many white matter disorders, prompt treatment of this disorder holds the promise of more salutary results.

Hydrocephalus Ex Vacuo

An increase in CSF volume is regularly seen on neuroimaging scans of individuals with brain atrophy. This observation, often called hydrocephalus ex vacuo, is one of the most common neuroradiologic findings in the older population (Fig. 14-2).

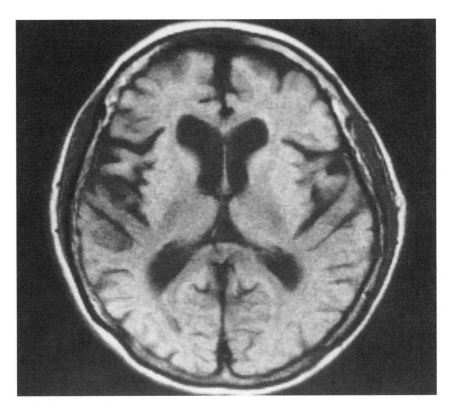

Figure 14-2. T1-weighted MRI scan of hydrocephalus ex vacuo in a 65-year-old woman with Alzheimer's disease. The brain shows volume loss that results primarily from gray matter atrophy.

Often striking in its severity, hydrocephalus ex vacuo is nevertheless nonspecific because it can be present with many degenerative diseases or with normal aging. While the utility of this term has been questioned, it does serve to point out how excessive water within the cranium may simply result from the normal or abnormal loss of brain tissue.

In many cases, hydrocephalus ex vacuo is due primarily to the cortical cell loss that occurs in Alzheimer's disease (AD). In this disease, massive cortical neuronal dropout is characteristic, and the brain atrophy that occurs does not imply significant white matter loss (Double et al., 1996). However, as pointed out in Chapter 3, normal aging also results in decreased brain weight and size (Creasey and Rapoport, 1985). Much of this decline, if not the majority, is caused by white matter loss (Double et al., 1996). Thus, it is worth recalling that atrophy does not necessarily imply gray matter loss, and hydrocephalus ex vacuo can imply a normal attrition of cerebral white matter. Clinically, the importance of this insight is that the normal white matter loss of aging can complicate the interpretation of neuroimaging scans because it typically coexists with many neurologic disorders that occur in the elderly. Another implication is that the popular term "cortical atrophy"—often used to describe brain atrophy in aging—would be better replaced by the less committal but more accurate "cerebral atrophy."

Normal Pressure Hydrocephalus

Few entities in clinical neurology produce such diagnostic, pathophysiologic, and therapeutic perplexity as normal pressure hydrocephalus (NPH). Since the first description of the disease in the 1960s (Adams et al., 1965), NPH has alternately been heralded as a reversible form of dementia and an entity whose very existence is open to debate. The opportunity to detect and effectively treat a cause of dementia is appealing, but the risks of treatment are not insubstantial. When patients present with symptoms and signs indicating possible NPH, the clinician is therefore challenged to decide upon which individuals might be likely to benefit from treatment. In this section, the continuing clinical conundrum of NPH is discussed as a disorder of cerebral white matter.

Normal pressure hydrocephalus presents with the classic clinical triad of dementia, gait disorder, and incontinence (Adams et al., 1965). The dementia has been noted to have frontal features, with cognitive slowing and apathy, and the gait disorder and incontinence also seem to stem from frontal lobe damage (Adams et al., 1965). Some cases are thought to follow meningitis, traumatic brain injury, or subarachnoid hemorrhage, but many remain idiopathic (Graff-Radford, 1999). Computed tomography (CT) scans show enlarged ventricles and relatively normal cortical gyri without sulcal enlargement (Fig. 14-3), but these findings are subjective and the scans are often difficult to distinguish from those representing other neuropathologic conditions and normal aging.

Magnetic resonance imaging scans may often show additional high signal lesions in the deep cerebral white matter (Fig. 14-4), and some have suggested that

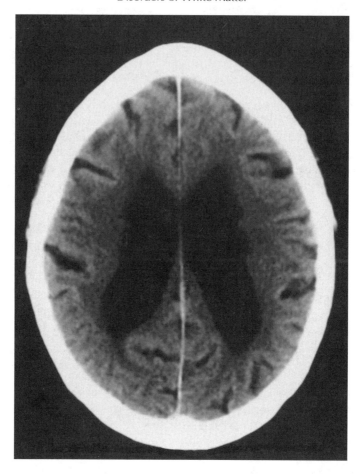

Figure 14-3. Computed tomography scan of a 78-year-old man with NPH. There is ventriculomegaly with relatively normal cortical sulci, but the white matter is not well seen.

this transpendymal CSF flow is a clue to a good outcome with shunting (Jack et al., 1987). Other investigations, however, have not been consistent in supporting this claim (Graff-Radford, 1999). More recent studies showing a low magnetization transfer ratio in the normal appearing white matter of patients with NPH (Hähnel et al., 2000) may further assist in demonstrating white matter damage and in improving clinical management. The diagnosis is presently made by identifying the clinical triad, finding a consistent neuroimaging pattern, and ruling out other etiologic possibilities; many also perform a high volume CSF "tap test" because a temporary improvement in gait and sometimes cognition may help predict a good surgical outcome (Fisher, 1978).

The pathophysiology of NPH has continued to be an enigma. Adams and colleagues (1965) offered the first and still most familiar theory, which holds that ob-

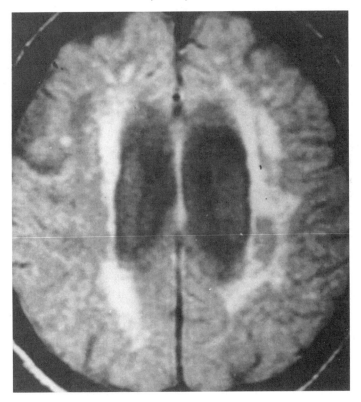

Figure 14-4. Mildly T2-weighted MRI scan of a patient with NPH. The scan shows the changes seen on CT (Fig. 14-3) as well as additional periventricular white matter hyperintensity. (Reprinted with permission from Atlas SW, ed. Magnetic resonance imaging of the brain and spine. 2nd ed. Philadelphia: Lippincott-Raven, 1996.)

struction of CSF outflow causes ventricular enlargement without cortical atrophy; the assumption is that the outflow obstruction is at the level of the arachnoid villi. The CSF pressure remains normal because of Pascal's Law (Force = Pressure × Area), which predicts that with an increased ventricular wall area, the force applied to the brain can be high while pressure is still normal (Adams et al., 1965). This explanation has been questioned by several investigators. Symon and colleagues (1972) demonstrated episodes of raised intracranial pressure throughout the night in patients with NPH, and suggested that a better term for the disorder might be "episodically raised pressure hydrocephalus." Geschwind (1968) challenged the theory of Adams and colleagues on physical grounds, and argued that the properties of the ventricular wall need to be considered in formulating the pathogenesis of NPH. These ideas helped generate another major competing hypothesis, which is that ischemia and infarction in the cerebral white matter may lead to ventriculomegaly, and the reduced tensile strength of the white matter could cause further ventricular enlargement under the stress of intraventricular pulse pressure (Earnest et al., 1974). In support of this hypothesis are studies showing increased severity of periventricular and deep white matter lesions in NPH compared to age-matched controls (Krauss et al., 1997). This theory thus suggests that there may be an overlap of NPH with Binswanger's disease (BD), or even that the two may in fact be the same disease. Most authorities, however, favor the existence of NPH as a distinct entity, recognizing that it may coexist with other neuropathologic processes. A recent report, for example, identified a subgroup of NPH patients who had simultaneous vascular white matter disease, and found that they had a less favorable outcome after shunt surgery (Boon et al., 1999). The validity of distinguishing between NPH and BD was also supported by recent CSF studies demonstrating elevated neurofilament triplet protein and normal sulfatide in the former, and the opposite pattern in the latter (Tullberg et al., 2000). These findings imply a neuropathologic distinction between ongoing axonal involvement in NPH as opposed to active demyelination in BD (Tullberg et al., 2000). From a clinical perspective, the beneficial response to surgery seen in many individuals with NPH seems to justify the conclusion that the disease may exist in isolation, but that white matter ischemia and infarction can often be present as well and therefore limit its reversibility.

Regardless of the mechanism of NPH, the neuropathologic findings are generally consistent with primary involvement of white matter. Whereas details of the neuropathology are debated, the white matter of the cerebrum seems to bear the brunt of the damage (Di Rocco et al., 1977; Akai et al., 1987; Del Bigio, 1993). There is evidence both for direct mechanical compression of the periventricular white matter (Di Rocco et al., 1977) and for ischemic demyelination and infarction (Akai et al., 1987). Gray matter, both of the subcortical nuclear structures and the cortex, is less affected, although with severe and prolonged hydrocephalus there may be some neuronal damage in these areas (Del Bigio, 1993). As is true of the white matter, however, unrelated neuropathology in the cortex can be found in patients suspected of having NPH. A recent study found that 10 out of 38 patients thought clinically to have NPH actually had biopsy-proven AD (Bech et al., 1997). These data further highlight the difficulty in diagnosing NPH, suggest that cortical pathology may be present in many cases, and offer another explanation why some patients have a poor outcome after treatment.

The neurobehavioral profile of NPH has been studied in only a limited fashion. Derix (1994) reviewed the literature and concluded that NPH has neuropsychological features typical of subcortical dementia. There are prominent frontal signs including cognitive slowing, inattention, and perseveration, and memory loss occurs as well (Derix, 1994). Importantly, there is typically little or no aphasia, apraxia, or agnosia, with the exception of the gait disorder, which is sometimes called gait apraxia (Derix, 1994); this aspect of the disease is best considered a motor sign. Cognitive slowing has been noted to be prominent in patients with NPH (Gustafson and Hagberg, 1978). Gallassi and colleagues (1991) compared NPH with BD patients and found these groups to be similarly impaired in comparison to control subjects. In contrast, Iddon and colleagues (1999) were able to show selective executive function deficits in patients with NPH that were not present in AD patients with comparable dementia severity. In light of these findings and the neuropathology of the disease, NPH has been classified as a white matter dementia (Filley, 1998).

When surgical treatment of NPH is undertaken, a diversionary shunt is placed in the brain to reduce ventricular volume. Shunts of this type are flexible tubes with one-way valves that can be positioned to provide ventriculoperitoneal, ventriculoatrial, or lumboperitoneal CSF drainage. The critical issue revolves around the decision as to which patients are most likely to benefit from a shunt procedure. This determination is not trivial because of the high incidence of shunt complications including anesthesia reactions, hemorrhage, and infection (Vanneste et al., 1992). Although clinicians have differing preferences, it is reasonable to refer for surgery only those patients who have the full clinical triad, consistent neuroimaging studies, a positive tap test, no evidence of other cerebral diseases, and no prohibitive surgical risk. Graff-Radford (1999) has suggested that additional favorable prognostic signs are the presence of dementia for fewer than 2 years, the gait abnormality preceding the dementia, and a known cause of NPH. Despite some skepticism that less favorable studies of outcome and shunt complications have generated (Vanneste et al., 1992), and the continuing confusion about the pathophysiology of the disease, NPH appears to be a dementia primarily caused by cerebral white matter damage that can be treated successfully in some patients.

References

Adams RD, Fisher CM, Hakim S, et al. Symptomatic occult hydrocephalus with "normal" cerebrospinal-fluid pressure. N Engl J Med 1965; 273: 117–126.

Akai K, Uchigasaki S, Tanaka U, Komatsu A. Normal pressure hydrocephalus. Neuropathological study. Acta Pathol Jpn 1987; 37: 97–110.

Bech RA, Juhler M, Waldemar G, et al. Frontal brain and leptomeningeal biopsy specimens correlated with cerebrospinal fluid outflow resistance and B-wave activity in patients suspected of normal-pressure hydrocephalus. Neurosurgery 1997; 40: 497–502.

Boon AJ, Tans JT, Delwel EJ, et al. Dutch normal-pressure hydrocephalus study: the role of cerebrovascular disease. J Neurosurg 1999; 90: 221–226.

Creasey H. Rapoport SI. The aging human brain. Ann Neurol 1985; 17: 2–10.

Del Bigio MR. Neuropathological changes caused by hydrocephalus. Acta Neuropathol 1993; 85: 573–585.

Del Bigio MR, da Silva MC, Drake JM, Tuor UI. Acute and chronic cerebral white matter damage in neonatal hydrocephalus. Can J Neurol Sci 1994; 21: 299–305.

Dennis M, Fitz CR, Netley CT, et al. The intelligence of hydrocephalic children. Arch Neurol 1981: 38: 607–615.

Dennis M, Hendrick EB, Hoffman HJ, Humphreys RP. Language of hydrocephalic children and adolescents. J Clin Exp Neuropsychol 1987; 9: 593–621.

Derix MMA. Neuropsychological differentiation of dementia syndromes. Lisse: Swets and Zeitlinger, 1994.

Di Rocco C, Di Trapani G, Maira G, et al. Anatomo-clinical correlations in normotensive hydrocephalus. J Neurol Sci 1977; 33: 437–452.

Double KL, Halliday GM, Kril JJ, et al. Topography of brain atrophy during normal aging and Alzheimer's Disease. Neurobiol Aging 1996; 17: 513–521.

Earnest MP, Fahn S, Karp JH, Rowland LP. Normal pressure hydrocephalus and hypertensive cerebrovascular disease. Arch Neurol 1974; 31: 262–266.

Filley CM. The behavioral neurology of cerebral white matter. Neurology 1998; 50: 1535–1540.

Fisher CM. Communicating hydrocephalus. Lancet 1978; 1: 37.

Fishman RA. Cerebrospinal fluid in diseases of the nervous system. 2nd ed. Philadelphia: W.B. Saunders, 1992.

Fletcher JM, Bohan TP, Brandt ME, et al. Cerebral white matter and cognition in hydrocephalic children. Arch Neurol 1992; 49: 818–824.

Fletcher JM, Bohan TP, Brandt ME, et al. Morphometric evaluation of the hydrocephalic brain: relationships with cognitive development. Childs Nerv Sys 1996a; 192–199.

Fletcher JM, McCauley SR, Brandt ME, et al. Regional brain tissue composition in children with hydrocephalus. Relationships with cognitive development. Arch Neurol 1996b; 53: 549–557.

Gallassi R, Morreale A, Montagna P, et al. Binswanger's Disease and normal-pressure hydrocephalus. Clinical and neuropsychological comparison. Arch Neurol 1991; 48: 1156–1159.

Geschwind N. The mechanism of normal pressure hydrocephalus. J Neurol Sci 1968; 7: 481–493.

Graff-Radford NR. Normal pressure hydrocephalus. Neurologist 1999; 5: 194–204.

Graff-Radford NR, Godersky JC. Symptomatic congenital hydrocephalus in the elderly simulating normal pressure hydrocephalus. Neurology 1989; 39: 1596–1600.

Gustafson L, Hagberg B. Recovery in hydrocephalic dementia after shunt operation. J Neurol Neurosurg Psychiatry 1978; 41: 940–947.

Hähnel S, Freund M, Münkel K, et al. Magnetisation transfer ratio is low in normal-appearing cerebral white matter in patients with normal pressure hydrocephalus. J Neurol 2000; 42: 174–179.

Hoon AH, Melhem ER. Neuroimaging: applications in disorders of early brain development. J Dev Behav Pediatr 2000; 21: 291–302.

Iddon JL, Pickard JD, Cross JJL, et al. Specific patterns of cognitive impairment in patients with idiopathic normal pressure hydrocephalus and Alzheimer's disease: a pilot study. J Neurol Neurosurg Psychiatry 1999; 67: 723–732.

Jack CR, Mokri B, Laws ER, et al. MR findings in normal-pressure hydrocephalus: significance and comparison with other forms of dementia. J Comput Assist Tomogr 1987; 11: 923–931.

Kirkinen P, Serlo W, Jouppila P, et al. Long-term outcome in fetal hydrocephaly. J Child Neurol 1996; 11: 189–192.

Krauss JK, Regel JP, Vach W, et al. White matter lesions in patients with idiopathic normal pressure hydrocephalus and in an age-matched control group: a comparative study. Neurosurgery 1997; 40: 491–496.

Mataró M, Poca, MA, Sahuquillo J, et al. Cognitive changes after cerebrospinal fluid shunting in young adults with spina bifida and arrested hydrocephalus. J Neurol Neurosurg Psychiatry 2000; 68: 615–621.

Resch B, Gedermann A, Maurer U, et al. Neurodevelopmental outcome of hydrocephalus following intra-/periventricular hemorrhage in preterm infants: short- and long-term results. Childs Nerv Syst 1996; 12: 27–33.

Scott MA, Fletcher JM, Brookshire BL, et al. Memory functions in children with early hydrocephalus. Neuropsychology 1998; 12: 578–589.

Symon L, Dorsch NWC, Stephens RJ. Pressure waves in so-called low-pressure hydrocephalus. Lancet 1972; 2: 1291–1292.

Tullberg M, Månsson J-E, Fredman P, et al. CSF sulfatide distinguishes between normal pressure hydrocephalus and subcortical arteriosclerotic encephalopathy. J Neurol Neurosurg Psychiatry 2000; 69: 74–81.

van der Knaap, Valk J, Bakker CJ, et al. Myelination as an expression of the functional maturity of the brain. Dev Med Child Neurol 1991; 33: 849–857.

Vanneste J, Augustijn P, Dirven C, et al. Shunting normal-pressure hydrocephalus: do the benefits outweigh the risks? A multicenter study and literature review. Neurology 1992; 42: 54–59.

III

WHITE MATTER AND HIGHER FUNCTION

15

Cognitive Dysfunction and Dementia

The disorders covered in Part II of this book collectively demonstrate that damage to the white matter of the brain can disrupt higher functions. The review of these individual disorders forms a basis for considering the many neurobehavioral syndromes they may produce. These syndromes are described primarily in case reports and case series, in which there is a variable amount of clinical detail. For some disorders, more comprehensive information is available from systematic studies using neuropsychological testing and magnetic resonance imaging (MRI) correlation. The goal in Part III is to discuss these syndromes in detail as a prelude to developing a behavioral neurology of white matter, to be presented in Chapter 18.

Cognitive impairment emerges as the most frequent neurobehavioral syndrome in patients with white matter disorders. This disturbance may range from a mild attention or concentration deficit to severe dementia or the vegetative state. The apparent primacy of cognitive impairment, however, needs to be taken as tentative. An important point is that many reports of individuals with white matter disorders focus on etiologic or elemental neurologic aspects of the case rather than neurobehavioral phenomena, and hence the details of mental status are often incomplete. Of all mental changes, clinicians are probably most adept at detecting cognitive impairment, whereas focal neurobehavioral syndromes or neuropsychiatric dysfunction may not be as readily appreciated. Thus, future investigation examining white matter disorders may disclose that other neurobehavioral syndromes are more prominent than they appear at present.

Cognitive Dysfunction

Cognitive dysfunction is a term that can be widely and diversely interpreted. For the purposes of this discussion, it will be considered a variable syndrome of relatively mild disturbance across a range of higher functions that may include attention, memory, language, visuospatial skills, complex cognition, and emotion or personality. This formulation thus excludes cases of severe cognitive impairment—dementia—which is addressed later in this chapter. Cognitive dysfunction implies a meaningful decline from a normal level of competence, but not to a point where independent living is precluded. Both cognitive dysfunction and dementia are also to be distinguished from cases in which the clinical picture is dominated by focal neurobehavioral syndromes, such as amnesia (Chapter 16), or isolated neuropsychiatric presentations, such as psychosis (Chapter 17).

One of the important insights in behavioral neurology to emerge in the last decade is the appreciation of a category of cognitive loss that does not reach the level of dementia. It is increasingly recognized that cognitive impairment is not an all-or-none phenomenon, and that many individuals have deficits intermediate in severity between normal cognition and dementia as formally defined (Cummings and Benson, 1994). In clinical practice, for example, it is common to encounter mild degrees of cognitive loss that do not meet criteria for dementia but which are often troubling to the patient. Perhaps the most useful descriptor for this problem is the recently defined "mild cognitive impairment" (MCI; Petersen et al., 1999), which can be detected in many older people and may indicate a feature of normal aging or an early clinical manifestation of Alzheimer's disease (AD). Mild cognitive impairment is a worrisome syndrome to patients and their physicians, but it does not represent the widespread and disabling deficits implied by the term dementia.

Cognitive dysfunction can thus be meaningfully differentiated from dementia, and in the context of this discussion, the distinction is particularly relevant. Individuals with multiple sclerosis (MS), for example, often experience subtle cognitive loss that may not be detected by clinicians (Franklin et al., 1990), as may individuals with other white matter disorders (Filley, 1998). In the realm of vascular disease, a similar category of "vascular cognitive impairment without dementia" has recently been proposed (Rockwood et al., 2000), which can be used to describe the cognitive loss experienced by individuals with many kinds of cerebrovascular disease, including white matter ischemia and infarction. Similar cognitive loss is a regular feature of other white matter disorders, as reviewed in Part II.

Despite the growing recognition that cognitive dysfunction can be a feature of white matter disorders, patients with this syndrome are frequently not identified. Because of the influence of traditional teaching that white matter disease only minimally impacts cognition, cognitive concerns may be overlooked in busy neurology clinics where motor, sensory, and visual deficits may be more apparent. This relative lack of ascertainment can also be attributed to other factors. First, from studies of MS it is apparent that the degree of physical disability is not well correlated with cognitive status (Franklin et al., 1989). Thus, a patient may have significant cognitive loss even if elemental neurologic function is well preserved.

Second, studies of MS demonstrate that routine clinical mental status testing by neurologists does not reliably detect cognitive dysfunction (Heaton et al., 1985). Office mental status tests were developed as relatively brief screening tests for dementia, and cannot be expected to be sensitive to all the subtle deficits that are produced by white matter disorders. Third, clinicians may be misled by the fact that language is largely spared in white matter disorders (Filley, 1998). Language testing is a cornerstone of office testing, and screening of linguistic function that detects no abnormality may falsely suggest intact cognition. Moreover, standardized mental status examinations such as the Mini-Mental State Examination (MMSE: Folstein et al., 1975) heavily weigh language function, so that reliance on such instruments may again be misleading in white matter disorders (Filley, 1998). Finally, a less tangible but still probable reason for the underdetection of cognitive dysfunction in white matter disorders is the clinician's reluctance to risk demoralizing the patient who may already be obliged to deal with major neurologic disability. Franklin and colleagues (1990) pointed out the belief of many clinicians that the identification of presumably irreversible cognitive disturbances in MS adds needlessly to the psychological burden of affected patients.

Regardless of these concerns, cognitive impairment in white matter disorders is not trivial. Patients with this level of impairment can often be helped by the recognition of the problem in terms of counseling and rehabilitation, and significant relief can come from the understanding that a cognitive difficulty originates from structural lesions in the brain and not from what may have been labelled a psychiatric problem. Perhaps even more important in the years ahead is the prospect of effective therapy for neurobehavioral syndromes in the white matter disorders that will permit early treatment of cognitive dysfunction. To continue with the example of MS, it is conceivable that the use of immunomodulatory agents (Pliskin et al., 1996; Fischer et al., 2000) may forestall the onset of more severe cognitive loss or even restore normal cognition in some cases. Another example is leukoaraiosis, in which the control of hypertension and the use of antiplatelet agents may be especially important to prevent dementia or slow its progress (Rockwood et al., 2000).

The pathogenesis of cognitive dysfunction in white matter disorders likely involves neuropathologic changes that are relatively mild in comparison to those that produce dementia. Although the range of neuropathologic change is broad, a trend emerges from considering parallel literatures. In MS, for example, Rao and colleagues (1989a) found that a lesion area of >30 cm^2 predicted cognitive impairment, implying that the burden of disease determines the severity of cognitive change. A similar observation was made by Boone and colleagues in patients with leukoaraiosis (1992), who found that a lesion area of >10 cm^2 predicted cognitive impairment. In toluene abuse, the severity of white matter change on MRI correlates with the degree of cognitive loss (Filley et al., 1990), and a general tendency exists for toxic leukoencephalopathy from any cause to exhibit the same pattern (Filley, 1999). It can still be debated at what level of white matter involvement clinically meaningful impairment begins, and the answer to this question undoubtedly implicates many factors such as the method of measuring cognitive function, the neuroradiologic assessment of white matter lesions, the nature of the white matter neuropathology (i.e., with or without axonal loss), and the premorbid cognitive profile of the individual. However, the weight of evidence supports a general relationship between white matter involvement and cognitive loss.

An interesting approach that may apply to cognitive dysfunction in white matter disorders has been offered from a neuropsychological perspective. The nonverbal learning disability (NLD) syndrome is a clinical model developed from observations of children who appear to have deficits and assets similar to those of adults with acquired right hemisphere neuropathology (Rourke, 1995). According to this model, the NLD syndrome consists of a profile of deficits in tactile perception, visual perception, complex psychomotor skills, dealing with novelty, tactile attention, visual attention, exploratory behavior, tactile memory, visual memory, concept formation, problem solving, and prosody. Most aspects of language and verbal memory are preserved (Rourke, 1995). The problems experienced by these children in turn compromise arithmetic ability, visuospatial skills, and social relationships, and the subsequent social withdrawal and anxiety that result can lead to depression and suicide (Rourke, 1987; Cleaver and Whitman, 1998). Because evidence exists for the presence of proportionally more white matter in the right hemisphere (Gur et al., 1980), Rourke (1995) has hypothesized that the NLD syndrome may be associated with white matter dysfunction. Examination of this model discloses some clinical similarities to descriptions of cognitive dysfunction with white matter neuropathology advanced herein, as the NLD syndrome appears to included aspects of attentional dysfunction, frontal lobe impairment, visuospatial dysfunction, psychiatric disability, and spared language. Moreover, Rourke has presented provocative reviews of suggestive relationships between the NLD model and white matter disorders including metachromatic leukodystrophy (MLD), MS, toxic leukoencephalopathy, traumatic brain injury (TBI), and early hydrocephalus (1995). Thus, it is conceivable that white matter dysfunction underlies many cases of the NLD syndrome, and that this model can be used to characterize individuals with known white matter pathology.

However, the NLD syndrome remains a theoretical construct, and there is little documentation of right hemisphere damage in white (or gray) matter among children with this disability (Semrud-Clikeman and Hynd, 1990). The essential step required to establish the validity of the NLD syndrome as a descriptor of white matter dysfunction would therefore be to correlate aspects of the syndrome with data from neurologic subjects who have well-defined white matter alterations as demonstrated neuropathologically or neuroradiologically. Until then, the relevance of the NLD syndrome to the behavioral neurology of white matter must remain conjectural.

White Matter Dementia

Individuals with white matter disorders may also develop dementia, a disabling syndrome that represents a more florid manifestation of cognitive impairment. This concept immediately seems counterintuitive to many, as it is widely held that dementia represents exclusively cortical neuropathology. Whereas it is true that

cortical tissue loss accounts for cognitive decline in AD, the most common degenerative dementia (Mouton et al., 1998), involvement of white matter may have
similar results. Vascular disease involving 25% or more of the cerebral white
matter, for example, has been suggested to be sufficient to cause dementia (Román
et al., 1993). Tissue loss or dysfunction in white matter regions can thus lead to
dementia as surely as does AD, although the specific clinical features of affected
individuals may be strikingly different.

For our purposes, the most useful definition of dementia is that of Cummings
and Benson (1994), who define dementia as an acquired and persistent disorder of
intellectual function with deficits in at least three of the following: memory, language, visuospatial skills, complex cognition, and emotion or personality. It is important to note that this definition differs from that of the widely cited American
Psychiatric Association Diagnostic and Statistical Manual (DSM-IV; 1994), which
emphasizes aphasia, apraxia, and agnosia as core disturbances. Careful analysis of
white matter disorder patients with dementia discloses that whereas disabling deficits in various domains do arise, the cortical syndromes of aphasia, apraxia, and
agnosia are encountered only exceptionally. Thus, the DSM-IV definition, based
as it is on the cognitive profile of cortical dementias such as AD, is less useful than
the more inclusive definition by Cummings and Benson (1994).

Dementia in individuals with white matter disorders has been recognized for
many years. This syndrome, however, has not attracted the attention given to cortical dementias, or even to subcortical dementias such as Parkinson's disease and
Huntington's disease (HD). When white matter disorders have been formally considered, the dementias that occur have usually been classified as subcortical, and
indeed many similarities have been noted that would support this claim (Cummings, 1990). However, evidence exists to indicate that the white matter disorders
may deserve to be separated from other categories and classified as a distinct group.

In 1988, the idea of white matter dementia was first introduced (Filley et al.,
1988). At that time, the notion was based on clinical experience with selected
white matter disorders and a literature review of many others that suggested neurobehavioral features common to all. In particular, patients with MS (Franklin et al.,
1988, 1989) and toluene abuse (Hormes et al., 1986; Rosenberg et al., 1988) provided two plausible examples of this phenomenon, as severe and unequivocal dementia was evident in both. These two disorders shared the feature of neuropathology essentially confined to white matter, and thus presented the opportunity to
study secondary neurobehavioral manifestations in two different clinical populations. The idea of white matter dementia was put forth as a hypothesis in hopes of
stimulating further work that could assist in the understanding and treatment of
many neurologic disorders, and more generally in advancing knowledge of the operations of the human brain.

This initial formulation was derived from a consideration of subcortical dementia, with which the syndrome is closely associated (Chapter 1). In general,
white matter dementia was thought to be characterized by inattention, forgetfulness,
emotional changes, and the absence of aphasia, apraxia, and a movement disorder
(Filley et al., 1988). This profile is of course similar to that of subcortical dementia (Cummings, 1990). However, two clinical features seemed sufficiently promi-

nent to support the creation of a separate dementia category. The first was the saliency of attentional dysfunction, which was felt to be closely allied with cognitive slowing. The second was the typical absence of a movement disorder, which distinguished white matter dementia from subcortical dementias that regularly feature an extrapyramidal component.

In the years since this proposal, further investigation has been conducted that pertains to this hypothesis (Filley et al., 1989, 1990; Merriam et al., 1989, 1990; Filley and Gross, 1992; Rao et al., 1993; Shapiro et al., 1994; Yamanouchi et al., 1997; Filley et al., 1999; Riva et al., 2000; Mendez et al., 2000), and critical reviews have dealt with conceptual issues (Rao, 1993, 1996; Feinstein, 1999). Although systematic study of the distinctions between these dementia categories has been undertaken only rarely (Rao et al., 1993), many relevant observations have illuminated this topic. As a result, a further refinement of the idea has been facilitated.

One clinically helpful point is the tendency for the differentiating aspects of the dementias to be most evident in the early and middle stages of the disease. This feature is particularly useful in that it assists in the clinical diagnosis of dementia when the greatest opportunity for treatment is still present. Specific patterns of cognitive deficit may even persist late into the disease course. Paulsen and colleagues (1995) used the Dementia Rating Scale (Mattis, 1988) to show that profiles of cortical and subcortical deficits were evident in patients with AD and HD, respectively, even when the dementia was rated as severe. However, as the dementing illness progresses in most cases, the accumulation of neuropathology usually results in a clinical picture of neurobehavioral and neurologic disability that appears increasingly uniform. In the most severe and terminal stages, little if any distinction between cortical, subcortical gray, or white matter dementia can be detected.

Bearing in mind that the defining clinical features of dementia are most evident in early stages, a more complete profile of deficits and preserved strengths in white matter dementia can be proposed. Based on a review of the existing literature, Table 15-1 presents the neurobehavioral details of dementia in 10 prominent white matter disorders representing the neuropathologic categories covered in Part II. Relying heavily on the terminology of Cummings and Benson (1994), this summary represents the current state of the clinical evidence regarding dementia in these disorders. Although incomplete, this tabulation supports the concept that white matter dementia may be a consistent clinical syndrome.

The general portrait of white matter dementia shown in Table 15-1 is a useful beginning, but further information can be gleaned from a careful reading of the literature. Attention and memory, for example, are not unitary concepts, and the exact characterization of attentional and memory dysfunction is crucial to the concept as a whole. The various domains listed in Table 15-1 are discussed in detail below.

Sustained Attention Deficit

Attention is a problematic term in behavioral neurology and neuropsychology. While useful in that it designates important mental operations, the meaning of attention depends on the context in which it is used. In its most general sense, attention refers to the ability to focus on some stimuli while competing distractors

Table 15-1. Characteristics of Dementia in Selected White Matter Disorders

Disorder	Attention	Memory	Language	Visuo-spatial Skills	Complex Cognition	Emotions & Personality	Extra-pyramidal Function
MLD	↓	↓	N	↓	↓	↓	N
MS	↓	↓	N	↓	↓	↓	N
AIDS dementia complex	↓	↓	N	↓	↓	↓	±
SLE	↓	↓	N	↓	↓	↓	±
Toluene dementia	↓	↓	N	↓	↓	↓	N
Cobalamin deficiency	↓	↓	N	↓	↓	↓	N
BD	↓	↓	N	↓	↓	↓	±
TBI	↓	↓	N	↓	↓	↓	N
NPH	↓	↓	N	↓	↓	↓	N
Gliomatosis cerebri	↓	↓	N	?	↓	↓	N

N, normal; MLD, metachromatic leukodystrophy; MS, multiple sclerosis; AIDS, acquired immunodeficiency syndrome; SLE, systemic lupus erythematosus; BD, Binswanger's disease; TBI, traumatic brain injury; NPH, normal pressure hydrocephalus.

are present; this capacity, often called selective attention, operates over a period of seconds, and is commonly tested by the digit span (Mesulam, 2000). When selective attention operates over a period of minutes, sustained attention, also known as concentration or vigilance, is engaged, and a variety of continuous performance tasks are suitable for assessment (Mesulam, 2000).

To test the idea that attentional disturbances are prominent in white matter disorders, a comparison of neuropsychological features in MS and AD was conducted, revealing that sustained attention was markedly affected in the former while relatively normal in the latter (Filley et al., 1989). This study, the first to compare white matter and cortical disease directly from a neurobehavioral perspective, demonstrated contrasting profiles of attention and concentration dysfunction in patients with MS versus memory and language impairment in those with AD, and it was proposed that these two diseases may represent prototype white matter and cortical dementias (Filley et al., 1989). Attention and concentration deficits were also found to be more common in Binswanger's disease (BD) than in AD (Doody et al., 1998), further supporting this distinction. These results are usefully interpreted in light of a neuropsychological comparison of subcortical gray with subcortical white matter disease (Caine et al., 1986); in this study, patients with MS and HD had similar cognitive impairment, but memory dysfunction was generally more severe in HD, and MS patients showed normal cognitive strategies but lowered mental efficiency. Thus, in these respects MS differs from both AD and HD.

The neuroanatomy of sustained attention is not well established, although it is likely that a network of interconnected structures mediates this capacity. Many lines of evidence implicate the frontal lobes and their connections to more posterior structures (Mesulam, 2000), and it is conceivable that the right frontal lobe is particularly specialized for sustained attention (Rueckert and Grafman, 1996). It also appears likely that the white matter of the frontal lobes, especially the right, contributes to this capacity (Filley, 1995). In one study, for example, children with attention deficit disorder with hyperactivity had a smaller volume of the right frontal lobe white matter than normal control subjects, and poorer performance on sustained attention tasks was associated with reduced right hemisphere white matter volume (Semrud-Clikeman et al., 2000). Additional evidence exists for a role of the anterior corpus callosum, which joins the frontal lobes. Studies in normal subjects support a role of the corpus callosum in sustained attention (Rueckert et al., 1994, 1999). Consistent with these observations, patients with lesions of the corpus callosum have deficits in sustained attention. In MS, for example, an impairment of vigilance is correlated with reduced size of the corpus callosum as measured by MRI (Rao et al., 1989b). Similar reductions in corpus callosum size have been reported in children with attention deficit hyperactivity disorder (Giedd et al., 1994). In TBI patients, dichotic listening experiments reveal a left ear suppression of information suggesting impaired callosal transfer from the right to the left hemisphere (Levin et al., 1989; Benavidez et al., 1999).

In considering the phenomenon of attention in white matter disorders, a factor that impacts performance dramatically is slowing of cognitive speed. This deficit has been emphasized as a cardinal feature of subcortical dementia (Cummings, 1990), and slowed information processing has also been noted in white matter disorders such as MS (Litvan et al., 1988; Demaree et al., 1999). Impaired cognitive speed will most often be evident in everyday tasks dependent on rapid information processing, and patients may complain of being overwhelmed with the burden of multiple tasks that may be present in a work setting. Some evidence exists to suggest that "cognitive fatigue" in MS patients may contribute to poor performance on tasks requiring sustained attention (Schwid et al., 2000; Krupp and Elkins, 2000). In a neuropsychology laboratory setting, this deficit will be apparent on vigilance tests, and an increase in reaction time may coexist with a deficit in sustained attention (Rueckert and Grafman, 1996). Indeed, some have suggested that impairments in vigilance are explained entirely by cognitive slowing (Spikman et al., 1996). Whatever its mechanism(s), cognitive slowing is a common impairment that often dominates the behavioral repertoire of patients with white matter disorders of any origin. In the context of white matter dementia, cognitive slowing is best considered a nonspecific deficit that can become manifest in the performance of attentional and other tasks.

Memory Retrieval Deficit with Normal Procedural Memory

Memory, like attention, is a difficult yet fundamental concept in clinical neuroscience. Many different forms of memory have been postulated, which are derived from clinical examples in which specific deficits in memory can follow documented brain lesions. For our purposes, two distinctions will prove most useful.

The first is between declarative and procedural memory, which in essence refers to the difference between fact and skill memory. Declarative memory is the variety regularly tested in neurologic encounters, and this process is a mainstay of the mental status examination; procedural memory, however, must presently be evaluated by special neuropsychological tests that tap motor learning. The second distinction lies within the category of declarative memory and involves the separable processes of encoding versus retrieval. The clinician has some capacity to evaluate these aspects of memory by determining if the recall of items that cannot be recalled after a delay can be improved by one of two methods: *(1)* cueing the patient with the provision of semantic clues that may trigger a memory, and *(2)* providing a list of items in which the desired ones are included. If either of these procedures results in improved recall, the patient can be said to have encoded the information but has been deficient in its retrieval. In the practice of behavioral neurology, it is sometimes possible to establish this distinction during the evaluation, but as a rule, neuropsychological testing offers a more thorough assessment of this distinction, and the data on memory retrieval have been primarily derived from this approach.

In this light, it is pertinent to review some neuropsychological studies of memory that have suggested a unique pattern in patients with white matter disorders. Individuals with MS were first evaluated with this objective in mind, and were found to have a retrieval deficit in declarative memory (Rao et al., 1984) but a preservation of procedural memory (Rao et al., 1993). As mentioned in Chapter 6, some studies have presented data supporting an alternative idea that the declarative memory deficit of MS patients is more related to difficulty with the acquisition of information than its retrieval (DeLuca et al., 1994, 1998). However, retrieval deficits have been documented in several other diseases with white matter involvement, including the AIDS dementia complex (ADC; White et al., 1997; Jones and Tranel, 1991), Lyme encephalopathy (Kaplan and Jones-Woodward, 1997), radiation leukoencephalopathy (Armstrong et al., 1995), ischemic vascular dementia (Lafosse et al., 1997; Libon et al., 1998), subcortical stroke (Reed et al., 2000), and TBI (Timmerman and Brouwer, 1999), suggesting that this pattern of declarative memory loss may be generalizable to all the white matter disorders. The preservation of procedural memory has been confirmed in MS (Lafosse et al., 2001), and has also been observed in the ADC (White et al., 1997; Jones and Tranel, 1991) and in TBI (Timmerman and Brouwer, 1999), although in ischemic vascular dementia it was found to be impaired (Libon et al., 1998). Despite some inconsistent data, the neuropsychological results thus far generally support a specific pattern of memory loss proposed for white matter dementia. This pattern stands in contrast to patterns of memory loss seen both in cortical disease, in which there is an encoding deficit in declarative memory and normal procedural memory, and in subcortical gray matter diseases, in which there is a retrieval deficit but impaired procedural memory (Filley, 1998; Table 15-2).

Although these distinctions are subtle, they indicate the possibility that white matter disorders may disturb memory in a specific and reproducible fashion. Presumably this pattern relates to the selective involvement of white matter tracts, which disrupts memory retrieval but not encoding, and the sparing of subcortical gray matter regions responsible for procedural memory. An intriguing hypothesis

Table 15-2. Memory Dysfunction in Cortical, White Matter, and Subcortical Dementia

	Cortical	White Matter	Subcortical
Declarative	Encoding deficit	Retrieval deficit	Retrieval deficit
Procedural	Normal	Normal	Impaired

bearing upon this topic has been presented by Markowitsch (1995), who suggested on the basis of clinical reports and functional neuroimaging data that the uncinate fasciculus (Fig. 2-2) is responsible for memory retrieval. According to this notion, memory retrieval requires the engagement of working memory systems in the frontal lobes to recall information stored in the temporal lobes, and the essential tract connecting these regions is the uncinate fasciculus (Markowitsch, 1995). Furthermore, the theory proposes that episodic memories are retrieved by this system in the right hemisphere, whereas semantic memories are retrieved in the left (Markowitsch, 1995). This idea is particularly important in that it posits a specific cognitive role for a white matter tract that has not heretofore had any neurobehavioral affiliation, and invites further study with modern neuroimaging technology applied to a variety of white matter disorders in which memory is affected.

As in the case of attentional dysfunction, the retrieval deficit seen in patients with white matter disorders can be seen as a problem with cognitive slowing. In clinical practice, these patients will often produce the correct answer to a question if sufficient time is provided, implying that the information is encoded but not easily retrieved. Thus, the delay in providing the correct answer may be interpreted as slowed cognition rather than a memory deficit. In other words, the patient is indeed cognitively slow, but the reason for this slowing is a failure of memory retrieval. As intimated above, cognitive slowing, although important as a general observation, can be analyzed in more detail and interpreted in terms of cognitive dysfunction. The delineation of specific deficits, most obviously in attention and memory, that contribute to cognitive slowing is an important neuropsychological issue deserving further study.

Normal Language

One of the most robust observations in the white matter disorders is that language is usually well preserved. In this respect, the clinical lore of classical neurology is entirely accurate. In MS, for example, aphasia is indeed rare, but can appear as an isolated syndrome related to a focal plaque in an eloquent white matter tract such as the arcuate fasciculus (Arnett et al., 1996). With detailed testing, minor deficits in language can be detected in MS (Kujala et al., 1996), but these are typically not evident in ordinary discourse or even on routine mental status testing. In comparison to patients with AD, MS patients have little linguistic difficulty (Filley et al., 1989). Aphasia is rarely encountered in other white matter disorders, although impaired verbal fluency may be seen (Derix, 1994).

Speech disorders, however, are frequent in white matter disorders. Dysarthria is well known in MS, and can sometimes assume a scanning quality. Articulation deficits are also described in the ADC (Navia et al., 1986), toluene dementia (Hormes et al., 1986), and BD (Babikian and Ropper, 1986). In these disorders, involvement of corticobulbar tracts subserving articulation is likely.

Visuospatial Dysfunction

Visuospatial function has only lately received attention, and what studies are available suggest an impairment. In MS patients, scores on the performance subtests of the Wechsler Adult Intelligence Scale are about 10 points lower than those of the verbal subtests (Rao, 1996), and specific visuospatial deficits have been shown on a variety of standard tests of right hemisphere function (Heaton et al., 1985; Rao et al., 1991). Further studies of solvent-induced leukoencephalopathy have confirmed that nonverbal abilities are more impaired than verbal skills in patients with toluene dementia (Yamanouchi et al., 1997). This nonverbal–verbal neuropsychological discrepancy has also been observed in patients with MLD (Shapiro et al., 1994).

Frontal Lobe Impairment

Many mental operations can be reasonably subsumed under the heading of complex cognition in Table 15-1, but most important are those commonly labelled frontal lobe functions. Deficits in tests that measure executive function have been noted in MS patients (Heaton et al., 1985), and MRI studies have correlated these deficits with plaques in the frontal lobe white matter (Arnett et al., 1994). Apathy is a prominent feature of toluene dementia, and probably stems from frontal lobe myelin loss (Hormes et al., 1986). In patients with MLD, a frontal lobe syndrome with poor attentional function has been documented neuropsychologically (Shapiro et al., 1994). More recently, Iddon and colleagues (1999) compared patients with NPH to those with AD, and found that a pattern of executive dysfunction related to frontal lobe involvement distinguished the former from the latter. Executive dysfunction is further discussed in Chapter 16.

Psychiatric Disturbance

Emotional and personality aspects of white matter dementia have also received more attention. Psychosis as an early feature of adult-onset MLD was noted as a frequent trend (Filley and Gross, 1992; Hyde et al., 1992), and the development of this syndrome was interpreted as an early component of a sequential progression to dementia seen in these patients (Filley and Gross, 1992; Shapiro et al., 1994). Depression in MS received considerable scrutiny (Minden and Schiffer, 1990), and the lethality of this problem was better appreciated as a high risk for suicide was documented (Sadovnick et al., 1991). Depression has been reported to be more common in BD patients than in AD patients who are comparably demented (Bennett et al., 1994). In vascular white matter dementia, the severity of delusions and hallucinations, aggression, irritability, aberrant motor behavior, nighttime behavior, and appetite changes has been correlated with cognitive decline, whereas no such correlations were found in AD (Aharon-Peretz et al., 2000). These data suggest that white matter ischemia and infarcts have a direct impact on psychosis and behavioral dysfunction. Chapter 17 addresses the neuropsychiatry of white matter disorders in greater detail.

Normal Extrapyramidal Function

An initial criticism of the white matter dementia hypothesis questioned the usefulness of the absence of movement disorders based on the observation that these phenomena may be encountered in white matter diseases (Merriam et al., 1990). However, despite exceptions to the rule, white matter disorders generally do not involve significant disorders of movement, at least early in the clinical course. Tranchant and colleagues (1995), for example, found that movement disorders related to basal ganglia dysfunction were rare in MS. Movement disorders reflecting basal ganglia involvement can occasionally occur in white matter disorders that have reached a late stage, as in the case of myoclonus in the ADC (Navia et al., 1986), or when the leukoencephalopathy is sufficiently widespread to involve the white matter of the basal ganglia, as exemplified by parkinsonism from severe carbon monoxide poisoning (Sohn et al., 2000).

Summary

The clinical and experimental observations made in the last decade in various white matter disorders have thus prompted a reconsideration and refinement of the original hypothesis (Filley, 1998). On the basis of this new information, the most likely neurobehavioral profile of white matter dementia now appears to be a combination of deficits in sustained attention, memory retrieval, visuospatial skills, frontal lobe function, and psychiatric status, with preserved language, procedural memory, and extrapyramidal function (Filley, 1998; Table 15-3). An interesting feature of this profile is that it represents the pattern that might be expected from the prominence of white matter in the frontal lobes (Filley, 1996) and in the right hemisphere (Gur et al., 1980). That is, because there appears to be proportionally more white matter in the frontal lobes and in the right hemisphere, disorders that

Table 15-3. Neurobehavioral Features of White Matter Dementia

Sustained attention deficit
Memory retrieval deficit with normal procedural memory
Normal language
Visuospatial dysfunction
Frontal lobe impairment
Psychiatric disturbance
Normal extrapyramidal function

diffusely affect the white matter would be predicted to cause primary deficits in functions mediated by these regions. This prediction has been upheld thus far.

Why a New Syndrome?

The proposal of a new syndrome in neurology is fraught with potential hazards. One need only recall the proposal of subcortical dementia in the 1970s (Chapter 1) to encounter a lively controversy stimulated by criticisms of the concept (Whitehouse, 1986; Brown and Marsden, 1988). Indeed, the notion of white matter dementia, like subcortical dementia, suffers from both clinical imprecision and a degree of neuropathologic overlap with other syndromes. Moreover, even if the legitimacy of subcortical dementia is accepted, it can be maintained that white matter disorders causing dementia are simply additional entries on this list, as some have maintained (Cummings, 1990). However, the delineation of a separate syndrome offers both practical and heuristic advantages that render such a venture worthwhile.

First, in clinical terms, concepts that organize thinking in medicine can improve diagnostic accuracy and overall patient care. The idea of white matter dementia can serve as a reminder that significant cognitive impairment attends many, perhaps all white matter disorders of the brain seen in clinical practice. This admonition would seem to be a useful one, given the often demonstrated failure of clinicians to make accurate observations of neurobehavioral deficits in these patients. Even if no specific profile emerges with further investigation, the heightened clinical awareness that this idea generates would be beneficial for many affected individuals. Classic neurologic teaching is notably deficient in presenting the details of neurobehavioral impairment of this type, a deficiency that made the background literature search for this text considerably more challenging than anticipated.

Second, in theoretical terms, the concept of white matter dementia is also intended to provide a stimulus for considering the role of white matter in the higher functions of the brain. Whereas this goal has been pursued with a modicum of enthusiasm lately, it must be acknowledged that the events taking place in the gray matter—particularly cortical gray matter—attract far more interest among neurologists and neuroscientists in general. One of the major goals of this book is to demonstrate how white matter plays a crucial role in the distributed neural networks that are recognized to mediate all aspects of cognitive and emotional function (Mesulam, 1990, 1998). Thus, white matter dementia serves to inform a more general behavioral neurology of white matter that is discussed in the last chapter of this book.

The idea of white matter dementia is therefore still put forth in the spirit of its original purpose, which is to stimulate clinical interest and promote research on the most common neurobehavioral syndrome in individuals with disorders of the brain white matter. From this admittedly speculative notion, it is hoped that patients with many different dementing diseases and injuries will receive more informed and appropriate care, and that meaningful study of the contribution of white matter disorders to the problem of dementia can proceed. Substantial support for the legitimacy of the proposal has appeared, both from the analysis of individual white matter disorders and from studies comparing these disorders with the cortical and subcortical gray matter diseases. Although more research is clearly needed, the evidence increasingly compels the view that a classification of dementia that neglects nearly half the volume of the brain cannot presume to provide a complete understanding of this common syndrome.

References

Aharon-Peretz J, Kliot D, Tomer R. Behavioral differences between white matter lacunar dementia and Alzheimer's Disease: a comparison on the Neuropsychiatric Inventory. Dement Geriatr Gogn Disord 2000; 11: 294–298.

American Psychiatric Association. Diagnostic and statistical manual. 4th ed. Washington, D.C.: American Psychiatric Association Press, 1994: 134–135.

Armstrong C, Ruffer J, Corn B, et al. Biphasic patterns of memory deficits following moderate-dose partial brain irradiation: neuropsychologic outcome and proposed mechanisms. J Clin Oncol 1995; 13: 2263–2271.

Arnett PA, Rao SM, Bernardin L, et al. Relationship between frontal lobe lesions and Wisconsin Card Sorting Test performance in patients with multiple sclerosis. Neurology 1994; 44: 420–425.

Arnett PA, Rao SM, Hussain M, et al. Conduction aphasia in multiple sclerosis: a case report with MRI findings. Neurology 1996; 47: 576–578.

Babikian V, Ropper AH. Binswanger's disease: a review. Stroke 1986; 18: 2–12.

Benavidez DA, Fletcher JM, Hannay HJ, et al. Corpus callosum damage and interhemispheric transfer of information following closed head injury in children. Cortex 1999; 35: 315–336.

Bennett DA, Gilley DW, Lee S, Cochran EJ. White matter changes: neurobehavioral manifestations of Binswanger's disease and clinical correlates in Alzheimer's Disease. Dementia 1994; 5: 148–152.

Boone KB, Miller BL, Lesser IM, et al. Neuropsychological correlates of white-matter lesions in healthy elderly subjects. Arch Neurol 1992; 49: 549–554.

Brown RG, Marsden CD. "Subcortical dementia": The neuropsychological evidence. Neuroscience 1988; 25: 363–387.

Caine ED, Bamford KA, Schiffer RB, et al. A controlled neuropsychological comparison of Huntington's disease and multiple sclerosis. Arch Neurol 1986; 43: 249–254.

Cleaver RL, Whitman RD. Right hemisphere, white-matter learning disabilities associated with depression in an adolescent and young adult psychiatric population. J Nerv Ment Dis 1998; 186: 561–565.

Cummings JL, ed. Subcortical dementia. New York: Oxford University Press, 1990.

Cummings JL, Benson DF. Dementia: a clinical approach. 2nd ed. Boston: Butterworths, 1994.

DeLuca J, Barbieri-Berger S, Johnson SK. The nature of memory acquisition in multiple sclerosis: acquisition versus retrieval. J Clin Exp Neuropsychol 1994; 16: 183–189.

DeLuca J, Gaudino EA, Diamond BJ, et al. Acquisition and storage deficits in multiple sclerosis. J Clin Exp Neuropsychol 1998; 20: 376–390.

Demaree HA, DeLuca J, Gaudino EA, Diamond BJ. Speed of information processing as a key deficit in multiple sclerosis: implications for rehabilitation. J Neurol Neurosurg Psychaitry 1999; 67: 661–663.

Derix MMA. Neuropsychological differentiation of dementia syndromes. Lisse: Swets and Zeitlinger, 1994.

Doody RS, Massman PJ, Mawad M, Nance M. Cognitive consequences of subcortical magnetic resonance imaging changes in Alzheimer's Disease: comparison to small vessel ischemic vascular dementia. Neuropsychiatry Neuropsychol Behav Neurol 1998; 11: 191–199.

Feinstein A. The clinical neuropsychiatry of multiple sclerosis. Cambridge: Cambridge University Press, 1999.

Filley CM. Neurobehavioral anatomy. Niwot, CO: University Press of Colorado, 1995.

Filley CM. Neurobehavioral aspects of cerebral white matter disorders. In: Fogel BS, Schiffer RB, Rao SM, eds. Neuropsychiatry. Baltimore: Williams and Wilkins, 1996: 913–933.

Filley CM. The behavioral neurology of cerebral white matter. Neurology 1998; 50: 1535–1540.

Filley CM. Toxic leukoencephalopathy. Clin Neuropharmacol 1999; 22: 249–260.

Filley CM, Franklin GM, Heaton RK, Rosenberg NL. White matter dementia: clinical disorders and implications. Neuropsychiatry Neuropsychol Behav Neurol 1988; 1: 239–254.

Filley CM, Gross KF. Psychosis with cerebral white matter disease. Neuropsychiatry Neuropsychol Behav Neurol 1992; 5: 119–125.

Filley CM, Heaton RK, Nelson LM, et al. A comparison of dementia in Alzheimer's disease and multiple sclerosis. Arch Neurol 1989; 46: 157–161.

Filley CM, Rosenberg NL, Heaton RK. White matter dementia in chronic toluene abuse. Neurology 1990; 40: 532–534.

Filley CM, Thompson LL, Sze C-I, et al. White matter dementia in CADASIL. J Neurol Sci 1999; 163: 163–167.

Fischer JS, Priore RL, Jacobs LD, et al. Neuropsychological effects of interferon b-1–a in relapsing multiple sclerosis. Ann Neurol 2000; 48: 885–892.

Folstein MF, Folstein SE, McHugh PR. "Mini-Mental State": a practical method for grading the cognitive state of patients for the clinician. J Psychiat Res 1975; 12: 189–198.

Franklin GM, Heaton RK, Nelson LM, et al. Correlation of neuropsychological and magnetic resonance imaging findings in chronic/progressive multiple sclerosis. Neurology 1988; 38: 1826–1829.

Franklin GM, Nelson LM, Filley CM, Heaton RK. Cognitive loss in multiple sclerosis. Case reports and review of the literature. Arch Neurol 1989; 46: 162–167.

Franklin GM, Nelson LM, Heaton RK, Filley CM. Clinical perspectives in the identification of cognitive impairment. In: Rao SM, ed. Neurobehavioral aspects of multiple sclerosis. New York: Oxford University Press, 1990: 161–174.

Giedd JN, Castellanos FX, Casey BJ, et al. Quantitative morphology of the corpus callosum in attention deficit hyperactivity disorder. Am J Psychiatry 1994; 151: 665–669.

Gur RC, Packer IK, Hungerbuhler JP, et al. Differences in the distribution of gray and white matter in the human cerebral hemispheres. Science 1980; 207: 1226–1228.

Heaton RK, Nelson LM, Thompson DS, et al. Neuropsychological findings in relapsing-remitting and chronic-progressive multiple sclerosis. J Consul Clin Psychol 1985; 53: 103–110.

Hormes JT, Filley CM, Rosenberg NL. Neurologic sequelae of chronic solvent vapor abuse. Neurology 1986; 36: 698–702.

Hyde TM, Ziegler JC, Weinberger DR. Psychiatric disturbances in metachromatic leukodystrophy: insights into the neurobiology of psychosis. Arch Neurol 1992; 49: 401–406.

Iddon JL, Pickard JD, Cross JJL, et al. Specific patterns of cognitive impairment in patients with idiopathic normal pressure hydrocephalus and Alzheimer's disease: a pilot study. J Neurol Neurosurg Psychiatry 1999; 67: 723–732.

Jones RD, Tranel D. Preservation of procedural memory in HIV-positive patients with subcortical dementia. J Clin Exp Neuropsychol 1991; 13: 74.

Kaplan RF, Jones-Woodward L. Lyme encephalopathy: a neuropsychological perspective. Semin Neurol 1997; 17: 31–37.

Krupp L, Elkins LE. Fatigue and declines in cognitive functioning in multiple sclerosis. Neurology 2000; 55: 934–939.

Kujala P, Portin R, Ruutianen J. Language functions in incipient cognitive decline in multiple sclerosis. J Neurol Sci 1996; 141: 79–86.

Lafosse J, Reed BR, Mungas D, et al. Fluency and memory differences between ischemic vascular dementia and Alzheimer's disease. Neuropsychology 1997; 11: 514–522.

Lafosse JM, Corboy JR, Leehey MA, et al. Neuropsychological distinction between subcortical white and gray matter dementia. J Int Neuropsychol Soc 2001; 7: 195.

Levin HS, High WM, Williams DL, et al. Dichotic listening and manual performance in relation to magnetic resonance imaging after closed head injury. J Neurol Neurosurg Psychiatry 1989; 52: 1162–1169.

Libon DJ, Bogdanoff B, Cloud BS, et al. Declarative and procedural learning, quantitative measures of the hippocampus, and subcortical white matter alterations in Alzheimer's disease and ischaemic vascular dementia. J Clin Exp Neuropsychol 1998; 20: 30–41.

Litvan I, Grafman J, Vendrell P, Martinez JM. Slowed information processing in multiple sclerosis. Arch Neurol 1988; 45: 281–285.

Markowitsch HJ. Which brain regions are critically involved in the retrieval of old episodic memory? Brain Res Rev 1995; 21: 117–127.

Mattis S. Dementia rating scale. Professional manual. Odessa, FL: Psychological Assessment Resources, 1988.

Mendez MF, Perryman KM, Bronstein YL. White matter dementias: neurobehavioral aspects and etiology. J Neuropsychiatry Clin Neurosci 2000; 12: 133.

Merriam AE, Hegarty A, Miller A. A proposed etiology for psychotic symptoms in white matter dementia. Neuropsychiatry Neuropsychol Behav Neurol 1989; 2: 225–228.

Merriam AE, Hegarty AM, Miller A. The mental disabilities of metachromatic leukodystrophy: implications concerning the differentiation of cortical, subcortical, and white matter dementias. Neuropsychiatry Neuropsychol Behav Neurol 1990; 3: 217–225.

Mesulam M-M. Large-scale neurocognitive networks and distributed processing for attention, memory, and language. Ann Neurol 1990; 28: 597–613.

Mesulam M-M. From sensation to cognition. Brain 1998; 121: 1013–1052.

Mesulam M-M. Attentional networks, confusional states, and neglect syndromes. In: Mesulam M-M, ed. Principles of behavioral and cognitive neurology. 2nd ed. New York: Oxford University Press, 2000: 174–256.

Minden SL, Schiffer RB. Affective disorders in multiple sclerosis. Review and recommendations for clinical research. Arch Neurol 1990; 47: 98–104.

Mouton PR, Martin LJ, Calhoun ME, et al. Cognitive decline strongly correlates with cortical atrophy in Alzheimer's dementia. Neurobiol Aging 1998; 19: 371–377.

Navia BA, Jordan BD, Price RW. The AIDS dementia complex: I. Clinical features. Ann Neurol 1986; 19: 517–524.

Paulsen JS, Butters N, Sadek JR, et al. Distinct cognitive profiles of cortical and subcortical dementia in advanced illness. Neurology 1995; 45: 951–956.

Petersen RC, Smith GE, Waring SC, et al. Mild cognitive impairment: clinical characterization and outcome. Arch Neurol 1999; 56: 303–308.

Pliskin NH, Hamer DP, Goldstein DS, et al. Improved delayed visual reproduction test performance in multiple sclerosis patients receiving interferon beta-1b. Neurology 1996: 47: 1463–1468.

Rao SM. White matter dementias. In: Parks RW, Zec RF, Wilson RS, eds. Neuropsychology of Alzheimer's disease and other dementias. New York: Oxford University Press, 1993: 438–456.

Rao SM. White matter disease and dementia. Brain Cogn 1996; 31: 250–268.

Rao SM, Bernardin L, Leo GJ, et al. Cerebral disconnection in multiple sclerosis: relationship to atrophy of the corpus callosum. Arch Neurol 1989b; 46: 918–920.

Rao SM, Grafman J, DiGiulio D, et al. Memory dysfunction in multiple sclerosis: its relation to working memory, semantic encoding, and implicit learning. Neuropsychology 1993; 7: 364–374.

Rao SM, Hammeke TA, McQuillen MP, et al. Memory disturbance in chronic-progressive multiple sclerosis. Arch Neurol 1984; 41: 625–631.

Rao SM, Leo GJ, Bernardin L, Unverzagt F. Cognitive dysfunction in multiple sclerosis. I. Frequency, patterns, and prediction. Neurology 1991; 41: 685–691.

Rao SM, Leo GJ, Haughton VM, et al. Correlation of magnetic resonance imaging with neuropsychological testing in multiple sclerosis. Neurology 1989a; 39: 161–166.

Reed BR, Eberling JL, Mungas D, et al. Memory failure has different mechanisms in subcortical stroke and Alzheimer's Disease. Ann Neurol 2000; 48: 275–284.

Riva D, Bova SM, Bruzzone MG. Neuropsychological testing may predict early progression of asymptomatic adrenoleukodystrophy. Neurology 2000; 54: 1651–1655.

Rockwood K, Wentzel C, Hachinski VC, et al. Prevalence and outcomes of vascular cognitive impairment. Neurology 2000; 54: 447–451.

Román GC, Tatemichi TK, Erkinjuntti T, et al. Vascular dementia: diagnostic criteria for research studies. Report of the NINDS-AIREN International Workshop. Neurology 1993; 43: 250–260.

Rosenberg NL, Kleinschmidt-DeMasters BK, Davis KA, et al. Toluene abuse causes diffuse central nervous system white matter changes. Ann Neurol 1988; 23: 611–614.

Rourke BP. The syndrome of nonverbal learning disabilities: the final common pathway of white matter disease/dysfunction? Clin Neuropsychol 1987; 2: 209–234.

Rourke BP. Syndrome of nonverbal learning disabilities. New York: Guilford Press, 1995.

Rueckert L, Grafman J. Sustained attention deficits in patients with right frontal lesions. Neuropsychologia 1996; 34: 953–963.

Rueckert L, Baboorian D, Stavropoulos K, Yasutake C. Individual differences in callosal efficiency: correlation with attention. Brain Cogn 1999; 41: 390–410.

Rueckert LM, Sorenson L, Levy J. Callosal efficiency is related to sustained attention. Neuropsychologia 1994; 32: 159–173.

Sadovnick AD, Eisen K, Ebers GC, Paty DW. Cause of death in patients attending multiple sclerosis clinics. Neurology 1991; 41: 1193–1196.

Schwid SR, Weinstein A, Scheid EA, Goodman AD. Cognitive fatigue measured during a test of sustained attention in multiple sclerosis patients. Ann Neurol 2000; 48: 478.

Semrud-Clikeman M, Hynd GW. Right hemisphere dysfunction in nonverbal learning disabilities: social, academic, and adaptive functioning in adults and children. Psychol Bull 1990; 107: 196–209.

Semrud-Clikeman M, Steingard RJ, Filipek P, et al. Using MRI to examine brain-behavior relationships in males with attention deficit disorder with hyperactivity. J Am Acad Child Adolesc Psychiatry 2000; 39: 477–484.

Shapiro EG, Lockman LA, Knopman D, Krivit W. Characteristics of the dementia in late-onset metachromatic leukodystrophy. Neurology 1994; 44: 662–665.

Sohn YH, Jeong Y, Kim HS, et al. The brain lesion responsible for parkinsonism after carbon monoxide poisoning. Arch Neurol 2000; 57: 1214–1218.

Spikman JM, van Zomeren AH, Deelman BG. Deficits of attention after closed-head injury: slowness only? J Clin Exp Neuropsychol 1996; 18: 755–767.

Timmerman ME, Brouwer WH. Slow information processing after very severe closed head injury: impaired access to declarative knowledge and intact application and acquisition of procedural knowledge. Neuropsychologia 1999; 37: 467–478.

Tranchant C, Bhatia KP, Marsden CD. Movement disorders in multiple sclerosis. Mov Disord 1995; 10: 418–423.

White DA, Taylor MJ, Butters N, et al. Memory for verbal information in individuals with HIV-associated dementia complex. HNRC Group. J Clin Exp Neuropsychol 1997; 19: 357–366.

Whitehouse PJ. The concept of cortical and subcortical dementia: another look. Ann Neurol 1986; 19: 1–6.

Yamanouchi N, Okada S, Kodama K, et al. Effects of MRI abnormalities on WAIS-R performance in solvent abusers. Acta Neurol Scand 1997; 96: 34–39.

16

Focal Neurobehavioral Syndromes

As the information in Chapter 15 indicates, cognitive dysfunction and dementia are the most frequently recognized neurobehavioral syndromes encountered in patients with white matter disorders of the brain. In contrast, focal syndromes are relatively rare. Three major factors help explain these observations. First, the neuropathologic involvement of most diseases and injuries of the white matter tends to be diffuse or multifocal, so that isolated lesions that might give rise to focal syndromes are relatively uncommon. Second, the neurobehavioral syndrome might occur only transiently and never come to clinical attention, and the patient recovers before a precise clinical–pathologic correlation can be made. Finally, focal syndromes, even when present, may be underappreciated because of the attention focused on other clinical and basic aspects of the disorder.

Focal neurobehavioral syndromes, however, can develop in patients with white matter disorders. These syndromes have been recognized for many years, but with the advent of magnetic resonance imaging (MRI), their identifications have been accelerated substantially. Most of the available cases are found in descriptions of multiple sclerosis (MS), cerebrovascular disease, and tumors, but other neuropathologic processes occasionally are found to be responsible. Whereas it is unlikely that focal syndromes will be found to surpass diffuse syndromes in frequency, they are likely be appear more often with further clinical and neuroradiologic sophistication. Newer structural MRI techniques (Chapter 4) in particular promise to play a major role in the search for such cases in the future. Table 16-1 lists the focal neurobehavioral syndromes of white matter that are adequately documented in the literature.

Table 16-1. Focal Neurobehavioral Syndromes
of White Matter

Amnesia	Developmental dyslexia
Aphasia	Gerstmann's syndrome
Broca's	Agnosia
Transcortical motor	Visual
Conduction	Auditory
Wernicke's	Neglect
Global	Visuospatial dysfunction
Mixed transcortical	Akinetic mutism
Apraxia	Executive dysfunction
Alexia	Callosal disconnection
Pure alexia	
Alexia with agraphia	

Amnesia

Memory impairment in white matter disorders may take many forms. The complaint of memory loss is one of the most common in the practice of neurology, and the clinician's task is to determine the nature and origin of this symptom so that appropriate treatment can begin. In Chapter 15, the specific form of memory disturbance postulated to characterize white matter cognitive dysfunction and dementia was considered, and it was pointed out that this retrieval deficit in declarative memory is typically embedded within an array of associated impairments in attention and other functions. Amnesia, however, is a different type of memory disturbance. Traditional usage considers amnesia a disorder of new learning, implying that the encoding of information, rather its than retrieval, is primarily deficient (Filley, 1995).

Isolated amnesia has been observed in the setting of white matter involvement. Although there are few well-described cases, the location of lesions in available reports clusters around the medial temporal–diencephalic–basal forebrain region known to be associated with amnesia (Filley, 1995). One controversial question has been whether damage to the fornix can produce amnesia, because despite its importance as a connecting tract in the limbic system (Chapter 2), lesions confined to the fornix are uncommon. However, support for this idea comes from reports of recent memory disturbance following damage to the fornices from neoplasms (Heilman and Sypert, 1977; Tucker et al., 1988; Aggleton et al., 2000), trauma (D'Esposito et al., 1995), infarction (Park et al., 2000; Moudgil et al., 2000), and surgical section (Gaffan and Gaffan, 1991; Calabrese et al., 1995). In the case of Tucker and colleagues (1988), the verbal memory loss observed with a left-sided lesion is consistent with current theories on the lateralization of verbal and nonverbal memory in the cerebral hemispheres (Filley, 1995). The disruption of a circuit such as this, dedicated to a specific neurobehavioral domain, argues for the importance of white matter tracts in the organization of these networks.

Amnesia has also been noted in several individuals after infarction of the internal capsule, particularly the genu (Kooistra and Heilman, 1988; Tatemichi et al., 1992). In these cases, the lesion was interpreted as interfering with the connections of the declarative memory system while not directly damaging any of its gray matter components. Tatemichi and colleagues (1992) concluded that the amnesia was caused by interruption of the inferior and anterior thalamic peduncles that traverse the internal capsule in the region of the genu. This lesion in turn disconnected the limbic system from the ipsilateral frontal cortex, presumably preventing the storage of memory (Tatemichi et al., 1992). Similar to the cases of fornical damage described above, in these patients verbal memory loss occurred with left capsular infarction and visuospatial memory loss with right capsular infarction (Tatemichi et al., 1992).

Aphasia

Aphasia, a disturbance of language resulting from acquired brain damage, is the quintessential cortical syndrome. A large body of literature supports the localization of language to specific perisylvian zones, and the left hemisphere is primarily implicated in most individuals (Damasio, 1992). However, as recognized by classical neurologists for over a century (Geschwind, 1965), white matter lesions are also capable of producing this syndrome. With the advent of modern neuroimaging (Chapter 4), a growing number of observations has confirmed this assertion. White matter structures are now understood to play a central role in the organization of language. To underscore this point, Alexander and colleagues (1987), after collecting data from a large series of unilateral left hemisphere strokes and an extensive literature review, came to the conclusion that white matter pathways were crucial for all aspects of aphasia.

Broca's Aphasia

In parallel with the resurgence of the concept of subcortical dementia, an entity called subcortical aphasia has been postulated in the last 2 decades (Alexander and LoVerme, 1980; Damasio et al., 1982). This term refers to aphasia in the setting of various lesions affecting the deep gray and white matter of the left hemisphere. Cerebrovascular disease has provided much of the data for this discussion, even though the relative rarity of isolated white matter infarcts renders study of the question more difficult. In general, however, vascular white matter lesions seem to be capable of producing Broca's aphasia. Although some investigators have used regional cerebral blood flow data to suggest that cortical hypoperfusion can explain Broca's aphasia from subcortical lesions (Skyhøj-Olsen et al., 1986), comprehensive computed tomography (CT) studies of left hemisphere stroke patients have concluded that white matter areas—specifically the subcallosal fasciculus (a branch of the superior occipitofrontal fasciculus) and the periventricular white matter— are essential for language fluency (Naeser et al., 1989). Remarkably, a similar pattern of white matter involvement has also been reported using CT to examine the brain of Leborgne—Broca's original patient who had severe nonfluency—140 years after the onset of his stroke (Naeser et al., 1989).

Demyelinative disease has also provided useful information on aphasia in white matter disorders. Typically these cases reflect acute exacerbations of the disease that produce transient language deficits. The most common type of aphasia reported in MS is Broca's aphasia, alternatively referred to as motor aphasia (Olmos-Lau et al., 1977; Achiron et al., 1992; Devere et al., 2000). Magnetic resonance imaging studies may show large lesions in the left frontal white matter (Achiron et al., 1992).

Transcortical Motor Aphasia

Infarction of the left anterior periventricular white matter has been observed with transcortical motor aphasia (Freedman et al., 1984). In this syndrome, the initiation of speech is compromised, and the responsible lesion can be in the white matter connections between the left supplementary motor area and the perisylvian language zone. Subsequent studies with more stroke patients and detailed CT localizations have been consistent with this notion (Alexander et al., 1987). Transcortical motor aphasia has also been noted with MS (Devere et al., 2000).

Conduction Aphasia

Since the time of Wernicke, classical neurologic thinking has held that a lesion in the arcuate fasciculus underlying the left inferior parietal cortex is responsible for conduction aphasia (Geschwind, 1965). This localization has been debated, however, because lesions that cause conduction aphasia, the great majority of which are ischemic infarctions, typically damage overlying perisylvian cortex as well as the arcuate fasciculus (Damasio, 1992). However, several observations have supported the notion of white matter disconnection in the pathogenesis of conduction aphasia. One MS patient who developed the syndrome had an MRI-proven large plaque in the white matter underlying the left supramarginal gyrus (Arnett et al., 1996). Conduction aphasia was also noted in a patient with an infarct of the left parietal lobe that spared the cortex on MRI (Poncet et al., 1987). Other stroke cases have suggested that conduction aphasia may also follow damage to the left extreme capsule, which contains additional fibers connecting the temporal and frontal lobes (Damasio and Damasio, 1980).

Wernicke's Aphasia

This syndrome appears thus far to be rare in the setting of white matter disorders. One case of fluent aphasia with impaired comprehension and repetition was reported by Day and colleagues (1987) in a patient with MS. The MRI scan of this individual showed a large area of demyelination in the left temporoparietal region. With treatment of MS the syndrome significantly improved.

Global Aphasia

A case has been reported in which an MS patient had global aphasia with right hemiparesis and homonymous hemianopia, and a CT scan demonstrated a large white matter lesion in the left periventricular region (Friedman et al., 1983). The authors concluded it was likely that the arcuate fasciculus and all connections from Broca's and Wernicke's areas were affected to produce this syndrome, which was substantially improved 1 year later (Friedman et al., 1983).

Mixed Transcortical Aphasia

This aphasia has rarely been described with neuropathology of any kind, but one case has been reported in a patient with a left subangular white matter lesion that followed a left parietal hemorrhage (Pirozzolo et al., 1981). The lesion was interpreted as disconnecting the left auditory cortex from other cortical regions where semantic information is represented (Pirozzolo et al., 1981). Mixed transcortical aphasia has also been observed in MS (Devere et al., 2000).

Apraxia

Disorders of learned movement are traditionally ascribed to cortical lesions, but apraxia may also occur with white matter involvement. As reviewed by Geschwind (1965), bilateral ideomotor apraxia was classically associated with lesions of the left arcuate fasciculus. Consistent with this hypothesis, a case report with MRI lesion localization confirmed that a single white matter infarct in the left parietal lobe can produce bilateral ideomotor apraxia (Poncet et al., 1987). Unilateral (left hand) ideomotor apraxia may also occur with callosal lesions (see below).

Alexia

Acquired disorders of reading have been recognized for over a century, and the enduring works of Dejerine established the now accepted distinction between alexia with agraphia and pure alexia (Geschwind, 1965). Pure alexia is a classic disconnection syndrome stemming from strategically placed white matter damage, and alexia with agraphia may also occur from appropriately placed white matter lesions.

Pure Alexia

The usual cause of pure alexia is cerebrovascular disease, and the presence of a left occipital lesion combined with another in the splenium of the corpus callosum is widely thought to be responsible (Geschwind, 1965). One of the most elegant neurobehavioral syndromes, pure alexia represents a disconnection between the visual and language systems that disturbs reading but not the capacity to write (Filley, 1995). Recently, cases of pure alexia have been described in MS (Doğulu et al., 1996; Jónsdóttir et al., 1998). Both of the patients in these reports had widespread MRI lesions in the cerebral white matter; the case of Doğulu and colleagues (1996) had plaques specifically within the left occipital lobe and the splenium.

Alexia with Agraphia

The patient studied by Day and colleagues (1987) mentioned above also experienced an acquired disorder of reading and writing. The large plaque in the left temporoparietal white matter was therefore responsible both for fluent aphasia and alexia with agraphia. Thus, the single white matter lesion produced a clinical picture similar to that which is often seen after a lesion in the temporoparietal cortex immediately overlying this area.

Developmental Dyslexia

This disorder, which affects about 10% of children, is an impairment of the ability to read despite adequate intelligence and access to instruction (Shaywitz, 1998). Although recent findings have suggested a genetic basis for the syndrome (Pennington et al., 1991), it has been difficult to detect robust structural changes in the brains of dyslexic individuals by conventional neuroimaging (Pennington et al., 1999). Advanced neuroimaging techniques focusing on the white matter may clarify the neuroanatomy of dyslexia. In a recent study using diffusion tensor MRI, Klingberg and colleagues (2000) found a significant correlation between reading scores and lower anisotropy in the left temporoparietal white matter of dyslexic adults. This study is particularly important in that it exploits a new MRI technique to support the role of white matter in a specific neurobehavioral domain, and its conclusions converge with Dejerine's original ideas on the neuroanatomy of reading (Filley, 1995).

Gerstmann's Syndrome

The tetrad of agraphia, acalculia, finger agnosia, and right–left confusion has been associated with left inferior parietal lesions since Gertsmann's first description of this syndrome (Filley, 1995). These lesions are typically ischemic infarcts of the parietal cortex. Recently, a case of Gerstmann's syndrome was described in a patient with a pure subangular white matter lesion (Mayer et al., 1999). As is apparent with many focal syndromes, the white matter lesion is neuroanatomically related to the cortical region classically associated with the deficit.

Agnosia

Agnosia is a modality-specific disorder of recognition that has most often been ascribed to damage in relevant areas of sensory association cortex (Filley, 1995). With the advent of MRI, it has also been possible to detect agnosic syndromes patients with white matter lesions.

Visual Agnosia

In three cases of visual object agnosia with alexia presented by Feinberg and colleagues (1994), CT scan analysis revealed that the left inferior longitudinal (occipitofrontal) fasciculus was the critical structure involved. These cases support the idea that associative visual agnosia can represent a unilateral left temporal disconnection syndrome involving selective damage to white matter. A case of visual form agnosia in a patient with MS was described by Okuda and colleagues (1996). This patient had bilateral occipitotemporal and callosal lesions that were interpreted as interrupting the ventral stream of the visual association system.

Auditory Agnosia

This syndrome has been divided into two categories: auditory verbal agnosia (pure word deafness) and auditory sound agnosia (Filley, 1995). A case of pure word deafness from a left thalamic hemorrhage damaging white matter fibers of the auditory system has been reported (Takahashi et al., 1992). In this instance, the lesion was interpreted as interrupting the auditory input from both primary auditory regions to Wernicke's area (Takahashi et al., 1992). Auditory sound agnosia from a white matter lesion has not been described. However, a case of cortical deafness in MS has been observed, suggesting that bilateral temporal white matter lesions have the capacity to disconnect Heschl's gyri from auditory input (Tabira et al., 1981). In light of this case, the term cortical deafness needs revision, as the cortex itself is structurally normal; cerebral deafness would better serve to designate this syndrome.

Neglect

The literature on neglect generally points to cortical lesions of the right hemisphere as responsible, and the right parietal lobe is most often implicated (Vallar and Perani, 1986). However, more detailed formulations of neglect have postulated a distributed right hemisphere network for directed attention that includes the parietal lobe, frontal cortex, cingulate gyrus, and subcortical regions (Mesulam, 1981). White matter tracts are implicated because of the connections linking these areas. Left hemineglect may occur in MS patients who have large right hemisphere demyelinative lesions (Graff-Radford and Rizzo, 1987). This syndrome has been also described in patients with right internal capsule infarcts that were thought to deactivate the ipsilateral parietal and frontal cortices (Bogousslavsky et al., 1988). The related syndrome of anosognosia, in which there is unawareness of neurologic deficit, has also been studied in this context. A CT study of patients with right hemisphere infarcts found that those with denial of hemiplegia had significantly more involvement of the white matter, particularly the corona radiata (Small and Ellis, 1996). These studies argue for the presence of a multifocal attentional network in the right hemisphere in which white matter plays a key role.

Visuospatial Dysfunction

Visuospatial dysfunction has been observed in patients with right cerebral white matter lesions. A case of topographical disorientation was associated with an infarct in the posterior limb of the right internal capsule, which was thought to disrupt cortical metabolism in the overlying parietal lobe (Hublet and Demeurisse, 1992). In another report, spatial delirium with reduplicative paramnesia was ascribed to a white matter infarct in the right corona radiata that extended into the retrolenticular portion of the internal capsule (Nighoghossian et al., 1992).

Akinetic Mutism

Akinetic mutism has occasionally been related to white matter lesions. In one patient, the syndrome evolved after the removal of a tumor in the anterior hypothalamus; this lesion destroyed the medial forebrain bundle (Ross and Stewart, 1981). Treatment with dopamine agonists was successful in alleviating this syndrome, which was thought to stem from dopamine depletion in the medial frontal lobes. In another case, a patient with MS developed transient akinetic mutism after the appearance of a midbrain plaque on MRI (Scott et al., 1995). Although the presence of cerebral demyelination complicated interpretation, involvement of dopaminergic transmission in the the medial forebrain bundle was also possible in this case. These observations introduce the possibility that isolated lesions of subcortical white matter tracts conveying neurotransmitters to the neocortex can result in specific neurobehavioral syndromes.

Executive Dysfunction

Executive dysfunction is most securely associated with frontal lobe lesions, including those confined to white matter. In MS for example, executive dysfunction can dominate the clinical picture and by itself cause major disability (Filley, 2000). Pursuing this idea experimentally, Arnett and colleagues (1994) examined the relationship between focal white matter involvement in MS and performance on the Wisconsin Card Sorting Test (WCST), a test of conceptual reasoning generally regarded as a measure of executive function. A significant correlation between frontal white matter lesion area and impaired WCST performance was found (Arnett et al., 1994). This study was an important attempt to establish the impact of regional white matter involvement in MS, and its results may generalize to other white matter disorders.

White matter lesions of other origin can interfere with frontal lobe function. In the cases reported by Tatemichi and colleagues (1992; see above), apathy, abulia, and other frontal lobe features occurred in the acute stages of capsular genu infarction that caused ipsilateral frontal lobe deactivation. A patient with traumatic brain injury (TBI) and a focal lesion in the ventral midbrain tegmentum had persistent executive dysfunction as a component of a frontal lobe syndrome, and interference with dopamine transmission from the brainstem to the frontal lobe via the medial forebrain bundle was suggested as an explanation (Goldberg et al., 1989). Another report described five patients with isolated brainstem stroke who each exhibited prominent executive dysfunction and other frontal lobe disturbances on neuropsychological testing (Hoffman and Watts, 1998). Although details of neuroanatomy were not provided, disruption of ascending neurotransmitter systems by damage to white matter tracts was also implied by these cases. The possibility that functional deactivation of frontal cortex may occur through interruption of white matter pathways deserves further investigation.

Callosal Disconnection

The corpus callosum is the largest white matter tract in the brain. Although its clinical importance is debated because of the relative paucity of significant neurobehavioral deficits in many individuals with corpus callosum lesions, examples of hemispheric disconnection have been described (Geschwind, 1965). Callosal agenesis is discussed in Chapter 5, and corpus callosotomy in Chapter 12; in this section, the effects of other callosal lesions are considered.

Cerebrovascular disease is a commonly reported cause of focal damage to the corpus callosum. In their seminal case report, Geschwind and Kaplan (1962) described a patient with the anterior four-fifths of the corpus callosum destroyed because of a left anterior cerebral artery infarct after surgery for a glioblastoma, and who had apraxia and agraphia of the left hand. Graff-Radford and Rizzo (1987) described a patient with callosal apraxia who had left hand apraxia after rupture of a pericallosal aneurysm. Studies of patients with infarction of the body of the corpus callosum have correlated this region with the alien hand phenomenon (Geschwind, 1995; Chan and Liu, 1999). Left hemialexia has been seen with vascular lesions of the splenium (Suzuki et al., 1998).

Demyelinative disease and TBI may also cause callosal disconnection. A report of an MS patient with callosal disconnection noted tactile anomia, agraphia, and apraxia affecting only the left hand (Schnider et al., 1993). In patients with TBI, corpus callosum damage was documented with the use of MRI and dichotic listening and tachistoscopic tests indicating disconnection in auditory and visual modalities (Levin et al., 1989; Benavidez et al., 1999).

References

Achiron A, Ziv I, Djaldetti R, et al. Aphasia in multiple sclerosis: clinical and radiologic correlations. Neurology 1992; 42: 2195–2197.

Aggleton JP, McMackin D, Carpenter K, et al. Differential cognitive effects of colloid cysts of the third ventricle that spare or compromise the fornix. Brain 2000; 123: 800–815.

Alexander MP, LoVerme SR. Aphasia after left hemispheric intracerebral hemorrhage. Neurology 1980; 30: 1193–1202.

Alexander MP, Naeser MA, Palumbo CL. Correlations of subcortical CT lesion sites and aphasia profiles. Brain 1987; 110: 961–991.

Arnett PA, Rao SM, Bernardin L, et al. Relationship between frontal lobe lesions and Wisconsin Card Sorting Test performance in patients with multiple sclerosis. Neurology 1994; 44: 420–425.

Arnett PA, Rao SM, Hussain M, et al. Conduction aphasia in multiple sclerosis: a case report with MRI findings. Neurology 1996; 47: 576–578.

Benavidez DA, Fletcher JM, Hannay HJ, et al. Corpus callosum damage and interhemispheric transfer of information following closed head injury in children. Cortex 1999; 35: 315–336.

Bogousslavsky J, Miklossy J, Regli F, et al. Subcortical neglect: neuropsychological, SPECT, and neuropathological correlates with anterior choroidal artery territory infarctions. Ann Neurol 1988; 23: 448–452.

Calabrese P, Markowitsch HJ, Harders AG, et al. Fornix and memory damage. A case report. Cortex 1995; 31: 555–564.

Chan JL, Liu AB. Anatomical correlates of alien hand syndromes. Neuropsychiatry Neuropsychol Behav Neurol 1999; 12: 149–155.

Damasio AR. Aphasia. N Engl J Med 1992; 326: 531–539.

Damasio AR, Damasio H, Rizzo M, et al. Aphasia with nonhemorrhagic lesions in the basal ganglia and internal capsule. Arch Neurol 1982; 39: 15–20.

Damasio H, Damasio AR. The anatomical basis of conduction aphasia. Brain 1980; 103: 337–350.

Day TJ, Fisher AG, Mastaglia FL. Alexia with agraphia in multiple sclerosis. J Neurol Sci 1987; 78: 343–348.

D'Esposito M, Verfaellie M, Alexander MP, Katz DI. Amnesia following traumatic bilateral fornix transection. Neurology 1995; 45: 1546–1550.

Devere TR, Trotter JL, Cross AH. Acute aphasia in multiple sclerosis. Arch Neurol 2000; 57: 1207–1209.

Doğulu CF, Kansu T, Karabudak R. Alexia without agraphia in multiple sclerosis. J Neurol Neurosurg Psychiatry 1996; 61: 528.

Feinberg TE, Schindler RJ, Ochoa E, et al. Associative visual agnosia and alexia without prosopagnosia. Cortex 1994; 30: 395–411.

Filley CM. Neurobehavioral anatomy. Niwot, CO: University Press of Colorado, 1995.

Filley CM. Clinical neurology and executive dysfunction. Semin Speech Lang 2000; 21: 95–108.

Freedman M, Alexander MP, Naeser MA. Anatomic basis of transcortical motor aphasia. Neurology 1984; 34: 409–417.

Friedman JH, Brem H, Mayeux R. Global aphasia in multiple sclerosis. Ann Neurol 1983; 222–223.

Gaffan D, Gaffan EA. Amnesia in man following transection of the fornix. A review. Brain 1991; 114: 2611–2618.

Geschwind DH, Iacoboni M, Mega M, et al. Alien hand syndrome: interhemispheric motor disconnection due to a lesion in the midbody of the corpus callosum. Neurology 1995; 45: 802–808.

Geschwind N. Disconnexion syndromes in animals and man. Brain 1965; 88: 237–294, 585–644.

Geschwind N, Kaplan E. A human cerebral deconnection syndrome: a preliminary report. Neurology 1962; 12: 675–685.

Goldberg E, Bilder RM, Hughes JEO, et al. A reticulo-frontal disconnection syndrome. Cortex 1989; 25: 687–695.

Graff-Radford NR, Rizzo M. Neglect in a patient with multiple sclerosis. Eur Neurol 1987; 26: 100–103.

Graff-Radford NR, Welsh K, Godersky J. Callosal apraxia. Neurology 1987; 37: 100–105.

Heilman KM, Sypert GW. Korsakoff's syndrome resulting from bilateral fornix lesions. Neurology 27: 1977: 490–493.

Hoffman M, Watts A. Cognitive dysfunction in isolated brainstem stroke: a neuropsychological and SPECT study. J Stroke Cerebrovasc Dis 1998; 7: 24–31.

Hublet C, Demeurisse G. Pure topographical disorientation due to a deep-seated lesion with cortical remote effects. Cortex 1992; 28: 123–128.

Jónsdóttir MK, Magnússon T, Kjartansson O. Pure alexia and word-meaning deafness in a patient with multiple sclerosis. Arch Neurol 1998; 55: 1473–1474.

Klingberg T, Hedehus M, Temple E, et al. Microstructure of temporo-parietal white matter as a basis for reading ability: evidence from diffusion tensor magnetic resonance imaging. Neuron 2000; 25: 493–500.

Kooistra CA, Heilman KM. Memory loss from a subcortical white matter infarct. J Neurol Neurosurg Psychiatry 1988; 51: 866–869.

Levin HS, High WM, Williams DL, et al. Dichotic listening and manual performance in relation to magnetic resonance imaging after closed head injury. J Neurol Neurosurg Psychiatry 1989; 52: 1162–1169.

Mayer E, Martory M-D, Pegna AJ, et al. A pure case of Gerstmann syndrome with a sub-angular lesion. Brain 1999; 122: 1107–1120.

Mesulam M-M. A cortical network for directed attention and unilateral neglect. Ann Neurol 1981; 10: 309–325.

Moudgil SS, Azzouz M, Al-Azzaz A, et al. Amnesia due to fornix infarction. Stroke 2000; 31: 1418–1419.

Naeser MA, Palumbo CL, Helm-Estabrooks N, et al. Severe nonfluency in aphasia. Role of the medial subcallosal fasciculus and other white matter pathways in recovery of spontaneous speech. Brain 1989; 112: 1–38.

Nighoghossian N, Trouillas P, Vighetto A, Philippon B. Spatial delirium following a right subcortical infarct with frontal deactivation. J Neurol Neurosurg Psychiatry 1992; 55: 334–335.

Okuda B, Tanaka H, Tachibana H, et al. Visual form agnosia in multiple sclerosis. Acta Neurol Scand 1996; 94: 38–44.

Olmos-Lau N, Ginsberg MD, Geller JB. Aphasia in multiple sclerosis. Neurology 1977; 27: 623–626.

Park SA, Hahn JH, Kim JI, et al. Memory deficits after bilateral fornix infarction. Neurology 2000; 54: 1379–1382.

Pennington BF, Filipek PA, Lefly D, et al. Brain morphometry in reading-disabled twins. Neurology 1999; 53: 723–729.

Pennington BF, Gilger JW, Pauls D, et al. Evidence for major gene transmission of developmental dyslexia. JAMA 1991; 266: 1527–1534.

Pirozzolo FJ, Kerr KL, Obrzut JE, et al. Neurolinguistic analysis of the language abilities of a patient with a "double disconnection syndrome": a case of subangular alexia in the presence of mixed transcortical aphasia. J Neurol Neurosurg Psychiatry 1981; 44: 152–155.

Poncet M, Habib M, Robillard A. Deep left parietal lobe syndrome: conduction aphasia and other neurobehavioral disorders due to a small subcortical lesion. J Neurol Neurosurg Psychiatry 1987; 50: 709–713.

Ross ED, Stewart RM. Akinetic mutism from hypothalamic damage: successful treatment with dopamine agonists. Neurology 1981; 31: 1435–1439.

Schnider A, Benson DF, Rosner LJ. Callosal disconnection in multiple sclerosis. Neurology 1993; 43: 1243–1245.

Scott TF, Lang D, Girgis RM, Price T. Prolonged akinetic mutism due to multiple sclerosis. J Neuropsychiatry Clin Neurosci 1995; 7: 90–92.

Shaywitz SE. Dyslexia. N Engl J Med 1998; 338: 307–312.

Skyhøj-Olsen T, Bruhn P, Öberg GE. Cortical hypoperfusion as a possible cause of "subcortical aphasia." Brain 1986; 109: 393–410.

Small M, Ellis S. Denial of hemiplegia: an investigation into the theories of causation. Eur Neurol 1996; 36: 353–363.

Suzuki K, Yamadori A, Endo K, et al. Dissociation of letter and picture naming resulting from callosal disconnection. Neurology 1998; 51: 1390–1394.

Tabira T, Tsuji S, Nagashima T, et al. Cortical deafness in multiple sclerosis. J Neurol Neurosurg Psychiatry 1981; 44: 433–436.

Takahashi N, Kawamura M, Shinotou H, et al. Pure word deafness due to left hemisphere damage. Cortex 1992; 28: 295–303.

Tatemichi TK, Desmond DW, Prohovnik I, et al. Confusion and memory loss from capsular genu infarction: a thalamocortical disconnection syndrome? Neurology 1992; 42: 1966–1979.

Tucker DM, Roeltgen DP, Tully R, et al. Memory dysfunction following unilateral transection of the fornix: a hippocampal disconnection syndrome. Cortex 1988: 24: 465–472.

Vallar G, Perani D. The anatomy of unilateral neglect after right-hemisphere stroke lesions. A clinical/CT-scan correlation study in man. Neuropsychologia 1986; 24: 609–622.

17

Neuropsychiatric Syndromes

Neurobehavioral manifestations of white matter disorders are not limited to cognitive syndromes. Emotional dysfunction can also be seen, often arising earlier in the course of the disorder and in some cases proving more problematic than cognitive impairment. In this respect, white matter disorders resemble the subcortical gray matter diseases, which also feature prominent neuropsychiatric manifestations (Salloway and Cummings, 1994). The most comprehensive information on this kind of neuropsychiatric disturbance comes from study of multiple sclerosis (MS), but observations of other white matter disorders have also contributed to this topic. In this chapter, neuropsychiatric syndromes in selected white matter disorders are reviewed in view of their putative relationship to cerebral neuropathology.

Depression

In the combined literatures describing all the white matter disorders discussed in this book, depression appears to be the most common neuropsychiatric syndrome. That this is so should not be surprising, as many of the diseases and injuries of white matter have devastating neurologic consequences that can naturally generate depression as a psychological reaction. However, the emerging correlation of white matter neuropathology with cognitive dysfunction, reviewed in Part II, has helped stimulate interest in the possibility that depression might also be related to structural brain involvement. Preliminary observations suggest that whereas reactive depression is probably one contributory factor, white matter neuropathology is also likely to participate in the pathogenesis of depression. The etiology of this syndrome is complex, and further study will be required to establish the relative importance of the many factors involved.

To begin, it is noteworthy that depression is uncommon in dysmyelinative diseases, largely because many of these diseases begin early in life and are dominated throughout by devastating cognitive effects. Even with later onset cases, however, personality change and psychosis tend to be more prominent neuropsychiatric features (see below). In contrast, demyelination is strongly associated with depression. Depression in MS has been studied in considerable detail, and many studies have demonstrated that it is the most frequent neuropsychiatric syndrome in these patients (Feinstein, 1999). Estimates of the prevalence of depression in MS vary, but a range of 27%–54% has been cited (Minden and Schiffer, 1990) and a useful overall figure puts the lifetime prevalence of major depression in MS at 50% (Feinstein, 1999). Depression may be the chief complaint of MS patients (Young et al., 1976), and may even represent the initial presentation of the disease (Salloway et al., 1988). The functional impact of this syndrome is significant. Depression in MS is associated with cognitive impairment and social stress (Gilchrist and Creed, 1994), so that preexisting cognitive dysfunction or dementia may be exacerbated by the mood disorder. More urgent is the remarkable increase in the possibility of suicide in MS (Sadovnick et al.,1991; Stenager et al., 1992), which may imply a sevenfold increase in suicide risk compared to an age-matched normal population (Sadovnick et al., 1991).

The relationship of depression and demyelination in MS has generated considerable debate. Surridge (1969), after comparing MS patients with a group of muscular dystrophy patients and finding similar rates of depression, argued that depression in MS is purely a psychological reaction to the illness. However, Whitlock and Siskind (1980) noted a higher rate of depression in MS than in other disabling neurologic diseases, and maintained that the syndrome was likely caused by cerebral MS lesions. Supportive evidence for this notion came from studies of MS patients showing that those with cerebral involvement had more depression than those with mainly spinal cord disease (Schiffer et al., 1983). Furthermore, MS patients were found to have higher rates of affective disorder than patients with temporal lobe epilepsy and amyotrophic lateral sclerosis (Schiffer and Babigian, 1984). Rabins and colleagues (1986) concluded that both brain involvement and an emotional reaction contributed to depression in MS.

Although a firm relationship has yet to be demonstrated between MRI-proven white matter disease and depression in MS (Feinstein, 1999), evidence favoring this idea has been accumulating. In a small series, Honer and colleagues (1987) suggested an association of depression and temporal lobe lesions. Reischies and colleagues (1988) found a correlation between psychopathology and periventricular and frontal white matter lesions. Pujol and colleagues (1997) found that left suprainsular lesions, including the arcuate fasciculus, were correlated with depression. In contrast, other studies found no relationship between depression and white matter neuropathology in any region (Huber et al., 1987; Ron and Logsdail, 1989; Anzola et al., 1990). More recently, however, other investigations have again suggested that depression may relate to specific sites of neuropathology in MS. Sabatini and colleagues (1996) found a correlation between depression and perfusion abnormalities in the limbic system as determined by single photon emission computed tomography. Using conventional MRI, Bakshi and colleagues (2000) correlated severity of depression with frontal atrophy and with T1 hypointensities ("black holes") in the frontal, temporal, and parietal lobe white matter.

Treatment of depression in MS is typically successful if the syndrome is recognized. Psychotherapy, medications, and electroconvulsive therapy in resistant cases all have a place in treatment (Feinstein, 1999). Because of the potential lethality of depression in MS, vigorous treatment should not be avoided because of concerns of cognitive and other adverse effects. Only one controlled trial of antidepressant treatment in MS has been published, and the tricyclic antidepressant desipramine was found to be moderately effective (Schiffer and Wineman, 1990). Experience with the selective serotonin reuptake inhibitors suggests that these are preferable to tricyclic drugs because of fewer side effects (Feinstein, 1999). The efficacy of antidepressant treatment is compatible with either a psychological or structural explanation of depression in MS.

Depression also occurs in the infectious, inflammatory, toxic, and metabolic white matter disorders. About 10% of patients with human immunodeficiency virus (HIV) infection experience depression (Perry, 1994), and in those with the acquired immunodeficiency syndrome (AIDS) dementia complex (ADC), depression commingled with cognitive impairment can produce a complex clinical picture. In many cases, apathy dominates the mental status of HIV patients, and it is difficult to determine whether depression is in fact present (Castellon et al., 1998). Both stimulant medications and antidepressants may be helpful in HIV-infected patients (Perry, 1994), however, implying that apathy and depression can coexist. The role of white matter neuropathology in the depression of ADC is as yet undefined, but a causative role of leukoencephalopathy affecting limbic function has been suggested (Schiffer, 1990). In systemic lupus erythematosus (SLE), depression is reported to be the most common of many neuropsychiatric syndromes (Wekking, 1993). The pathogenesis of depression in SLE is no better understood than that of dementia, but a combination of vascular and immunologic abnormalities affecting white matter regions may be involved (Schiffer, 1990). Depression has been noted in toluene abusers, and the initiation of drug abuse by young persons was initially interpreted as a result of the mood disorder (Masterson, 1979). However, other investigators found that some abusers have no premorbid psychiatric history, suggesting that the depression may be a consequence, rather than a cause, of the drug abuse (Zur and Yule, 1990). Depression has also been observed as a significant feature of both cobalamin (Penninx et al., 2000) and folate (Hutto, 1997) deficiency. The pathogenesis of depression in both disorders remains speculative, but white matter involvement is a likely contributor.

The relationship between depression and vascular white matter changes in older people has been studied intensively. In patients with Binswanger's disease

(BD), depression is more frequent than in comparably demented patients with Alzheimer's disease (AD; Bennett et al., 1994). Other observers found depression in BD to be reversible, suggesting that disruption of ascending monoaminergic pathways may be causative (Venna et al., 1988). Depression may also occur as a prominent feature of cerebral autosomal dominant arteriopathy with subcortical infarcts and leukoencephalopathy (CADASIL), sometimes preceding cognitive impairment and dementia (Harris and Filley, 2001). Many reports have also focused on depression in individuals with leukoaraiosis. As reviewed in Chapter 11, this finding is very common in older persons, and in many cases these lesions exert no apparent clinical effect. Nevertheless, a plethora of studies beginning in the late 1980s documented an association between geriatric depression and white matter changes on neuroimaging scans (Jeste et al., 1988; Krishnan et al., 1988; Coffey et al., 1990; Zubenko et al., 1990; Lesser et al., 1991; Salloway et al., 1996; Hickie et al., 1997; Greenwald et al., 1998; Kramer-Ginsberg et al., 1999). In one intriguing case, Lesser and colleagues (1993) described a medically healthy man who developed major depression in temporal association with an increase in the number and size of MRI white matter lesions. Using another approach, O'Brien and colleagues (1998) found that elderly depressed patients with severe white matter change on MRI had a poorer psychiatric prognosis. In AD patients, Lopez and colleagues (1997) found that depressive symptomatology correlated with severity of MRI white matter lesions, particularly when they occurred in the frontal lobes. Among patients with AD, vascular dementia, and dementia with Lewy bodies, frontal lobe white matter hyperintensities were found to be associated with depression irrespective of disease diagnosis (O'Brien et al., 2000). Greenwald and colleagues (1998) found that left frontal and left putaminal lesions significantly predicted depression, consistent with considerable evidence from the stroke literature that left frontal lesions in general are related to depression (Starkstein and Robinson, 1989). A comprehensive review of neuroimaging studies in patients with mood disorders concluded that the best replicated structural brain abnormality in depression was an increased rate of white matter and periventricular hyperintensities (Soares and Mann, 1997). Because these changes likely result from cerebral ischemia, the term vascular depression was proposed as a subtype of mood disorder (Steffens and Krishnan, 1998).

A depressed mood may also afflict individuals with traumatic brain injury (TBI), tumors of the white matter, and normal pressure hydrocephalus (NPH). Depressive symptoms of varying severity are common in the aftermath of TBI (McAllister, 1992). A recent review concluded that major depression was the most common psychiatric disorder following TBI, occurring in 44% of patients across many studies (van Reekum et al., 2000). Depression is a major source of disability in both severe TBI and in the common postconcussion syndrome. Tumors of the cerebral white matter may be associated with depression, and the fact that mood change can appear before the diagnosis is made indicates that cerebral neuropathology may be causative (Galasko et al., 1988). Depression and other neuropsychiatric syndromes are more likely when the tumor involves the frontal or temporal lobes (Filley and Kleinschmidt-DeMasters, 1995). A tendency for depression with neoplasms of the corpus callosum has also been noted (Nasrallah and McChesney, 1981). Finally, depression can be seen as a presenting or prominent feature of NPH (Rice and Gendelman, 1973; Moss et al., 1987). This syndrome may be difficult to distinguish from the apathy or abulia that more often chararacterizes NPH patients. However, reports documenting improvement of depression after shunt procedures for NPH (Rice and Gendelman, 1973) indicate that depression in this disease may result from damage to cerebral white matter tracts compromised by hydrocephalus.

Mania

Mania, or the full syndrome of bipolar disorder, is often reported in individuals with white matter disorders. The etiology of these syndromes is unknown, as the possibility exists that they coexist with white matter disorders by chance alone. However, the association of mania and bipolar disorder with white matter dysfunction may imply an etiologic connection, and offers a new perspective on the neurobiology of mood disorders.

As is true of depression, mania has not been noted in many cases of dysmyelinative diseases. An exception to this rule is adult-onset adrenoleukodystrophy, in which features of mania were commonly observed at the time of presentation in one series of patients examined psychiatrically (Rosebush et al., 1999). Both mania and bipolar disorder, however, often have been observed in patients with demyelinative disease. Epidemiologic data indicate a higher than expected occurrence of bipolar disorder in patients with MS (Schiffer et al., 1986), and one study found a prevalence of bipolar disorder in MS to be more than 10 times than expected (Joffe et al., 1987). Bipolar disorder can be the presenting manifestation of MS (Kellner et al., 1984), and in one autopsy-verified case, a woman had bipolar disorder as the dominant syndrome of MS for more than 30 years (Casanova et al., 1996). Mania may also complicate acute disseminated encephalomyelitis (Paskavitz et al., 1995).

Manic behavior has also been observed with greater than chance frequency in patients with AIDS (Kieburtz et al., 1991). A consecutive series of patients with HIV infection and mania found that the mood disorder could occur early in the disease course, when cognition was normal, or later, when psychomotor slowing or dementia was present (Lyketsos et al., 1997). Another study found that zidovudine therapy was protective against the development of mania in individuals with HIV infection, suggesting that AIDS neuropathology may produce mania (Mijch et al., 1999). Mania or hypomania develops in some patients with SLE, although good prevalence figures are unavailable (West, 1994). In toxic disorders, mania is not commonly observed, but the syndrome appears fairly often in metabolic disorders. Manic features are among the psychiatric presentations of both cobalamin and folate deficiency (Hutto, 1997).

In the realm of vascular disease, many observations suggest that bipolar disorder is associated with ischemic white matter changes on neuroimaging scans. As in the case of depression, bipolar disease frequently has been associated with white matter lesions of this kind (Soares and Mann, 1997). Dupont and colleagues (1995) found an association of frontally predominant white matter changes in young patients with bipolar disorder in comparison to those with unipolar mood disorder and normal control subjects. However, some investigators have not found a link between white matter lesions and bipolar disorder (Krabbendam et al., 2000). Despite this uncertainty, the term vascular mania has been proposed as a subtype of mood disorder that can result from white matter involvement (Steffens and Krishnan, 1998). Additional insight into this issue may be possible with the use of newer MRI techniques that permit the imaging of normal appearing white matter. Mania may be explainable in part by the interruption of cerebral white matter tracts in the frontal and temporal lobes subserving mood regulation.

In patients with TBI, mania can occur either as an isolated feature or as part of bipolar disorder (McAllister, 1992). The review by van Reekum and colleagues (2000) found a strong association of TBI with bipolar affective disorder, such that 4% of TBI patients could be expected to develop this mood disorder compared to fewer than 1% in the general population. Some studies have suggested that secondary mania after TBI may preferentially involve the right frontal and temporal regions (McAllister, 1992), but the diffuse neuropathology of TBI renders this observation difficult to verify. Mania has also been observed with neoplastic involvement of the temporal lobe white matter with glioblastoma multiforme (Filley and Kleinschmidt-Demasters, 1995). The coexistence of gray matter neuropathology complicates interpretation of most tumor cases, but because gliomas typically originate in white matter areas, mania as a first symptom seems plausible. Normal pressure hydrocephalus is uncommonly associated with mania, but this syndrome has been observed as an initial presentation (Kwentus and Hart, 1987). Improvement with neurosurgical intervention suggests that structural injury to white matter was responsible.

Psychosis

A link between psychosis and the cerebral white matter has been demonstrated in a variety of different contexts. One clue to this association comes from a recent study that was the first to compare personality variables with neuroimaging findings in normal individuals (Matsui et al., 2000). In this report, the scales of the Minnesota Multiphasic Personality Inventory (MMPI) were analyzed in comparison to MRI volumetric measurements, and among many correlations found, the highest was between the schizophrenia scale and lower frontal lobe white matter volume in men (Matsui et al., 2000). Although clearly preliminary, this study raises the possibility that personality in healthy people is determined in part by the structure of frontal lobe white matter. Furthermore, these data suggest that subtle changes in frontal white matter may predispose to psychosis, and that, as discussed below, more severe frontal white matter involvement may be the direct cause of this clinical syndrome.

Psychotic behavior has been observed in many cerebral white matter disorders. In the dysmyelinative category, one of the most frequent early presentations of adult-onset metachromatic leukodystrophy (MLD) is psychosis. This syndrome often precedes cognitive impairment and dementia in the clinical course (Filley and Gross, 1992; Hyde et al., 1992), in some cases leading to diagnostic confusion and delayed recognition of the disease. At a time when the cerebral white matter is not affected in a widespread fashion, and presumably the integrity of axons is relatively well preserved, MLD may produce psychosis without dementia. Temporal and/or frontal lobe involvement has been implicated in the psychosis of MLD (Filley and Gross, 1992). Merriam and colleagues (1989) have hypothesized that damage to ascending white matter tracts produces psychosis in MLD by causing disinhibition of limbic catecholaminergic systems, and that this mechanism may also apply to other white matter disorders.

Psychosis is less often a feature of demyelinative, infectious, inflammatory, toxic, and metabolic diseases. In MS, psychosis may not occur with any greater than chance frequency (Feinstein, 1999), but a figure of 5% has been cited (Grant, 1986). As in the case of mania, psychosis can occasionally be the initial manifestation of the disease (Matthews, 1979; Awad, 1983). The presence of psychotic symptoms has been linked with bilateral temporal lobe plaques on MRI scans (Feinstein et al., 1992). Although florid mania may occur, psychosis is also rare in HIV infection (Navia et al., 1986). In SLE, however, psychosis can be seen in 5%–15% of patients (West, 1994). Paranoid psychosis has been noted as a persistent problem in some individuals with toluene abuse (Byrne et al., 1991), although neuroimaging data on this issue are not available. Other investigators have speculated that toluene abuse may be causally connected with schizophrenia (Lewis et al., 1981). Psychosis has been observed in cobalamin deficiency and pernicious anemia, and a recent review concluded that folate deficiency may actually be associated more closely with psychosis than with cobalamin deficiency (Hutto, 1997).

Late-onset psychosis has often been noted in association with vascular white matter disease. In BD, psychosis may appear as an early clinical feature, preceding the onset of dementia (Lawrence and Hillam, 1995). Leukoaraiosis has also been associated with psychosis by some (Breitner et al., 1990; Miller et al., 1991) but not all (Howard et al., 1995; Symonds et al., 1997) investigators. Whether white matter changes in older people are potential contributors to psychosis or simply coincidental findings cannot be determined with currently available information. In TBI, there appears to be little increased risk of psychosis as a late sequel (van Reekum et al., 2000). However, psychotic symptoms may occur in the acute recovery period after TBI, and discrete psychotic episodes may also occur in the postacute phase (McAllister, 1992). Cerebral tumors have often been associated with psychosis, again most often associated with frontal and temporolimbic sites of origin (Galasko et al., 1988; Filley and Kleinschmidt-DeMasters, 1995). Prominent features of psychosis are delusions, typically simple and with a paranoid component, and hallucinations, which are most likely in the visual modality (Galasko et al., 1988). Finally, psychosis, again with a paranoid flavor, can be seen in patients with NPH (Rice and Gendelman, 1973; Lying-Tunnell, 1979). Shunt placement has been reported to effect complete or substantial recovery from psychosis in patients with this disease (Rice and Gendelman, 1973; Lying-Tunnell, 1979), implying that injury to cerebral white matter may be pathogenetically important.

These various findings are of interest in view of increasing evidence of cerebral white matter abnormalities in patients with schizophrenia. Although establishing the neuropathology of schizophrenia has proven to be a remarkably elusive goal, a disorder of connectivity within and between cortical and subcortical regions is currently being considered (Harrison, 1999; Pearlson, 2000). Thus, although alterations in gray matter are also likely, a fundamental abnormality of white matter is an attractive possibility. Many decades ago, Elvidge and Reed (1938) observed swollen oligodendrocytes in schizophrenic brains studied post-mortem. The MRI era stimulated further observations in this area. Keshavan and colleagues (1996) noted a significant burden of MRI hyperintensities in the right posterior white matter of older schizophrenics, and Sachdev and Brodaty (1999) found increased periventricular hyperintensities in late-onset schizophenia. In these studies, however, the confounding issue of age raised the possibility that the white matter lesions might be of vascular origin. This problem was addressed by the application of advanced MRI techniques in young schizophrenic patients. With the use of diffusion tensor MRI, changes have been detected in the corpus callosum (Foong et al., 2000b), and diffusely in the white matter of the hemispheres (Lim et al., 1999). Moreover, magnetic resonance spectroscopy study of the white matter in schizophrenics detected a reduction in N-acetyl aspartate, a marker of axonal integrity (Lim et al., 1998). Evidence of more focal white matter disturbance has also appeared. Studies using conventional (Breier et al., 1992) and diffusion tensor MRI (Buchsbaum et al., 1998) have found white matter abnormalities in the frontal lobes, which may be attributable to a developmental migration defect (Akbarian et al., 1996) or delayed myelination (Benes et al., 1994). In addition, with the use of magnetization transfer imaging, white matter abnormalities have been observed in the temporal lobes (Foong et al., 2000a), Taken together, these findings are consistent with a disorder of cerebral white matter in schizophrenia that may be most evident in the frontal and temporal lobes. A disruption of connectivity may result to produce the clinical syndrome of psychosis. This notion has been elaborated by Crow (1998), who argued that schizophrenia is a transcallosal misconnection syndrome affecting the normal interaction of the language hemisphere with the nonlanguage hemisphere that represents the associated meanings of linguistic expression.

Personality Change

Although a difficult term to define, the concept of personality generally refers to the characteristic repertoire of behavioral responses used by an individual to deal with everyday situations (Filley, 1995). As with many other cerebral lesions, a change in personality can occur with white matter disorders. These symptoms and signs are often vague and nonspecific, and the best efforts by informants may yield only the description that a person not his or her "normal self." Apathy, irritability, lassitude, inattention, drowsiness, memory lapses, and emotional lability may all contribute to this picture. As is apparent from Part II of this book, these and related symptoms may characterize all of the disorders of white matter, particularly in their early stages before more specific symptoms and signs develop. The clinician is thus well advised to recall that a personality change, especially in adulthood, may require prompt investigation regardless of whether other neurologic features can be detected.

Personality changes with more recognizable implications, however, may also be seen in white matter disorders. One of these is emotional incontinence, also called pathologic laughter and crying or pseudobulbar affect, which is recognized by neurologists as a component of the syndrome of pseudobulbar palsy. In this disorder of emotional control, patients are plagued by uncontrollable laughter or crying that is out of proportion to the degree of happiness or sadness that they experience. The exaggerated and disproportional expression of affect is disturbing to patients and their families, and complicates the assessment of mood in those affected (Mahler, 1992). Emotional incontinence is seen in patients with MS, as well as in those with advanced BD and CADASIL. The syndrome may also appear in patients with amyotrophic lateral sclerosis, indicating that it is not necessarily associated with cognitive impairment. Classical teaching holds that emotional incontinence is caused by bilateral damage to the corticobulbar tracts, lesions of which presumably release brainstem motor centers from frontal cortical control. However, no definitive studies confirming this belief are as yet available. In MS, emotional incontinence is generally associated with more severe cognitive impairment, implying that affected patients have greater white matter involvement (Feinstein, 1999), but the exact locations of responsible lesions is unknown. Treatment however, can be gratifying because amitriptyline (Schiffer et al., 1985), fluoxetine, and dopaminergic agents have all been shown to be effective (Feinstein, 1999).

Euphoria is another personality change, encountered mainly in patients with MS. This syndrome is one of the more striking in behavioral neurology. Seen mainly in individuals with advanced MS, euphoria is a state of remarkable unconcern and even elation that arises in the setting of severe physical disability. As such, euphoria has much in common with the lack of insight that typifies patients with frontal lobe disease from any etiology (Filley, 1995). Euphoria also resembles mania in some respects, but it is of interest that whereas corticosteroid therapy may precipitate mania in MS patients (Minden et al., 1987), it does not appear to be a risk factor for euphoria (Mahler, 1992). Structural neuroimaging studies have been consistent in correlating this syndrome with white matter disease burden. Rabins and colleagues (1986) found that euphoric MS patients, in comparison to those without euphoria, were more likely to have cerebral involvement, enlarged ventricles on CT, more severe cognitive impairment, worse neurologic function, and greater social disability. Ron and Logsdail (1989) found that elation correlated with the presence of widespread MRI white matter changes. Later, correlations were observed between euphoria and frontal (Reischies et al., 1993) and frontotemporal (Diaz-Olavarrieta et al., 1999) white matter lesion burden on MRI.

Fatigue

Fatigue is a ubiquitous symptom in clinical medicine. A great variety of disorders affecting the brain and many other organs can produce fatigue, and its nonspecificity as a symptom is one of the barriers to its successful study. Fatigue may reflect chronic systemic disease, neuromuscular dysfunction, structural involvement of the brain, or many psychological issues, and more than one of these factors often coexist in an individual patient. Although not usually considered a standard neuropsychiatric problem, fatigue deserves comment in this chapter because of suggestions that it is associated with both white matter disorders and psychological distress. These questions are illustrated by two disorders in which fatigue is prominent: MS and the chronic fatigue syndrome (CFS). In each, white matter lesions have been proposed to be important determinants of fatigue, but it is unclear how much psychological and other factors contribute.

In MS, fatigue is a common and frequently disabling symptom. Little is known, however, about the origin of this complaint, which may occur independently of disease relapses. Three possible causes of fatigue in MS have been proposed: depression, motor dysfunction, and cognitive impairment. Krupp and colleagues (1988) found no relationship between fatigue and depression, but Feinstein (1999) expressed reservations about whether fatigue could exist in isolation from psychiatric symptoms. Motor dysfunction has been suggested by Colombo and colleagues (2000), who found that fatigue correlated with MRI plaque burden in descending motor tracts. However, several studies have shown that white matter lesion burden and cerebral atrophy as demonstrated by conventional MRI do not correlate with fatigue severity (van der Werf et al., 1998; Mainero et al, 1999; Bakshi et al., 1999). A relationship with cognitive impairment is suggested by the amelioration of fatigue in some MS patients with amantadine (Rosenberg and Appenzeller, 1988; Sailer et al., 2000), although other investigators have found no correlation between fatigue and cognitive dysfunction and no improvement in fatigue with stimulant drugs (Geisler et al., 1996). Some support for "cognitive fatigue" has appeared recently in studies of MS patients who demonstrate a significant decline in neuropsychological performance during a test of sustained attention (Schwid et al., 2000) or after a continuous effortful cognitive task (Krupp and Elkins, 2000). The origin of fatigue in MS thus remains uncertain, and several factors may play a role. Because it is conceivable that white matter disease burden could underlie all the proposed etiologies of fatigue, further study with newer MRI techniques in MS and other white matter disorders would be of interest to explore these possible relationships in more detail.

Still more uncertainty surrounds the neurobiological aspects of CFS (Goshorn, 1998). This syndrome is characterized by unexplained and persistent fatigue (Fukuda et al., 1994), and because there exists no satisfactory clinical assessment scale, established pathology, or laboratory test to assist with diagnosis, debate has centered on whether this disorder is medical or psychiatric in origin (Tiersky et al., 1997). Also referred to by some as Epstein-Barr virus infection, convincing evidence has not appeared to suggest that CFS has a viral or other infectious etiology, and similarities to other vague clinical entities such as fibromyalgia and the nineteenth century syndrome neurasthenia have been noted (Tiersky et al., 1997). Support for brain dysfunction in CFS has come mainly from neuropsychological and MRI studies. Despite methodological limitations, a fairly consistent pattern of impaired complex information processing speed and efficiency emerges in CFS patients (Tiersky et al., 1997). Several MRI studies have found a higher incidence of white matter hyperintensities in CFS patients (Tiersky et al., 1997), including one demonstrating excessive frontal lobe white matter changes in CFS patients who did not have a coexisting psychiatric diagnosis (Lange et al., 1999). However, it must be recognized that some CFS patients have neither cognitive dysfunction nor white matter changes (Cope et al., 1995), and that, when present, both subtle neuropsychological and MRI findings can have alternative explanations. Many studies of CFS patients report a high frequency of preexisting psychiatric disorders, primarily depression (Tiersky et al., 1997), and some evidence suggests a higher likelihood of malingering as well (van der Werf et al., 2000). In summary, whereas it is plausible that a subset of CFS patients may have frontal lobe white matter changes contributing to their complaints (Lange et al., 1999), the demonstration that CFS involves the brain white matter, or indeed is a distinct disease entity at all, remains to be made.

References

Akbarian S, Kim JJ, Potkin SG, et al. Maldistribution of interstitial neurons in prefrontal white matter of the brains of schizophrenic patients. Arch Gen Psychiatry 1996; 53: 425–436.

Anzola GP, Bevilacqua L, Cappa SF, et al. Neuropsychological assessment in patients with relapsing-remitting multiple sclerosis and mild functional impairment: correlation with magnetic resonance imaging. J Neurol Neurosurg Psychiatry 1990; 53: 142–145.

Awad AG. Schizophrenia and multiple sclerosis. J Nerv Ment Dis 1983; 171: 323–324.

Bakshi R, Czarnecki D, Shaikh ZA, et al. Brain MRI lesions and atrophy are related to depression in multiple sclerosis. Neuroreport 2000; 11: 1153–1158.

Bakshi R, Miletich RS, Henschel K, et al. Fatigue in multiple sclerosis: cross-sectional correlation with brain MRI findings in 71 patients. Neurology 1999; 53: 1151–1153.

Benes FM, Turtle M, Khan Y, Farol P. Myelination of a key relay zone in the hippocampal formation occurs in the human brain during childhood, adolescence, and adulthood. Arch Gen Psychiatry 1994; 51: 477–484.

Bennett DA, Gilley DW, Lee S, Cochran EJ. White matter changes: neurobehavioral manifestations of Binswanger's disease and clinical correlates in Alzheimer's Disease. Dementia 1994; 5: 148–152.

Breier A, Buchanan RW, Elkashef A, et al. Brain morphology and schizophrenia. A magnetic resonance imaging study of limbic, prefrontal cortex, and caudate structures. Arch Gen Psychiatry 1992; 49: 921–926.

Breitner JCS, Husain MM, Figiel GS, et al. Cerebral white matter disease in late-onset paranoid psychosis. Biol Psychiatry 1990; 28: 266–274.

Buchsbaum M, Chang CY, Peled S, et al. MRI white matter diffusion anisotropy and PET metabolic rate in schizophrenia. Neuroreport 1998; 9: 425–430.

Byrne A, Kirby B, Zibin T, Ensminger S. Psychiatric and neurological effects of chronic solvent abuse. Can J Psychiatry 1991; 36: 735–738.

Casanova MF, Kruesi M, Mannheim G. Multiple sclerosis and bipolar disorder: a case report with autopsy findings. J Neuropsychiatry Clin Neurosci 1996; 8: 206–208.

Castellon SA, Hinkin CH, Wood S, Yarema KT. Apathy, depression, and cognitive performance in HIV-1 infection. J Neuropsychiatry Clin Neurosci 1998; 10: 320–329.

Coffey CE, Figiel GS, Djang WT, et al. Subcortical hyperintensity on magnetic resonance imaging: a comparison of normal and elderly depressed subjects. Am J Psychiatry 1990; 47: 187–189.

Colombo B, Boneschi FM, Rossi P, et al. MRI and motor evoked potential findings in nondisabled multiple sclerosis patients with and without symptoms of fatigue. J Neurol 2000; 247: 506–509.

Cope H, Pernet A, Kendall B, David A. Cognitive functioning and magnetic resonance imaging in chronic fatigue. Br J Psychiatry 1995; 167: 86–94.

Crow TJ. Schizophrenia as a transcallosal misconnection syndrome. Schizophr Res 1998; 10: 111–114.

Diaz-Olavarrieta C, Cummings JL, Velasquez J, de la Cadena CG. Neuropsychiatric manifestations of multiple sclerosis. J Neuropsychiatry Clin Neurosci 1999; 11: 51–57.

Dupont RM, Jernigan TL, Heindel W, et al. Magnetic resonance imaging and mood disorders. Localization of white matter and other subcortical abnormalities. Arch Gen Psychiatry 1995; 52: 747–755.

Elvidge AR, Reed GE. Biopsy studies of cerebral pathologic changes in schizophrenia and manic-depressive psychosis. Arch Neurol Psychiatry 1938; 40: 227–268.

Feinstein A. The clinical neuropsychiatry of multiple sclerosis. Cambridge: Cambridge University Press, 1999.

Feinstein A, du Boulay G, Ron MA. Psychotic illness in multiple sclerosis. A clinical and magnetic resonance imaging study. Br J Psychiatry 1992; 161: 680–685.

Filley CM. Neurobehavioral anatomy. Niwot, CO: University Press of Colorado, 1995.

Filley CM, Gross KF. Psychosis with cerebral white matter disease. Neuropsychiatry Neuropsychol Behav Neurol 1992; 5: 119–125.

Filley CM, Kleinschmidt-DeMasters BK. Neurobehavioral presentations of brain neoplasms. West J Med 1995; 163: 19–25.

Foong J, Maier M, Barker GJ, et al. In vivo investigation of white matter pathology in schizophrenia with magnetisation transfer imaging. J Neurol Neurosurg Psychiatry 2000a; 68: 70–74.

Foong J, Maier M, Clark CA, et al. Neuropathological abnormalities of the corpus callosum in schizophrenia: a diffusion tensor imaging study. J Neurol Neurosurg Psychiatry 2000b; 68: 242–244.

Fukuda K, Straus SE, Hickie I, et al. The chronic fatigue syndrome: A comprehensive approach to its definition and study. Ann Int Med 1994; 121: 953–959.

Galasko D, Yuen K-O, Thal L. Intracranial mass lesions associated with late-onset psychosis and depression. Psychiatric Clin N Am 1988; 11: 151–166.

Geisler MW, Sliwinski M, Coyle PK, et al. The effects of amantadine and pemoline on cognitive functioning in multiple sclerosis. Arch Neurol 1996; 53: 185–188.

Gilchrist AC, Creed FH. Depression, cognitive impairment and social stress in multiple sclerosis. J Psychosom Res 1994; 38: 193–201.

Goshorn RK. Chronic fatigue syndrome: a review for clinicians. Semin Neurol 1998; 18: 237–242.

Grant I. Neuropsychological and psychiatric disturbances in multiple sclerosis. In: McDonald WI, Silberberg D, eds. Multiple sclerosis. London: Butterworths, 1986: 134–152.

Greenwald BS, Kramer-Ginsburg E, Krishnan RR, et al. Neuroanatomic localization of magnetic resonance imaging signal hyperintensities in geriatric depression. Stroke 1998; 29: 613–617.

Harris JG, Filley CM. CADASIL: neuropsychological findings in three generations of an affected family. J Int Neuropsychol Soc 2001; 7: 768–774.

Harrison PJ. The neuropathology of schizophrenia. A critical review of the data and their interpretation. Brain 1999; 122: 593–624.

Hickie I, Scott E, Wilhelm K, Brodaty H. Subcortical hyperintensities on magnetic resonance imaging in patients with severe depression—a longitudinal evaluation. Biol Psychiatry 1997; 42: 367–374.

Honer WG, Hurwitz T, Li DKB, et al. Temporal lobe involvement in multiple sclerosis patients with psychiatric disorders. Arch Neurol 1987; 44: 187–190.

Howard R, Cox T, Almeida O, et al. White matter signal hyperintensities in the brains of patients with late paraphrenia and the normal community-living elderly. Biol Psychiatry 1995; 38: 86–91.

Huber SJ, Paulsen GW, Shuttleworth EC, et al. Magnetic resonance imaging correlates of dementia in multiple sclerosis. Arch Neurol 1987; 44: 732–736.

Hutto BR. Folate and cobalamin in psychiatric illness. Comp Psychiatry 1997; 38: 305–314.

Hyde TM, Ziegler JC, Weinberger DR. Psychiatric disturbances in metachromatic leukodystrophy. Insights into the neurobiology of psychosis. Arch Neurol 1992; 49: 401–406.

Jeste D, Lohr JB, Goodwin FK. Neuroanatomical studies of major affective disorders: a review and suggestions for further research. Br J Psychiatry 1988; 153: 444–459.

Joffe RT, Lippert GP, Gray TA, et al. Mood disorder and multiple sclerosis. Arch Neurol 1987; 44: 376–378.

Kellner CH, Davenport Y, Post RM, Ross RJ. Rapidly cycling bipolar disorder and multiple sclerosis. Am J Psychiatry 1984; 141: 112–113.

Keshavan MS, Mulsant BH, Sweet RA, et al. MRI changes in schizophrenia in late life: a preliminary controlled study. Psychiatry Res 1996; 60: 117–123.

Kieburtz K, Zetelmaier AE, Ketonen L, et al. Manic syndrome in AIDS. Am J Psychiatry 1991; 148: 1068–1070.

Krabbendam L, Honig A, Wiersma J, et al. Cognitive dysfunctions and white matter lesions in patients with bipolar disorder in remission. Acta Psychiat Scand 2000; 101: 274–280.

Kramer-Ginsburg E, Greenwald BS, Krishnan KRR, et al. Neuropsychological functioning and MRI signal hyperintensities in geriatric depression. Am J Psychiatry 1999; 156: 438–444.

Krishnan KRR, Goli V, Ellinwood EH, et al. Leukoencephalopathy in patients diagnosed as a major depressive. Biol Psychiatry 1988; 23: 519–522.

Krupp LB, Alvarez LA, LaRocca NG, Scheinberg LC. Fatigue in multiple sclerosis. Arch Neurol 1988; 45: 435–437.

Krupp L, Elkins LE. Fatigue and declines in cognitive functioning in multiple sclerosis. Neurology 2000; 55: 934–939.

Kwentus JA, Hart RP. Normal pressure hydrocephalus presenting as mania. J Nerv Ment Dis 1987; 175: 500–502.

Lange G, DeLuca J, Maldjian JA, et al. Brain MRI abnormalities exist in a subset of patients with chronic fatigue syndrome. J Neurol Sci 1999; 171: 3–7.

Lawrence RM, Hillam JC. Psychiatric symptomatology in early-onset Binswanger's disease: two case reports. Behav Neurol 1995; 8: 43–46.

Lesser IM, Hill-Gutierrez E, Miller BL, Boone KB. Late-onset depression with white matter lesions. Psychosomatics 1993; 34: 364–367.

Lesser IM, Miller BL, Boone KB, et al. Brain injury and cognitive function in late-onset psychotic depression. J Neuropsychiatry Clin Neurosci 1991; 3: 33–40.

Lewis JD, Moritz D, Mellis LP. Long-term toluene abuse. Am J Psychiatry 1981; 138: 368–370.

Lim KO, Adalsteinson E, Spielman D, et al. Proton resonance spectroscopic imaging of cortical gray and white matter in schizophrenia. Arch Gen Psychiatry 1998; 55: 346–352.

Lim KO, Hedehus M, Moseley M, et al. Compromised white matter tract integrity in schizophrenia inferred from diffusion tensor imaging. Arch Gen Psychiatry 1999; 56: 367–374.

Lopez OL, Becker JT, Reynolds CF, et al. Psychiatric correlates of MR deep white matter lesions in probable Alzheimer's Disease. J Neuropsychiatry Clin Neurosci 1997; 9: 246–250.

Lying-Tunnell U. Psychotic symptoms in normal-pressure hydrocephalus. Acta Psychiatr Scand 1979; 59: 415–419.

Lyketsos CG, Schwartz J, Fishman M, Treisman G. AIDS mania. J Neuropsychiatry Clin Neurosci 1997; 9: 277–279.

Mahler ME. Behavioral manifestations associated with multiple sclerosis. Psychiat Clin N Am 1992; 15: 427–438.

Mainero C, Faroni J, Gasperini C, et al. Fatigue and magnetic resonance imaging activity in multiple sclerosis. J Neurol 1999; 246: 454–458.

Masterson G. The management of solvent abuse. J Adolescence 1979; 2: 66–75.

Matsui M, Gur RC, Turetsky BI, et al. The relation between tendency for psychopathology and reduced frontal brain volume in healthy people. Neuropsychiatry Neuropsychol Behav Neurol 2000; 13: 155–162.

Matthews WB. Multiple sclerosis presenting with acute remitting psychiatric symptoms. J Neurol Neurosurg Psychiatry 1979; 42: 859–863.

McAllister TW. Neuropsychiatric sequelae of head injuries. Psychiatric Clin N Am 1992; 15: 395–413.

Merriam AE, Hegarty A, Miller A. A proposed etiology for psychotic symptoms in white matter dementia. Neuropsychiatry Neuropsychol Behav Neurol 1989; 2: 225–228.

Mijch AM, Judd FK, Lyketsos CG, et al. Secondary mania in patients with HIV infection: are antiretrovirals protective? J Neuropsychiatry Clin Neurosci 1999; 11: 475–480.

Miller BL, Lesser IM, Boone KB, et al. Brain lesions and cognitive function in late-life psychosis. Brit J Psychiatry 1991; 158: 76–82.

Minden SL, Orav J, Reich P. Depression in multiple sclerosis. Gen Hosp Psychiatry 1987; 9: 426–434.

Minden SL, Schiffer RB. Affective disorders in multiple sclerosis. Review and recommendations for clinical research. Arch Neurol 1990; 47: 98–104.

Moss R, D'Amico S, Maletta G. Mental dysfunction as a sign of organic illness in the elderly. Geriatrics 1987; 42: 35–42.

Nasrallah HA, McChesney CM. Psychopathology of corpus callosum tumors. Biol Psychiatry 1981; 16: 663–669.

Navia BA, Jordan BD, Price RW. The AIDS dementia complex: I. Clinical features. Ann Neurol 1986; 19: 517–524.

O'Brien J, Ames D, Chiu E, et al. Severe deep white matter lesions and outcome in elderly patients with major depressive disorder: follow up study. Br Med J 1998; 317: 982–984.

O'Brien J, Perry R, Barber R, et al. The association between white matter lesions on magnetic resonance imaging and noncognitive symptoms. Ann NY Acad Sci 2000; 903: 482–489.

Paskavitz JF, Anderson CA, Filley CM, et al. Acute arcuate fiber demyelinating encephalopathy following Epstein-Barr virus infection. Ann Neurol 1995; 38: 127–131.

Pearlson G. Neurobiology of schizophrenia. Ann Neurol 2000; 48: 556–566.

Penninx BWJH, Guralnik JM, Ferrucci L, et al. Vitamin B$_{12}$ deficiency and depression in physically disabled older women: epidemiologic evidence from the Women's Health and Aging Study. Am J Psychiatry 2000; 157: 715–721.

Perry SW. HIV-related depression. Res Publ Assoc Res Nerv Ment Dis 1994; 72: 223–238.

Pujol J, Bello J, Deus J, et al. Lesions in the left arcuate fasciculus region and depressive symptoms in multiple sclerosis. Neurology 1997; 49: 1105–1110.

Rabins PV, Brooks BR, O'Donnell P, et al. Structural brain correlates of emotional disorder in multiple sclerosis. Brain 1986; 109: 585–597.

Reischies FM, Baum K, Brau H, et al. Cerebral magnetic resonance imaging findings in multiple sclerosis. Relation to disturbance of affect, drive and cognition. Arch Neurol 1988; 45: 1114–1116.

Reischies FM, Baum K, Nehrig C, Schörner W. Psychopathological symptoms and magnetic resonance imaging findings in multiple sclerosis. Biol Psychiatry 1993; 33: 676–678.

Rice E, Gendelman S. Psychiatric aspects of normal pressure hydrocephalus. JAMA 1973; 223: 409–412.

Ron MA, Logsdail SJ. Psychiatric morbidity in multiple sclerosis: a clinical and MRI study. Psychol Med 1989; 19: 887–895.

Rosebush PI, Garside S, Levinson AJ, Mazurek MF. The neuropsychiatry of adult-onset adrenoleukodystrophy. J Neuropsychiatry Clin Neuro Sci 1999; 11: 315–327.

Rosenberg GA, Appenzeller O. Amantadine, fatigue, and multiple sclerosis. Arch Neurol 1988; 45: 1104–1106.

Sabatini U, Pozzilli C, Pantano P, et al. Involvement of the limbic system in multiple sclerosis patients with depressive disorders. Biol Psychiatry 1996; 39: 970–975.

Sachdev P, Brodaty H. Quantitative study of signal hyperintensities on T2–weighted magnetic resonance imaging in late-onset schizophrenia. Am J Psychiatry 1999; 156: 1958–1967.

Sadovnick AD, Eisen K, Ebers GC, Paty DW. Cause of death in patients attending multiple sclerosis clinics. Neurology 1991; 41: 1193–1196.

Sailer M, Heinze HJ, Schoenfeld MA, et al. Amantadine influences cognitive processing in patients with multiple sclerosis. Pharmacopsychiatry 2000; 33: 28–37.

Salloway S, Cummings JL. Subcortical disease and neuropsychiatric illness. J Neuropsychiatry Clin Neurosci 1994; 6: 93–99.

Salloway S, Price LH, Charney DS, Shapiro M. Multiple sclerosis presenting as major depression: a diagnosis suggested by MRI but not CT scan. J Clin Psychiatry 1988; 49: 364–366.

Salloway S, Malloy P, Kohn R, et al. MRI and neuropsychological differences in early- and late-life—onset geriatric depression. Neurology 1996; 46: 1567–1574.

Schiffer RB. Depressive syndromes associated with diseases of the central nervous system. Semin Neurol 1990; 10: 239–246.

Schiffer RB, Babigian HM. Behavioral disorders in multiple sclerosis, temporal lobe epilepsy, and amyotrophic lateral sclerosis. An epidemiologic study. Arch Neurol 1984; 41: 1067–1069.

Schiffer RB, Caine ED, Bamford KA, Levy S. Depressive episodes in patients with multiple sclerosis. Am J Psychiatry 1983; 140: 1498–1500.

Schiffer RB, Herndon RM, Rudick RA. Treatment of pathologic laughing and weeping with amitriptyline. N Engl J Med 1985; 312: 1480–1482.

Schiffer RB, Wineman NM. Antidepressant pharmacotherapy of depression associated with multiple sclerosis. Am J Psychiatry 1990; 147: 1493–1497.

Schiffer RB, Wineman NM, Weitkamp LR. Association between bipolar affective disorder and multiple sclerosis. Am J Psychiatry 1986; 143: 94–95.

Schwid SR, Weinstein A, Scheid EA, Goodman AD. Cognitive fatigue measured during a test of sustained attention in multiple sclerosis patients. Ann Neurol 2000; 48: 478.

Soares JC, Mann JJ. The anatomy of mood disorders—review of structural neuroimaging studies. Biol Psychiatry 1997; 41: 86–106.

Starkstein SE, Robinson RG. Affective disorders and cerebral vascular disease. Br J Psychiatry 1989; 154: 170–182.

Steffens DC, Krishnan KRR. Structural neuroimaging and mood disorders: recent findings, implications for classification, and future directions. Biol Psychiatry 1998; 43: 705–712.

Stenager EN, Stenager E, Koch-Henriksen N, et al. Suicide and multiple sclerosis: an epidemiological investigation. J Neurol Neurosurg Psychiatry 1992; 55: 542–545.

Surridge D. An investigation into some psychiatric aspects of multiple sclerosis. Br J Psychaitry 1969: 115: 749–764.

Symonds LL, Olichney JM, Jernigan TL, et al. Lack of clinically significant gross structural abnormalities in MRIs of older patients with schizophrenia and related psychoses. J Neuropsychiatry Clin Neurosci 1997; 9: 251–258.

Tiersky LA, Johnson SK, Lange G, et al. Neuropsychology of chronic fatigue syndrome: a critical review. J Clin Exp Neuropsychol 1997; 19: 560–586.

van der Werf SP, Jongen PJ, Lycklama A Nijeholt GJ, et al. Fatigue in multiple sclerosis: interrelations between fatigue, cerebral MRI abnormalities and neurological disability. J Neurol Sci 1998; 160: 164–170.

van der Werf SP, Prins JB, Jongen PJ, et al. Abnormal neuropsychological findings are not necessarily a sign of cerebral impairment: a matched comparison between chronic fatigue syndrome and multiple sclerosis. Neuropsychiatry Neuropsychol Behav Neurol 2000; 13: 199–203.

van Reekum R, Cohen T, Wong J. Can traumatic brain injury cause psychiatric disorders? J Neuropsychiatry Clin Neurosci 2000; 12: 316–327.

Venna N, Mogocsi S, Jay M, et al. Reversible depression in Binswanger's Disease. J Clin Psychiatry 1988; 49: 23–26.

Wekking EM. Psychiatric symptoms in systemic lupus erythematosus: an update. Psychosom Med 1993; 55: 219–228.

West SG. Neuropsychiatric lupus. Rheum Dis Clin N Am 1994; 20: 129–158.

Whitlock FA, Siskind MM. Depression as a major symptom of multiple sclerosis. J Neurol Neurosurg Psychiatry 1980; 43: 861–865.

Young AC, Saunders J, Ponsford JR. Mental change as an early feature of multiple sclerosis. J Neurol Neurosurg Psychiatry 1976; 39: 1008–1013.

Zubenko GS, Sullivan P, Nelson JP, et al. Brain imaging abnormalities in mental disorders of late life. Arch Neurol 1990; 47: 1107–1111.

Zur J, Yule W. Chronic solvent abuse. 2. Relationship with depression. Child Care Heath Dev 1990; 16: 21–34.

18

The Behavioral Neurology
of White Matter

The foregoing chapters of this book are intended to elucidate various aspects of brain white matter and the afflictions to which it is vulnerable. The final remaining task is to assemble this diverse collection of details into a coherent whole. At present, the information at hand is essentially descriptive, derived as it is from basic scientific and clinical aspects of individuals with white matter disorders. As such, little detail regarding functional aspects of white matter is available. Much of this chapter, therefore, will necessarily be speculative. However, a large amount of clinical data can be invoked to inform a preliminary framework for developing more sophisticated understanding. The intent is to present a broad portrait of the white matter and its role in human behavior that can foster further interest and investigation. The many gaps in existing knowledge can serve to generate a wealth of testable hypotheses to stimulate further study of brain–behavior relationhips.

Clinical Implications

Behavioral neurology is a clinical discipline, and its first responsibility is to patients presenting with behavioral complaints presumably related to brain dysfunction. The study of white matter expands the clinical spectrum falling within the scope of behavioral neurology, and several practical implications can be derived from this pursuit.

One initial conclusion to be drawn from this book is that the term "higher cortical function" is inadequate to describe the neural basis of mental activity. Despite continuing and appropriate emphasis on the association and limbic cortices as substrates of cognitive and emotional capacities, it is now abundantly clear that subcortical structures, including both gray and white matter areas, are also centrally involved in the elaboration of the mind's activity. Thus, the term higher cerebral function would seem to be preferable (Filley, 1995). Even this term may need to be revisited as more information appears about possible contributions to mental processes from the brainstem (Katz et al., 1987; Price and Mesulam, 1987; Hofmann and Watts, 1998) and cerebellum (Schmahmann, 1991), but at present it can suffice to expand the focus of neuroscientists pursuing the details of human behavior.

The neurologic diseases and injuries discussed in Part II convincingly demonstrate that white matter disorders are regularly associated with specific neurobehavioral syndromes. Cognitive impairment is well documented, which may be diffuse, resulting in syndromes ranging from mild cognitive dysfunction to severe dementia, or focal, causing a variety of neurobehavioral syndromes that may closely resemble classic syndromes traditionally ascribed to cortical lesions. Emotional dysfunction also occurs, although clinical descriptions are less complete, and may take the form of many neuropsychiatric syndromes. Legitimate questions can be raised about the selectivity of white matter involvement in some of these conditions, and it is not always possible to rule out coexistent gray matter involvement in the pathogenesis of neurobehavioral dysfunction. Criticism may also arise from the uncertainty generated by the often impressionistic and nonstandardized assessments of clinical status that bedevil the existing literature. Still, the assignment of cognitive and emotional importance to the white matter is supported by an impressive number of diseases and injuries in which the common denominator of white matter neuropathology is associated with consistent and recognizable clinical manifestations. Just as cortical dysfunction produces recurrent clinical patterns, so do the many white matter disorders, and this conclusion becomes especially apparent when they are considered as a group. In short, a sufficient clinical database exists to justify a behavioral neurology of white matter (Filley, 1998).

Given that there is good reason to associate white matter lesions with neurobehavioral disturbances, the next issue concerns the correlation of these lesions with the clinical picture. The establishment of such correlations represents the best available method for determining the participation of white matter in a given function, although it must be remembered that correlation is not causation. The lesion method of behavioral neurology is appropriate as a means of addressing these issues. In general, the evidence to date indicates that correlations with cognitive syndromes are stronger than those with emotional disorders. Cognitive impairment and dementia are both increasingly correlated with the severity of white matter lesion burden, whether determined by neuroimaging or neuropathologic methods. Similarly, focal syndromes appear to correlate with white matter lesions that are either predicted by the findings of classic behavioral neurology or are neuroanatomically plausible.

In light of the recurring theme of cognitive impairment that characterizes the literature on white matter disorders, the concept of white matter dementia was formulated (Filley et al., 1988; Filley, 1998). The clinical and theoretical justifications for the creation of this category are advanced in Chapter 15, and it is hoped that the investigation this framework has provoked will continue in a useful manner. At the least, white matter dementia may invigorate thinking on brain–behavior relationships, and if so, its purpose will have been well served.

In clinical practice, the diagnosis of white matter disorders is a major concern. Previous chapters have demonstrated the subtlety of clinical features that may occur early in the course of the disorder when treatment may be most efficacious. Several points are useful for the clinician to recall at this stage. The first objective is to consider the possibility of a white matter disorder during the history-taking. Clues may be obvious, such as the infantile onset of the disease with a relevant family history, documented exposure to a leukotoxic substance, or significant traumatic brain injury (TBI), or less apparent, such as with the initial symptoms of multiple sclerosis (MS), human immunodeficiency virus (HIV) infection, or normal pressure hydrocephalus (NPH). Early clinical features of cerebral white matter involvement typically include confusion, inattention, memory dysfunction, and personality change. On neurologic examination, therefore, the careful testing of mental status is most revealing. Measures of attention, cognitive speed, memory retrieval, visuospatial skills, and executive function are likely to be most sensitive to subtle white matter dysfunction. In contrast to disorders primarily involving the cortex, higher cerebral functions such as language, praxis, and perception are uncommonly affected; the usual preservation of language is an important point because affected individuals may display normal language and thus appear cognitively intact, when in fact they have significant deficits in other neurobehavioral domains. Personality and emotional changes are common, often leading to the suspicion that the patient may suffer from a primary psychiatric disorder. Elemental neurologic findings such as hemiparesis and visual loss are uncommon initially unless the leukoencephalopathy is severe and associated with focal necrosis. In many cases, the office examination may not be sufficiently conclusive to document a neurobehavioral disorder, and the use of neuropsychological testing is then helpful. A magnetic resonance (MRI) scan of the brain is clearly required, as it is superior to computed tomography (CT) in its excellent visualization of the cerebral white matter and its ability to suggest one of the many possible etiologies of leukoencephalopathy. Conventional T2-weighted sequences have been the most useful for detecting white matter lesions, and newer MRI techniques may all improve the capacity to detect white matter neuropathology. The diagnosis is usually more straightforward with more extensive white matter involvement; somnolence, apathy, memory loss, and dementia then occur, and with severe damage, abulia, akinetic mutism, stupor, coma, the vegetative state, and death are possible.

Despite the frequent difficulty in their diagnosis, white matter disorders offer the refreshing prospect of a relatively good prognosis in many cases. Although the outcome of many disorders discussed in this book remains disappointingly poor, white matter disorders frequently have a less pervasive neuropathologic impact than gray matter disorders, including many neurodegenerative conditions such as Alzheimer's disease (AD) that produce far greater damage. Indeed, because neuronal elements other than myelin may be completely spared in white matter disorders, spontaneous recovery may be complete or nearly so if the neuropathologic process is identified and treated early enough in the course. Even if myelin is damaged, the frequent preservation of axons is noteworthy, and remyelination or other functional compensation can potentially occur in many disorders. If the axons are destroyed, there may be an opportunity for the brain to recover function through alternate white matter pathways that can reconnect relevant gray matter regions (Terayama et al., 1993; Alexander, 1996).

In the realm of treatment, again the prospects appear to be favorable. Prevention holds considerable promise because many white matter disorders are acquired through lifestyle, injury, or iatrogenesis. This approach may avert any significant white matter involvement, and recognition of the potential problem will assist in primary care and counseling. Major opportunities for clinical benefit are apparent in the prevention of HIV infection, vascular white matter disease, and TBI, among others. Even after early involvement has taken place, intervention to prevent further damage may often be successful, particularly if axonal loss has not occurred. When the syndrome is fully established, a wide range of treatment options are becoming available in the white matter disorders. These include modalities as diverse as bone marrow transplantation, gene therapy, immunomodulatory agents, stimulant drugs, and cognitive rehabilitation. The specific treatment possibilities depend on the detailed elucidation of neuropathology and pathogenesis, which is proceeding at a more rapid pace. As new treatments become available, the therapeutic armamentarium for these patients will substantially expand.

Distributed Neural Networks

In theoretical terms, the study of brain white matter leads naturally to the notion of distributed neural networks. This concept implies that a multitude of neural assemblies exist in the brain that are widely dispersed anatomically, yet structurally interconnected and functionally integrated to subserve a specific neurobehavioral role (Mesulam, 1990, 1998, 2000). By invoking the idea of such multifocal yet dedicated networks, this theory stands as a modern resolution of the familiar dispute in behavioral neurology between localizationists and equipotential theorists. In this time-worn controversy, those who believe higher functions to be strictly localized in specific brain regions differ from those who argue that the entire brain participates in organizing these activities. Despite much debate, evidence from the last several decades has suggested that a middle ground can be reasonably held; that is, whereas many higher functions are indeed represented to a variable extent in specific brain regions, these functions also depend on other areas that support the cognitive or emotional operation. From the arguments advanced in this book, it is clear that the white matter figures significantly in all of these networks.

Several neural networks can be plausibly identified, each of which subserves a distinct neurobehavioral domain (Mesulam, 2000). In humans, these networks are best known by their key gray matter structures, and the white matter tracts by which they are connected are not well defined. However, classical neuroanatomy and the results of human lesion analyses permit a preliminary listing of the white matter structures that participate in distributed neural networks. Table 18-1 displays the essential gray matter components of neural networks and the white matter tracts by which they are putatively interconnected.

First, arousal is dependent on the reticular activating system, which originates in the upper pons and midbrain and sends projections to the intralaminar nuclei of the thalamus or directly to the cortex. The neuroanatomy of these connections is complex, but the medial forebrain bundles and diffuse thalamocortical projections are prominently involved. Second, there is a spatial attention network, dominant in the right hemisphere, which includes the parietal cortex, prefrontal cortex (frontal eye field), and cingulate gyrus; the superior occipitofrontal fasciculus and the cingulum appear to interconnect these areas. Third, abundant evidence supports the existence of a medial temporal–diencephalic–basal forebrain network for recent memory. Connections here include the fornices, the mammillothalamic tracts, and the septohippocampal tracts. Fourth, the best known neural network is the language region, usually in the left hemisphere, in which Broca's and Wernicke's areas are connected by the arcuate fasciculus and the extreme capsule. Fifth, visuospatial function is subserved in most individuals by a network in the right hemisphere consisting of the parietal lobe and the frontal lobe, which are

Table 18-1. Distributed Neural Networks

Domain	Gray Matter Structures	Connecting Tracts
Arousal	Reticular activating system	Medial forebrain bundles
	Thalamus	Thalamocortical radiations
	Cerebral cortex	
Spatial attention	Parietal lobe (right)	Superior occipitofrontal fasciculus (right)
	Prefrontal cortex (right)	Cingulum (right)
	Cingulate gyrus (right)	
Memory	Medial temporal lobe	Fornices
	Diencephalon	Mammillothalamic tracts
	Basal forebrain	Septohippocampal tracts
Language	Broca's area	Arcuate fasciculus (left)
	Wernicke's area	Extreme capsule (left)
Visuospatial ability	Parietal lobe (right)	Superior occipitofrontal fasciculus (right)
	Frontal lobe (right)	
Recognition	Temporal lobes	Inferior occipitofrontal fasciculi
	Occipital lobes	
Executive function	Dorsolateral prefrontal cortices	Long association tracts
	Posterior cortices	
Emotions	Temporolimbic system	Medial forebrain bundles
and personality	Orbitofrontal cortices	Uncinate fasciculi

probably linked by the superior occipitofrontal fasciculus. Sixth, face and object recognition is organized by a number of cortical zones in the inferior temporal and occipital lobes joined by the inferior occipitofrontal fasciculi. Seventh, executive function can be envisioned as arising from a network including the dorsolateral prefrontal cortices and the posterior cortices connected by all the long association tracts. Lastly, an extensive network for emotion and personality can be conceived to include the temporolimbic system interacting with the orbitofrontal cortices. Prominent tracts in this network are the medial forebrain bundles and the uncinate fasciculi. These formulations of the architecture of cognition and emotion are of course largely speculative, and there is a pressing need for research in humans on the details of connectivity within these networks. Moreover, further understanding of functions such as sustained attention and memory retrieval (Chapter 15) may lead to a more complete description of the white matter components of neural networks.

A discussion of distributed neural networks would be incomplete without considering the corpus callosum and other cerebral commissures. Much has been written about the relevance of cerebral disconnection to the nature of consciousness, and the split-brain research does suggest the conclusion that the corpus callosum normally provides for the feeling of conscious integration that may "enable" the human condition (Gazzaniga, 2000). The corpus callosum and the other commissures can thus be seen to play a central role in consciousness, integrating all aspects of cognitive and emotional experience into a unified whole. In this sense, the commissural connections can be seen as somehow involved in all the constituent networks that collectively comprise the foundation of human consciousness. Yet, as we have seen heretofore, there is also much evidence to suggest that abnormalities of these tracts do not routinely disrupt consciousness, and resolution of this paradox presents an important research agenda in the neurosciences. Wherever the findings in this area may lead, the cerebral commissures and their role in interhemispheric communication provide yet more evidence of the importance of white matter in higher function.

Neural Network Disconnection

Disconnection of cerebral regions offers the most plausible organizing principle for the behavioral neurology of white matter. The idea of cerebral disconnection has an honored position in behavioral neurology (Geschwind, 1965), but details of the pathogenesis of this phenomenon are complex and poorly understood. An improved understanding of disconnection can clearly be achieved by a more directed emphasis on white matter dysfunction. Interference with the normal operations of distributed neural networks by white matter lesions may disturb all aspects of neurobehavioral function.

A discussion of the neuropathology of white matter lesions is critical as a first step. The specific process associated with each disorder is clearly important, as discussed in Part II. Many general aspects of neuropathology also influence the origin and clinical relevance of disconnection. It is thus important to consider whether the white matter lesion is *(1)* focal or diffuse, *(2)* static or progressive, *(3)* associated with edema or mass effect, *(4)* severe enough to cause axonal loss or frank necrosis, and *(5)* combined with significant cortical or subcortical gray matter pathology. These variables need all be included in the interpretation of the effects of white matter damage on neural network function.

At the microscopic level, the burden of white matter neuropathology may be conceptualized to involve one or more of five components: the myelin sheath, the oligodendrocyte, the axon, the vascular system, and the astrocyte (Fig. 18-1). Injury to these structures produces variable clinical effects, and although the diversity of neuropathologic lesions makes generalizations difficult, a range of major categories can be discerned (Table 18-2). At one end of this spectrum are mild changes of patchy intramyelinic edema without demyelination or axonal loss. This stage may be asymptomatic or associated with minimal clinical sequelae. Edema may be detected as scattered white matter hyperintensity or leukoaraiosis on neuroimaging scans, and MRI is considerably more sensitive to these changes than CT because it easily detects the presence of excess water in brain tissue. More

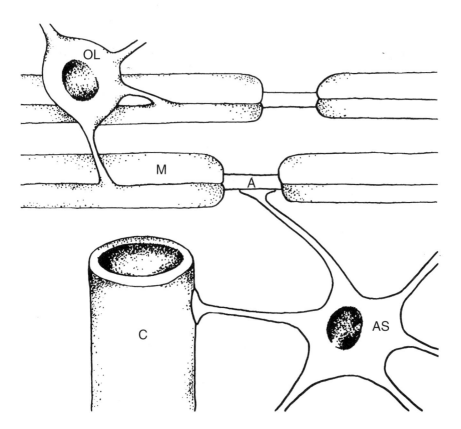

Figure 18-1. Schematic diagram of microscopic constituents of the white matter that are vulnerable to neuropathologic processes. (M, myelin sheath; OL, oligodendrocyte; A, axon; C, capillary; AS, astrocyte.)

Table 18-2. Neuropathology of White Matter Lesions

Degree	Neuropathologic Features	Neuroimaging Correlates
Mild	Patchy intramyelinic edema with preserved axons	Scattered white matter hyperintensity Leukoaraiosis
Moderate	Widespread edema	Confluent white matter hyperintensity
	Demyelination with preserved axons	Diffuse white matter hyperintensity
	Dysmyelination	
Severe	Axonal loss	Severe white matter hyperintensity
	Oligodendrocyte destruction	T1-weighted MRI "holes"
	Necrosis	Necrotic areas
	Infarction	Infarction

pronounced neuropathologic involvement takes the form of widespread edema with secondary demyelination, which may result from many neuropathologic processes, or the defective formation of myelin characteristic of dysmyelination. These changes produce more prominent clinical dysfunction. The neuroimaging appearance at this stage may involve confluent white matter changes or diffuse hyperintensity, often in specific patterns that have diagnostic utility. Finally, the most severe white matter injury involves axonal loss, oligodendrocyte destruction, necrosis, or infarction, all of which regularly result in marked and largely irreversible clinical deficits. These changes are typically widespread and dramatic on neuroimaging, manifesting as severe degrees of white matter hyperintensity, "holes" on T1-weighted MRI, or areas of necrosis and infarction visible on both CT and MRI. Astrocytes are implicated in many disorders, either because of their vulnerability to metabolic derangements or by virtue of their propensity to form gliotic scars in the area of white matter lesions.

The pathogenesis of disconnection caused by white matter dysfunction can be approached in light of available knowledge of the neuroanatomy of distributed neural networks and the neuropathologic changes that disrupt them. Several functional sequelae can be envisioned (Table 18-3). These processes are in many ways interrelated, and their effects in individual patients are not likely to be mutually exclusive.

Table 18-3. Pathogenesis of White Matter Disconnection

Slowed conduction
Absent conduction
Focal neural network disruption
Diaschisis
Wallerian degeneration
Transsynaptic degeneration

Slowed Conduction

First and most obviously, the conduction velocity of cerebral neurons may be reduced. Incomplete lesions of myelinated fibers may interfere with, but not completely eliminate, axonal conduction. This slowing of conduction may render the function of a neural network inefficient, but not impair the system to a point where it is completely inoperative. In clinical terms, this disturbance may thus mean that a patient will be able to complete a task accurately if given enough time to allow the effective engagement of the slowed neural network. Although there is a risk in reducing cognition directly to neurophysiology, considerable reason exists to believe that a slowing of central conduction velocity corresponds to a slowing of cognition in the individual. This type of change would logically apply to early stages of white matter involvement, including that associated with normal aging, and the potential for effective therapy would appear to be promising.

Absent Conduction

Another possibility is that the white matter lesion may be sufficiently severe to completely block axonal conduction. Marked demyelination and, of course, axonal loss could have this effect. In this instance, a distinct neurobehavioral deficit might emerge clinically that cannot be corrected by the provision of adequate time to complete the task. A change such as this would be expected in more advanced cases of white matter involvement, and the expectation of benefit from therapeutic interventions is likely to be less optimistic. In the usual case, slowed or absent conduction would both be expected to produce diffuse neurobehavioral syndromes because of the predilection of white matter disorders to affect widespread cerebral areas.

Focal Neural Network Disruption

Focal white matter involvement can produce specific effects on cerebral function by selectively interfering with the operations of distributed neural networks. A focal lesion in a white matter tract leading to an eloquent cortical zone can prevent incoming information from reaching the area where appropriate processing normally occurs. A good example of this phenomenon is auditory verbal agnosia (pure word deafness) from a left temporal white matter lesion (Chapter 16), a syndrome in which adequately perceived auditory input cannot be forwarded to the cortical area normally responsible for interpreting the meaning of the sounds. Alternatively, the white matter lesion can interrupt communication leaving a cortical area, so that adequately processed information does not reach its intended site. A classic example of this phenomenon is conduction aphasia, characterized by a prominent disturbance of the capacity to repeat language. In the traditional interpretation of this syndrome, a lesion in the connecting white matter separates the intact comprehension of language in Wernicke's area from the production of language mediated by Broca's area (Chapter 16).

Diaschisis

Disconnection of cerebral regions may also occur through the mechanism of diaschisis. This phenomenon, first described by von Monakow a century ago, has traditionally referred to the remote effects of an acute lesion on other regions of the brain (von Monakow, 1914). Because the remote area is itself intact, recovery from the acute insult eventually leads to partial or complete return of function in the temporarily deactivated region. The notion of diaschisis has thus been invoked to help explain why patients with marked disability after acute cerebral lesions may recover dramatically as the acute phase resolves. However, it has become clear that the concept of diaschisis can be applied to chronic lesions that cause lasting dysfunction of neural networks.

Many varieties of diaschisis are postulated, and whereas most implicate primary lesions in gray matter areas, white matter pathways are clearly involved in this phenomenon (Nguyen and Botez, 1998). When the primary lesion lies in a cortical region, the role of white matter most likely relates to the transient or permanent deafferentation that reduces the excitation of normal cortex, producing the "functional standstill" described by von Monakow (Feeney and Baron, 1986). In other words, there is an interruption of normal input travelling from one cortical region to another along white matter tracts. Modern physiological analysis has demonstrated that diaschisis produces a disruption of cerebral oxygen metabolism, glucose metabolism, and blood flow in the affected cortical area (Feeney and Baron, 1986; Meyer et al., 1993). The importance of white matter in this process was well recognized by von Monakow, who listed three types of diaschisis that correspond to the three major categories of cerebral white matter tracts: diaschisis cortico-spinalis, diaschisis commissuralis, and diaschisis associativa (Feeney and Baron, 1986).

More pertinent for this discussion, white matter lesions themselves have also been observed to produce diaschisis. In patients with MS, for example, studies with positron emission tomography have shown widespread cortical hypometabolism, particularly in the frontal lobes, attributed to diaschisis (Bakshi et al., 1998). Other studies succeeded in finding correlations between cortical hypometabolism, total T2-weighted lesion area, and cognitive dysfunction, implying that disruption of cortical metabolism by white matter lesions in MS interferes with cognitive function (Blinkenberg et al., 2000). Diaschisis from white matter lesions has also been investigated in individuals with cerebrovascular disease. Studies of patients with white matter ischemia and infarction indicate that these lesions may induce functional neuroimaging deficits in structurally normal but anatomically connected cortical regions (Metter et al., 1985; Sultzer et al., 1995). In a patient with Binswanger's Disease whose neocortex was normal at autopsy, persistent left hemineglect was ascribed to white matter ischemic demyelination that produced cortical deafferentation (Mayer et al., 1993). Most recently, a study of patients with multiple lacunar infarctions using diffusion-weighted MRI (DWMRI) and single photon emission computed tomography suggested that reduced diffusional anisotropy in the anterior corpus callosum was related to frontal cortical hypometabolism and cognitive dysfunction (Ishihara et al., 2000).

Wallerian Degeneration

The neurobehavioral effects of white matter lesions may also be related to Wallerian degeneration. This term refers to axonal injury in a white matter tract removed from the primary site of neuropathology (Waller, 1850), and the phenomenon is seen in a wide variety of demyelinative, vascular, degenerative, toxic, metabolic, and neoplastic diseases. Thus, a white matter lesion that is severe enough to injure axons at the site of the lesion may also produce damage in other regions of the tract. Wallerian degeneration may proceed distally through the length of the axon or proximally to the cell body, and the time course may be months to years. Magnetic resonance imaging studies have suggested that Wallerian degeneration can be seen after a variety of brain lesions, and its presence correlates with persistent functional disability (Sawlani et al., 1997). Using serial longitudinal MRI, Simon and colleagues (2000) have recently demonstrated Wallerian degeneration developing in appropriate regions within 12 to 18 months in individuals with demyelinative lesions. This finding may imply a scenario of an initial demyelinative plaque that proceeds to destroy the axons in the immediate vicinity and then causes subsequent degeneration of the tract. Wallerian degeneration may also occur in gray matter disorders. In AD, for example, the phenomemon has been suggested by studies with conventional MRI showing a high incidence of leukoaraiosis in that may be secondary to primary neuronal cell loss (Filley et al., 1989; Leys et al., 1991). More recently, a diffusion tensor MRI (DTI) study of AD patients demonstrated a significant reduction in the integrity of association and commissural fibers while the pyramidal tracts were normal (Rose et al., 2000). The clinical significance of this phenomenon needs further exploration, particularly with regard to its neurobehavioral effects. An important question, for example, is the extent to which Wallerian degeneration is associated with progressive dysfunction. It seems clear, however, that Wallerian degeneration from a white matter lesion can account for structural disruption of a neural network for a period long after the initial lesion occurs.

Transsynaptic Degeneration

A final possible result of white matter lesions is transsynaptic degeneration, in which secondary damage can be seen in neurons linked to those that undergo primary injury. This process can be considered to be allied with Wallerian degeneration because it involves a delayed loss of nervous tissue after a focal lesion, but it differs in that its effects extend beyond the initially damaged neurons to adjacent ones. Neuropathologically, transsynaptic degeneration refers to neuronal cell loss and reactive gliosis in neurons deprived of synaptic input by lesions in adjacent neurons (Adams et al., 1984). As a general phenomenon, transsynaptic degeneration may follow lesions in gray or white matter, and an essential requirement is that the primary damage is to axons or cell bodies. This phenomenon may occur in a retrograde or anterograde fashion, and is thought to evolve over many years or decades (Beatty et al., 1982). Transsynaptic degeneration has been well documented in the visual system, as both MRI (Uggetti et al., 1997) and neuropatho-

logic (Beatty et al., 1982) studies have shown neuronal loss in the lateral geniculate bodies that followed both anterograde (pregeniculate) or retrograde (post-
geniculate) lesions. In terms of neurobehavioral effects of transsynaptic degeneration, clinical examples have been presented (Medina et al., 1974), but because
transsynaptic degeneration has until recently been an exclusively neuropathologic
observation, the importance of this process in comparison to other mechanisms is
difficult to assess. As might be expected, neuroimaging studies now are appearing
that may contribute to this area. Conventional MRI studies of patients with subcortical ischemic vascular disease have found hippocampal and cortical atrophy
that could be a result of transsynaptic degeneration following primary subcortical
white matter injury (Fein et al., 2000). Similarly, studies using magnetic resonance
spectroscopy (MRS) in patients with ischemic vascular dementia have reported
cortical abnormalities that might represent transsynaptic degeneration (Capizzano
et al., 2000). However, it is possible in these studies that direct ischemia or coexistent AD could be responsible for these findings. Further studies of transsynaptic
degeneration are clearly needed, but the possibility of this mechanism helping to
explain neurobehavioral manifestations of white matter lesions is intriguing.

Summary

In most white matter disorders, it is likely that a combination of lesions and lesion
effects occurs that is unique to each patient. Unlike the discrete, localized, and uncomplicated lesions that are possible to produce under experimental conditions,
nature's experiments are not so easily interpretable. This reality introduces an im-
posing degree of complexity in interpretation of clinical data. For clinical observers, therefore, it is particularly important that attention be devoted to early and
mild white matter involvement that could prove informative about the effects of
isolated lesions. In the more typical case of multifaceted white matter dysfunction,
the challenge will be to disentangle the various contributions to neural network
disruption using all the tools currently available.

Future Directions

From the information available on the behavioral neurology of white matter, a
number of areas invite investigation into clinical and research aspects of the field.
At this point, there is enough information available at the descriptive level to point
out many areas for further work. Indeed, the white matter disorders represent a
largely untapped resource for productive clinical and basic research.

Neuroanatomy

At the level of neuroanatomy, many details of brain white matter are in need of
clarification. The fine structure of axonal tracts in the brain requires investigation
so that it can be determined which ones are or are not myelinated. These data will
be important for targeting efforts at remyelination now underway. At the gross

neuroanatomic level, more understanding of the origin, course, and destination of association and commissural fibers is clearly needed. Neuroanatomy textbooks are cautious in describing details of these tracts because little is known of them in humans. Such data can now be more readily gathered with the use of sophisticated neuroimaging techniques, and hence a more complete picture of the intricate connectivity of the brain can be developed. These investigations should not be confined to the cerebrum alone, as it is clear that white matter tracts originating in the brainstem participate in higher function, and the cerebellum may also contribute in important ways.

Armed with these insights, investigators can more precisely determine the clinical correlates of white matter lesions. Understanding how a white matter lesion interrupts cognition or emotion requires a knowledge of where the tract originates, its course through the brain, and where it terminates. Among many examples of areas in which neuroanatomic research can clarify clinical issues are the role of the left arcuate fasciculus in language repetition (Arnett et al., 1996), the participation of the fornix in memory encoding (D'Esposito et al., 1995), and the contribution of the uncinate fasciculi to memory retrieval (Markowitsch, 1995).

Neurophysiology

As the neuroanatomic details of cerebral white matter tracts become more clear, there will be a need for parallel research on functional aspects of these fiber systems. Although neurobehavioral domains have not been readily accessible to study with evoked potential or event-related potential techniques, continued refinement of these and similar methods may permit reliable assessment of white matter physiology. For example, it has recently been shown that the prefrontal regions are implicated in the origin of the P300 (Daffner et al., 1998), a feature that may render the use of this measure particularly well suited to the study of frontal lobe dysfunction in white matter disorders. In addition to this long latency evoked potential, the middle latency P50 may be applicable to the study of hippocampal white matter connections (Arciniegas et al., 2000). The kinds of analyses provided by electrophysiological techniques may permit the assessment of damaged tracts for clinical purposes, especially in conjunction with neuroimaging techniques that can help identify the neural structures responsible for generating the electrophysiological potential. Ultimately, this process will likely lead to an improved understanding of the functional architecture of distributed neural networks.

Clinical Assessment

One of the pressing needs in the clinical arena is for improved sensitivity to and recognition of mental status changes in patients with white matter disorders. As demonstrated many times in this book, these changes are often not obvious, as they typically are not manifest in the realm of language, may be confused with psychiatric disorders, and are frequently overshadowed by other manifestations of neurologic dysfunction. In addition, behavioral neurology and neuropsychology have tended to devote less attention to syndromes in which nonverbal dysfunction dominates the clinical picture (Filley, 1995). In clinical practice, an improvement in detection of these syndromes necessitates increased time for appropriate mental status examinations, a requirement made increasingly burdensome under the strictures of a managed care environment. However, the difficulty inherent in finding these disturbances should not mislead the clinician into believing they are clinically insignificant. In many disorders, cognitive or emotional syndromes comprise the principle or dominant source of overall disability (Hormes et al., 1986; Franklin et al., 1989; Janardhan and Bakshi, 2000).

Moreover, in the area of clinical trials, the importance of incorporating mental status and neuropsychological data into outcome assessments is increasingly recognized as a means of exploring the potential salutary effects of new drugs. The example of MS is most revealing in this context, as the cognitive benefits of immunomodulatory agents can only be recognized if neuropsychological data are collected and analyzed during the conduction of clinical trials (Chapter 6). Thus, neurobehavioral as well as elemental neurologic parameters should henceforth be used as markers of clinical response to therapy (Cutter et al., 1999).

Neuroimaging

Another field that will undoubtedly continue to show rapid progress is neuroimaging. Although the clinical encounter remains the cornerstone of neurologic practice, it is not an overstatement to assert that neuroimaging has revolutionized the clinical neurosciences in a remarkably short period of time. As repeatedly emphasized heretofore, advances in MRI have proven to be a major stimulus to the study of white matter and its many disorders. One area in need of further work is the standardization of visual rating scales for quantitating white matter lesions on conventional MRI scans (Mäntylä et al., 1997). Systematic efforts to develop topographic parcellations of cerebral white matter with standard MRI are underway and may provide a firmer basis for brain–behavior correlations (Meyer et al., 1999; Makris et al., 1999). Newer MRI techniques, including MRS, magnetization transfer imaging (MTI), DWMRI, and DTI, promise to provide ever more detailed views of the white matter, and in turn allow for increasingly accurate clinical-pathologic correlations. In many disorders, for example, abnormalities can be found in white matter that appears normal on conventional MRI, and the detection of these changes permits greater understanding of early pathogenetic events and their clinical correlates.

In a broader context, an exciting prospect is emerging with the use of combined neuroimaging techniques. Together with functional MRI, the newer structural MRI techniques offer the additional advantage of mapping out the white matter connectivity that completes the architecture of the brain's distributed neural networks (Conturo et al., 1999). An unprecedented opportunity is thus emerging to develop a more complete portayal of the brain in its mediation of all aspects of behavior.

Neuropathology

An essential foundation to the study of white matter disorders is neuropathology. It is obviously critical to establish the neuropathologic origin of the syndromes being considered so that their classification as white matter disorders can be supported. Among the many tasks lying ahead, one of the more challenging is to define more precisely the neuropathologic basis of white matter lesions seen on neuroimaging studies. The example of leukoaraiosis illustrates the complexity of documenting what the neuropathologic correlates of white matter changes may be. Another key imperative is to ascertain the relative impact on myelin, axons, glial cells, and vascular structures associated with each neuropathologic process. In general, improved knowledge of the neuropathology of all the white matter disorders will contribute significantly to meaningful brain–behavior correlations. This goal will be notably enhanced by the microscopic study of changes in white matter that can be seen with advanced MRI techniques but not conventional neuroimaging.

Another critical task is the ascertainment of the relative contribution of neuropathology in the white matter versus the subcortical gray matter in the pathogenesis of cognitive impairment and dementia. As discussed throughout this book, the subcortical dementias have been insufficiently examined with this question in mind, and the common failure to separate white and gray matter neuropathology obscures any potential distinctions that could come to light. Details of this kind will be essential for the assignment of neurobehavioral functions to the white matter, which can often only be estimated with currently available information.

Neuropharmacology

An area that has enjoyed little systematic investigation is the neuropharmacology of white matter. White matter conveys a number of important neurochemical projections—including cholinergic, dopaminergic, noradrenergic, and serotonergic fibers en route from subcortical sites to their destinations in the cerebral cortex and hippocampus—but much about these neurotransmitter systems remains obscure. Areas of uncertainty include the exact origin, course, and termination of white matter tracts, and the degree to which many ascending subcortical pathways are myelinated. The assumption that white matter lesions potentially disrupt neurotransmitter delivery is a reasonable one, and understanding the effects of various neuropathologic processes on neurotransmitter function will be revealing.

At present, the effects of white matter lesions on specific neurotransmitter systems can only be hypothesized. The recent findings of Selden and colleagues (1998) on the trajectories of cholinergic pathways in the white matter are a welcome development, and studies such as these could assist in the design of treatment regimens for patients with lesions of these tracts. Thus, the cholinergic agent donepezil may prove helpful for cognitive loss in MS (Krupp et al., 1999), TBI (Arciniegas et al., 1999), and other disorders of white matter. In the case of dopamine, evidence from acquired immunodeficiency syndrome dementia complex (ADC) patients that homovanillic acid is reduced in the cerebrospinal fluid raises the possibility that dopaminergic dysfunction plays a role in cognitive dysfunction from white matter involvement (Di Rocco et al., 2000). Growing experience with stimulant drugs such as methlyphenidate (Weitzner et al., 1995; Watanabe et al., 1999) and bromocriptine (Ross and Stewart, 1981) also suggests that dopaminergic systems are affected in white matter disorders. Rational attempts at pharmacology depend on a knowledge of these systems, and the potential for alleviating the symptoms of many neurobehavioral syndromes appears to be considerable.

Neuropsychology

The neurobehavioral profiles of individual white matter disorders require further elaboration, and neuropsychological study is an essential component of this process. The idea of white matter dementia has been proposed (Filley et al., 1988; Filley, 1998) to establish a clinical entity that captures the deficits of many individuals with diverse diseases and injuries (Chapter 15). Further investigation of this concept could proceed fruitfully with controlled neuropsychological and neuroimaging studies of different white matter disorders, and further comparisons of these conditions to cortical and subcortical disorders. The cognitive impact of white matter changes in aging also deserves further study, as suggested by the documentation of neuropsychological similarities between normal aged persons and those with the ADC (van Gorp et al., 1989). When feasible, studies of focal lesions can also contribute important information, as the lesion method has proven itself useful in the analysis of white matter disorders (Arnett et al., 1994). Newer MRI techniques with improved sensitivity to white matter abnormalites (Chapter 4) will allow better correlations between behavioral phenomena and white matter neuroanatomy and neuropathology.

The proposed NLD syndrome (Rourke, 1995) also deserves further investigation, as it may provide a useful model of the cognitive effects of white matter dysfunction in children and perhaps adults as well (Chapter 15). If the concept of the NLD syndrome is to prove useful in understanding the behavioral neurology of white matter disorders, a meaningful description of its clinical phenomenology is first necessary, followed by careful correlation with neuroradiologic or neuropathologic data to confirm or deny that white matter pathology is in fact present. Although the child and adult neurology and neuropsychology literatures often lack terminological consistency, an integrated approach to describing and investigating the white matter disorders over the entire life span is a laudable goal.

Clinical Outcomes

The care of patients with neurobehavioral syndromes will also be enhanced by more complete knowledge of the natural history and treatment of the white matter disorders. As an example of a recent advance in the understanding of natural history, Terayama and colleagues (1993) found that improvement of cognitive function correlated with restitution of white matter in patients with TBI and diffuse axonal injury. This report highlights the potential for spontaneous recovery of white matter function, and suggests important implications for rehabilitation. At the basic science level, important areas for further study are the processes by which axons can recover function once myelin has been damaged; preliminary information indicates that remyelination of denuded axons can occur in the brain (Ghatak et al., 1989), and that demyelinated axons can develop increased numbers of sodium channels in areas of myelin loss (England et al., 1991). A deeper understanding of these phenomena may lead to enhancement of clinical recovery by pharmacologic or other means.

In terms of treatment of the disease process itself, improved knowledge of the etiology and pathogenesis of white matter disorders can lead to more effective treatment that is specifically targeted to the neuropathologic process. Pharmacotherapy is but one of many approaches, which also include emerging treatments such as bone marrow transplantation (Krivit et al., 1999) and gene therapy (Leone et al., 2000) for genetic white matter disorders. Because the absence of a clear understanding of the mechanisms of many white matter disorders precludes curative treatment in most cases, more data are desirable on symptomatic treatment, so that more effective therapy for such symptoms as cognitive slowing, fatigue, inattention, memory loss, visuospatial impairment, executive dysfunction, and neuropsychiatric syndromes can be used in everyday practice. Stimulants, antidepressants with specific monoamine neurotransmitter effects, cholinergic agents, anticonvulsants, and antipsychotic drugs all need careful evaluation in double-blind, controlled studies to clarify their use in the white matter disorders. The increasing recognition of clinically significant syndromes that were previously overlooked in individuals with white matter disorders serves as an additional stimulus for rapid movement in this direction.

White Matter and the Mind

At the conclusion of this book, a return to the larger picture of the human mind is appropriate. A first observation is that the concept of the mind has but lately been admitted to the vocabulary of neuroscience. Long considered the province of philosophy, and later psychology and psychiatry, the idea that the mind can be meaningfully subjected to neuroscientific scrutiny has firmly taken hold only in recent decades (Kandel and Squire, 2000). Reflecting a remarkable shift in thinking, neuroscientists now commonly speak of the mind in terms of neurons, neurotransmitters, cortical gyri, and lobes. Symposia, conferences, and journals are increasingly devoted to the study of this topic. As the new millenium begins, the problem of the relation between mind and body can be seen to have evolved from a speculative philosophical issue to a legitimate scientific question (Searle, 1999).

This development does not mean, of course, that the ancient and thorny problem of defining the mind has been solved. As is the case with many of the terms used in discussing the qualities of human experience, the word continues to defy precise definition. Notwithstanding this difficulty, however, neuroscience is offering a fresh approach to exploring the neurobiological basis of mental life. In this context, a working definition of the mind becomes essential in the daily pursuit of its complexities. With apologies to those who approach this issue from other perspectives, neuroscientists must have a means of identifying in some practical sense what is being considered. In the language of behavioral neurology, then, the mind may be regarded as the totality of cognitive and emotional experience that comprises the foundation of the human behavioral repertoire (Filley, 1995).

In this book, the major proposition has been that white matter should be added to the list of brain regions regularly included in these discussions. In ways that can only be glimpsed at present, the white matter participates in the higher functions that Gall and Spurzheim once slavishly assigned to specific cortical areas under palpable landmarks on the skull. Correct as these early investigators were in identifying the presence of white matter deep in the brain, they were generally unaware of its importance for human behavior. Classical neurologists of the nineteenth century began to recognize the neurobehavioral significance of white matter, and Geschwind reaffirmed and expanded this growing awareness in the twentieth, but today the focus on the cerebral cortex continues to exert a dominant influence on neurologic thinking. The data now accumulated, albeit far from complete, are increasingly persuasive in compelling an alternative view (Filley, 1998). If the brain is the organ of the mind, an assumption that has proven to be of great theoretical and practical value, the importance of including its white matter in the study of mental activity seems not just reasonable but unquestionable.

References

Adams JH, Corsellis JAW, Duchen LW, eds. Greenfield's neuropathology. 5th ed. New York: Wiley, 1984: 20–22.

Alexander MP. Specific semantic memory loss after hypoxic-ischemic injury. Neurology 1997; 48: 165–173.

Arciniegas D, Olincy A, Topkoff J, et al. Impaired auditory gating and P50 nonsuppression after traumatic brain injury. J Neuropsychiatry Clin Neurosci 2000; 12: 77–85.

Arcinicgas DB, Adler LF, Topkoff J, et al. Attention and memory dysfunction after traumatic brain injury: cholinergic mechanisms, sensory gating, and a hypothesis for further investigation. Brain Injury 1999; 13: 1–13.

Arnett PA, Rao SM, Bernardin L, et al. Relationship between frontal lobe lesions and Wisconsin Card Sorting Test performance in patients with multiple sclerosis. Neurology 1994; 44: 420–425.

Arnett PA, Rao SM, Hussain M, et al. Conduction aphasia in multiple sclerosis: a case report with MRI findings. Neurology 1996; 47: 576–578.

Bakshi R, Miletich RS, Kinkel PR, et al. High-resolution fluorodeoxyglucose positron emission tomography shows both global and regional hypometabolism in multiple sclerosis. J Neuroimaging 1998; 8: 228–234.

Beatty RM, Sadun AA, Smith LEH, et al. Direct demonstration of transsynaptic degeneration in the human visual system: a comparison of retrograde and anterograde changes. J Neurol Neurosurg Psychiatry 1982; 45: 143–146.

Blinkenberg M, Rune K, Jensen CV, et al. Cortical cerebral metabolism correlates with MRI lesion load and cognitive dysfunction in MS. Neurology 2000; 54: 558–564.

Capizzano AA, Schuff N, Amend DL, et al. Subcortical ischemic vascular dementia: assessment with quantitative MR imaging and 1H MR spectroscopy. AJNR 2000; 21: 621–630.

Conturo TE, Lori NF, Cull TS, et al. Tracking neuronal fiber pathways in the living human brain. Proc Natl Acad Sci 1999; 96: 10422–10427.

Cutter GR, Baier ML, Rudick RA, et al. Development of a multiple sclerosis functional composite as a clinical trial outcome measure. Brain 1999; 122: 871–882.

Daffner KR, Mesulam M-M, Scinto LFM, et al. Regulation of attention to novel stimuli by frontal lobes: an event-related potential study. Neuroreport 1998; 9: 787–791.

D'Esposito M, Verfaellie M, Alexander MP, Katz DI. Amnesia following traumatic bilateral fornix transection. Neurology 1995; 45: 1546–1550.

Di Rocco A, Bottiglieri T, Dorfman D, et al. Decreased homovanilic acid in cerebrospinal fluid correlates with neuropsychologic function in HIV-1 infected patients. Clin Neuropharmacol 2000; 23: 190–194.

England JD, Gamboni F, Levinson SR. Increased numbers of sodium channels form along demyelinated axons. Brain Res 1991; 548: 334–337.

Feeney DM, Baron J-C. Diaschisis. Stroke 1986; 17: 817–830.

Fein G, Di Sclafani V, Tanabe J, et al. Hippocampal and cortical atrophy predict dementia in subcortical ischemic vascular disease. Neurology 2000; 55: 1626–1635.

Filley CM. Neurobehavioral anatomy. Niwot, CO: University Press of Colorado, 1995.

Filley CM. The behavioral neurology of cerebral white matter. Neurology 1998; 50: 1535–1540.

Filley CM, Franklin GM, Rosenberg NL, Heaton RK. White matter dementia. Clinical disorders and implications. Neuropsychiatry Neuropsychol Behav Neurol 1988; 1: 239–254.

Filley CM, Davis KA, Schmitz SP, et al. Neuropsychological performance and magnetic resonance imaging in Alzheimer's disease and normal aging. Neuropsychiatry Neuropsychol Behav Neurol 1989; 2: 81–91.

Franklin GM, Nelson LM, Filley CM, Heaton RK. Cognitive loss in multiple sclerosis. Case reports and review of the literature. Arch Neurol 1989; 46: 162–167.

Gazzaniga MS. Cerebral specialization and interhemispheric communication. Does the corpus callosum enable the human condition? Brain 2000; 123: 1293–1326.

Geschwind N. Disconnexion syndromes in animals and man. Brain 1965; 88: 237–294, 585–644.

Ghatak NR, Leshner RT, Price AC, Felton WL. Remyelination in the central nervous system. J Neuropathol Exp Neurol 1989; 48: 507–518.

Hoffman M, Watts A. Cognitive dysfunction in isolated brainstem stroke: a neuropsychological and SPECT study. J Stroke Cerebrovasc Dis 1998; 7: 24–31.

Hormes JT, Filley CM, Rosenberg NL. Neurologic sequelae of chronic solvent vapor abuse. Neurology 1986; 36: 698–702.

Ishihara M, Kumita S, Hayashi H, Kumazaki T. Loss of interhemispheric connectivity in patients with lacunar infarction reflected by diffusion-weighted MR imaging and single-photon emission CT. AJNR 2000; 20: 991–998.

Janardhan V, Bakshi R. Quality of life and its relationship to brain lesions and atrophy on magnetic resonance images in 60 patients with multiple sclerosis. Arch Neurol 2000; 57: 1485–1491.

Kandel ER, Squire LR. Neuroscience: breaking down scientific barriers to the study of brain and mind. Science 2000; 290: 1113–1120.

Katz DI, Alexander MP, Mandell AM. Dementia following strokes in the mesencephalon and diencephalon. Arch Neurol 1987; 44: 1127–1133.

Krivit W, Peters C, Shapiro EG. Bone marrow transplantation as effective treatment of central nervous system disease in globoid cell leukodystrophy, metachromatic leukodystrophy, adrenoleukodystrophy, mannosidosis, fucosidosis, aspartylglucosaminuria, Hurler, Maroteaux-Lamy, and Sly syndromes, and Gaucher disease type III. Curr Opin Neurol 1999; 12: 167–176.

Krupp LB, Elkins LE, Scheffer RS, et al. Donepezil for the treatment of memory impairments in multiple sclerosis. Neurology 1999 (suppl 2); 52: A137.

Leone P, Janson CG, Bilianuk L, et al. Aspartoacylase gene transfer to the mammalian central nervous system with therapeutic implications for Canavan's Disease. Ann Neurol 2000; 48: 27–38.

Leys D, Pruvo JP, Parent M, et al. Could Wallerian degeneration contribute to "leuko-araiosis" in subjects free of any vascular disorder? J Neurol Neurosurg Psychiatry 1991; 54: 46–50.

Makris N, Meyer JW, Bates JF, et al. MRI-based topographic parcellation of human cerebral white matter and nuclei II. Rationale and applications with systematics of cerebral connectivity. Neuroimage 1999; 9: 18–45.

Mäntylä R, Erkinjuntti T, Salonen O, et al. Variable agreement between visual rating scales for white matter hyperintensities on MRI. Comparison of 13 rating scales in a post-stroke cohort. Stroke 1997; 28: 1614–1623.

Markowitsch HJ. Which brain regions are critically involved in the retrieval of old episodic memory? Brain Res Rev 1995; 21: 117–127.

Mayer SA, Tatemichi TK, Hair LS, et al. Hemineglect and seizures in Binswanger's disease: clinical-pathological report. J Neurol Neurosurg Psychiatry 1993; 56: 816–819.

Medina JL, Rubino FA, Ross E. Agitated delirium caused by infarction of the hippocampal formation and fusiform and lingual gyri: a case report. Neurology 1974; 24: 1181–1183.

Mesulam M-M. Large-scale neurocognitive networks and distributed processing for attention, memory, and language. Ann Neurol 1990; 28: 597–613.

Mesulam M-M. From sensation to cognition. Brain 1998; 121: 1013–1052.

Mesulam M-M. Behavioral neuroanatomy. Large-scale neural networks, association cortex, frontal systems, the limbic system, and hemispheric specializations. In: Mesulam M-M. Principles of behavioral and cognitive neurology. 2nd ed. New York: Oxford University Press, 2000: 1–120.

Metter EJ, Mazziotta JC, Itabashi HH, et al. Comparison of glucose metabolism, x-ray CT, and postmortem data in a patient with multiple cerebral infarcts. Neurology 1985; 35: 1695–1701.

Meyer JS, Obara K, Muramatsu K. Diaschisis. Neurol Res 1993; 15: 362–366.

Meyer JW, Makris N, Bates JF, et al. MRI-based topographic parcellation of human cerebral white matter. Neuroimage 1999; 9: 1–17.

Nguyen DK, Botez MI. Diaschisis and neurobehavior. Can J Neurol Sci 1998; 25: 5–12.

Price BH, Mesulam M-M. Behavioral manifestations of central pontine myelinolysis. Arch Neurol 1987; 44: 671–673.

Rose SE, Chen F, Chalk JB, et al. Loss of connectivity in Alzheimer's disease: an evaluation of white matter tract integrity with colour coded MR diffusion tensor imaging. J Neurol Neurosurg Psychiatry 2000; 69: 528–530.

Ross ED, Stewart RM. Akinetic mutism from hypothalamic damage: successful treatment with dopamine agonists. Neurology 1981: 31: 1435–1439.

Rourke BP. Syndrome of nonverbal learning disabilities. New York: Guilford Press, 1995.

Sawlani V, Gupta RK, Singh MK, Kohli A. MRI demonstration of Wallerian degeneration in various intracranial lesions and its clinical implications. J Neurol Sci 1997; 146: 103–108.

Schmahmann JD. An emerging concept. The cerebellar contribution to higher function. Arch Neurol 1991; 48: 1178–1187.

Searle JR. The future of philosophy. Phil Trans R Soc Lond B 1999; 354: 2069–2080.

Selden NR, Gitelman DR, Salamon-Murayama N, et al. Trajectories of cholinergic pathways within the cerebral hemispheres of the human brain. Brain 1998; 121: 2249–2257.

Simon JS, Kinkel RP, Jacobs L, et al. A Wallerian degeneration pattern in patients at risk for MS. Neurology 2000; 54: 1155–1160.

Sultzer DL, Mahler ME, Cummings JL, et al. Cortical abnormalities associated with subcortical lesions in vascular dementia. Clinical and positron emission tomographic findings. Arch Neurol 1995; 52: 773–780.

Terayama Y, Meyer JS, Kawamura J, Weathers S. Cognitive recovery correlates with white-matter restitution after head injury. Surg Neurol 1993; 39: 177–186.

Uggetti C, Egitto MG, Fazzi E, et al. Transsynaptic degeneration of lateral geniculate bodies in blind children: in vivo demonstration. AJNR 1997; 18: 233–238.

Van Gorp WG, Mitrushina M, Cummings JL, et al. Normal aging and the subcortical encephalopathy of AIDS. A neuropsychological comparison. Neuropsychiatry Neuropsychol Behav Neurol 1989; 2: 5–20.

Von Monakow C. Diaschisis. (1914 article translated by Harris G). In: Pribram KH, ed. Brain and behavior I. Mood states and mind. Baltimore: Penguin Press, 1969: 27–36.

Waller AV. Experiments on the section of the glossopharyngeal and hypoglossal nerves of the frog, and observations of the alterations produced thereby in the structure of the of the primitive fiber. Philos Trans R Soc Lond [Biol] 1850; 140: 423–429.

Watanabe MD, Martin EM, DeLeon OA, et al. Successful methylphenidate treatment of apathy after subcortical infarcts. J Neuropsychiatry Clin Neurosci 1995; 7: 502–504.

Weitzner MA, Meyers CA, Valentine AD. Methylphenidate in the treatment of neurobehavioral slowing associated with cancer and cancer treatment. J Neuropsychiatry Clin Neurosci 1995; 7: 347–250.

Index

Abulia
  in Binswanger's disease, 147
  in carbon monoxide poisoning, 129
  in cerebral autosomal dominant
    arteriopathy with subcortical
    infarcts and leukoencephalopathy,
    151
  and executive dysfunction, 226
  in white matter disorders, 249
Acquired immunodeficiency syndrome,
  97, 181
Acquired immunodeficiency syndrome
  dementia complex, 10
  neurobehavioral features of, 97–101
  and depression, 233
  and dopamine, 261
  and mania, 235
  and memory, 209
  and normal aging, 262
Acquired immunodeficiency syndrome
  encephalopathy, 98
Acquired immunodeficiency syndrome-
  related dementia, 98
Action potential, 26, 27

Acute disseminated encephalomyelitis,
  89, 235
Acute hemorrhagic leukoencephalitis, 90
Acyclovir, 103
Adrenoleukodystrophy
  and mania, 235
  neurobehavioral features of, 63–65
  and toluene leukoencephalopathy, 124
Adrenomyeloneuropathy, 65
Aging, 28, 34–38, 262
Agnosia, 9, 205
  auditory, 220, 225, 255
  visual, 87, 88, 101, 220, 225
Akinetic mutism, 128, 220, 226
Albert, Martin, 9
Alcoholic dementia, 126
Alexander's disease, 66
Alexia, 9
  with agraphia, 87, 88, 220, 224
  pure, 87, 88, 101, 220, 223
Alien hand, 171, 227
Alzheimer's disease
  and aging, 35–37
  and cortical deficits, 206